Electrocardiography Review

A CASE-BASED APPROACH

Electrocardiography Review

A CASE-BASED APPROACH

Curtis M. Rimmerman, MD, MBA, FACC

Gus P. Karos Chair in Clinical Cardiovascular Medicine
Robert and Suzanne Tomsich Department of Cardiovascular Medicine
Cleveland Clinic
Cleveland, Ohio

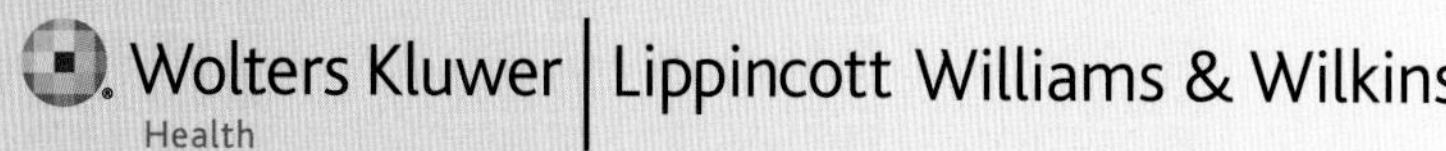

Philadelphia • Baltimore • New York • London
Buenos Aires • Hong Kong • Sydney • Tokyo

Acquisitions Editor: Frances DeStefano
Product Manager: Leanne Vandetty
Production Manager: Alicia Jackson
Senior Manufacturing Manager: Benjamin Rivera
Marketing Manager: Kimberly Schonberger
Design Coordinator: Stephen Druding
Production Service: SPi Global

Two Commerce Square
2001 Market Street
Philadelphia, PA 19103 USA
LWW.com

Printed in China

Library of Congress Cataloging-in-Publication Data

Rimmerman, Curtis M.
Electrocardiography review : a case-based approach / Curtis M. Rimmerman.
p. ; cm.
Includes bibliographical references and index.
ISBN-13: 978-1-4511-4947-0 (alk. paper)
ISBN-10: 1-4511-4947-6 (alk. paper)
I. Cleveland Clinic Foundation. II. Title.
[DNLM: 1. Electrocardiography—methods—Case Reports. 2. Electrocardiography—methods—Examination Questions. 3. Heart Diseases—diagnosis—Case Reports. 4. Heart Diseases—diagnosis—Examination Questions. WG 18.2]
616.1'207547—dc23

2011033742

To purchase additional copies of this book, call our customer service department at (800) 638-3030 or fax orders to (301) 223-2320. International customers should call (301) 223-2300.

Visit Lippincott Williams & Wilkins on the Internet: at LWW.com. Lippincott Williams & Wilkins customer service representatives are available from 8:30 am to 6 pm, EST.

10 9 8 7 6 5 4 3 2 1

RRS1112

Contents

Introduction

Electrocardiography is an indispensable tool in clinical medicine. An electrocardiogram can be obtained within a few minutes, is not harmful or painful, and is readily portable at a minimal cost. In addition to the history and physical examination, the electrocardiogram provides wonderful insight regarding underlying heart function and structure.

Additionally, electrocardiography is also an integral component to the American Board of Internal Medicine (ABIM) Cardiovascular Medicine Certifying Exam. A requisite to passing this examination is a passing score on the electrocardiography subsection.

To achieve a passing score on the ABIM Certifying Exam, it takes study and repetition. The best form of electrocardiogram learning is interpretation within the clinical context of your patient. Being able to synthesize the history and physical examination with the available electrocardiogram findings creates a body of evidence that can be applied to the diagnosis and management of your patient's condition. Like any test requiring interpretation, electrocardiogram findings can be both simple and complex. It's the most complex electrocardiograms that are the most informative, often preempting findings confirmed after invoking significantly more complex and invasive testing.

As we all know, patients and electrocardiograms do not arrive in a predetermined order. An acute myocardial infarction patient may be followed by a patient with recent-onset atrial fibrillation. That is why I am a huge proponent of case-based electrocardiography education, best approximating the unpredictability of clinical practice.

For this book targeting the ABIM Certifying Examinee and those electrocardiographers wishing to test and increase their electrocardiography knowledge, basic electrocardiogram interpretation skills are assumed to have been reasonably mastered. Once this has been accomplished, it is appropriate to begin learning from your patients. It is with this intent that I present 150 carefully selected electrocardiogram case studies. The electrocardiograms are chosen to maximize learning and ABIM Certifying Exam preparation, emphasizing concepts that are not traditionally taught in electrocardiogram courses or on the hospital wards. Using this approach, you will begin your journey toward achieving superior electrocardiogram interpretation skills.

Each case includes a clinical history, electrocardiogram interpretation, and key teaching points with clinically relevant commentary plus key clinical electrocardiogram diagnoses. I have also included a section on Certifying Exam coding tips with specific board exam diagnostic codes provided for each tracing as well as special chapters dedicated to Certifying Exam preparation and coding emphasizing keys to a passing score.

Lastly, for those needing concept reinforcement, I have also prepared a chapter outlining a recommended approach to electrocardiogram interpretation. It is with this case-based approach that your electrocardiogram acumen will improve and you will be well on your way to further benefiting your patients and achieving ABIM Cardiovascular Medicine Board Certification.

Curtis M. Rimmerman, MD, MBA, FACC
Gus P. Karos Chair in Clinical Cardiovascular Medicine
Robert and Suzanne Tomsich Department of Cardiovascular Medicine
Cleveland Clinic
Cleveland, Ohio

A Recommended Approach to Electrocardiogram Interpretation

To ensure accurate and consistent ECG interpretation, a systematic approach is required. Electrocardiogram interpretation is not an exercise in pattern recognition. To the contrary, employing a methodical strategy based on a thorough knowledge of the cardiac conduction sequence, cardiac anatomy, cardiac physiology, and cardiac pathophysiology can be applied to all electrocardiograms, regardless of the findings.

One systematic approach to each electrocardiogram is to ascertain the following in this recommended order:

1. Assess the standardization and identify the recorded leads accurately.
2. Determine the atrial and ventricular rates and rhythms.
3. Determine the P-wave axis and QRS-complex axis.
4. Measure all cardiac intervals.
5. Determine if cardiac chamber enlargement or hypertrophy is present.
6. Assess the P-wave, QRS-complex, and T-wave morphologies.
7. Draw conclusions and correlate clinically.

Cardiac pathology is manifest differently on the surface ECG, depending on which lead is interrogated. Each lead provides an "electrical window of opportunity" and, by this virtue, offers a unique electrical perspective. The experienced electrocardiographer amalgamates these different windows into a mental three-dimensional electrical assessment, drawing accurate conclusions pertaining to conduction system and structural heart disease. For example, precordial lead V_1 predominantly overlies the right ventricle, explaining why right ventricular cardiac electrical events are best observed in this lead. Likewise, precordial lead V_6 overlies the left ventricle. This lead optimally represents left ventricular cardiac electrical events.

1. Assess the Standardization and Identify the Recorded Leads Accurately

Standard ECG graph paper consists of 1-mm × 1-mm boxes divided by narrow lines, which are separated by bold lines into larger, 5-mm × 5-mm boxes. At standard speed (25 mm/s), each small box in the horizontal axis represents 0.040 second (40 milliseconds) of time and each large box represents 0.200 second (200 milliseconds). At standard calibration (1 mV/10 mm), each vertical small box represents 0.1 mV and each vertical large box represents 0.5 mV. One must be very careful to inspect the standardization square wave (1 mV in amplitude) at the left of each ECG to determine the calibration of the ECG. ECGs with particularly high or low voltages are often recorded at half-standard or twice standard, respectively. In these cases, the 1 mV square wave possesses an amplitude of either 5 or 20 mm. This distinction is important because it will impact the interpretation of all other voltage criteria. All further references to amplitude in this chapter will be under the assumption of the default or preset standardization (1 mV/10 mm).

2. Determine the Atrial and Ventricular Rates and Rhythms

The first step in determining the rate and rhythm is to identify atrial activity. If P waves are present, it is important to measure the P-wave to P-wave interval (P-P interval). This determines the rate of atrial depolarization. To estimate quickly either an atrial or a ventricular rate on a standard 12-lead ECG, one can count the number of 5-mm boxes in an interval and divide 300 by that number. For example, if there are four boxes between P waves, the rate is 300 divided by 4, or 75 complexes per minute.

Once the atrial activity and rate are identified, the P-wave frontal plane axis should be ascertained. A normal P-wave axis (i.e., –0 to 75 degrees) typically reflects a sinus node P-wave origin. A simple way of determining a normal P-wave axis is to confirm a positive P-wave vector in leads I, II, III, and aVF. An abnormal P-wave axis supports an ectopic or non–sinus node P-wave origin.

Several possible atrial and junctional rhythms are listed below. They are grouped by cardiac rhythm origin and subsequently subcategorized by atrial rate. Distinguishing features are italicized for emphasis.

Rhythms of Sinus Nodal and Atrial Origin

Normal Sinus Rhythm

Normal sinus rhythm (NSR) is defined as a *regular* atrial depolarization rate between *60 and 100 per minute* of *sinus node origin*, as demonstrated by a positive P-wave vector in leads I, II, III, and aVF.

Sinus Bradycardia

Sinus bradycardia is characterized by a *regular* atrial depolarization rate *less than 60 per minute of sinus node origin*, as demonstrated by a positive P-wave vector in leads I, II, III, and aVF. (This is similar to NSR, except the rate is slower.)

Sinus Tachycardia

Sinus tachycardia is characterized by a *regular* atrial depolarization rate *≥100 per minute* of *sinus node origin*, as demonstrated by a positive P-wave vector in leads I, II, III, and aVF. (This is similar to NSR, except the rate is faster.)

Sinus Arrhythmia

Sinus arrhythmia is characterized by an *irregular* atrial depolarization rate between *60 and 100 per minute* of *sinus node origin*, as demonstrated by a positive P-wave vector in leads I, II, III, and aVF. (This is similar to NSR, except there is *irregularity in the P-P interval >160 milliseconds.*)

Sinus Arrest or Pause

Sinus arrest or pause is characterized by a pause of >2.0 seconds without identifiable atrial activity. This may be caused by frank sinus arrest, or may be simply a sinus pause secondary to a non-conducted premature atrial complex (PAC), in which case a P wave can be seen deforming the T wave.

Sinoatrial (SA) block, which, like atrioventricular (AV) nodal block, has several forms.

First-degree SA block involves a fixed delay between the depolarizing SA node and the depolarization exiting the node and propagating as a P wave. Because the delay is fixed, this delay cannot be detected on the surface ECG.

Second-degree SA block has two varieties. In type I (Wenckebach) SA block, there is a progressive delay between SA nodal depolarization and exit of the impulse to the atrium. This is manifest as a progressive shortening of the P-P interval until there is a pause, reflecting an SA node impulse that was blocked from exiting the node. In Type II SA block, there is a constant P-P interval with intermittent pauses. These pauses also represent an SA node impulse that was blocked from exiting the node. However, in this case, the duration of the pause is a multiple of the basic P-P interval.

Third-degree SA block demonstrates no P-wave activity, as no impulses exit the sinus node. On the surface ECG, this is indistinguishable from sinus arrest, in which there is no sinus node activity.

Sinus Node Reentrant Rhythm

Sinus node reentrant rhythm is characterized by a *reentrant circuit involving the sinus node* and peri-sinus nodal tissues. Given the sinus origin, the *P-wave morphology and axis are normal and indistinguishable from a normal sinus P wave*. The rate is regular at a rate of *60 to 100 per minute*. (This is very similar to NSR, except characterized by abrupt onset and termination.)

Sinus Node Reentrant Tachycardia

Sinus node reentrant tachycardia is characterized by a *reentrant circuit involving the sinus node* and peri-sinus nodal tissues. Given the sinus origin, the *P-wave morphology and axis are normal and indistinguishable from a normal sinus P wave*. The rate is regular at a rate of *≥100 per minute*. (This is very similar to sinus tachycardia, except characterized by abrupt onset and termination.)

Ectopic Atrial Rhythm

Ectopic atrial rhythm is characterized by a *regular* atrial depolarization at a rate of *60 to 100 per minute* from a *single non-sinus origin*, as reflected by an abnormal P-wave axis. The PR interval may be shortened, particularly in the presence of a low ectopic atrial origin, closer to the AV node with a reduced intra-atrial conduction time. In the presence of slowed atrial conduction, the PR interval may be normal or even prolonged.

Ectopic Atrial Bradycardia

Ectopic atrial bradycardia is characterized by a *regular* atrial depolarization at a rate of *≤60 per minute* from a *single non-sinus origin*, as reflected by an abnormal P-wave axis. (This is similar to an ectopic atrial rhythm, except slower.)

Atrial Tachycardia

Atrial tachycardia is characterized by a *regular*, automatic tachycardia from a *single, ectopic atrial focus* typically with an atrial rate of *180 to 240 per minute*. The ventricular rate may be regular or irregular, depending on the AV conduction ratio. The P-wave axis is abnormal, given the ectopic atrial focus. (This is similar to an ectopic atrial rhythm, except faster.)

Wandering Atrial Pacemaker

A wandering atrial pacemaker (WAP) has a rate of *60 to 100 per minute* from multiple ectopic atrial foci, as evidenced by at least *three different P-wave morphologies* on the 12-lead ECG, possessing *variable P-P, PR, and R-R intervals*. Be careful not to confuse this dysrhythmia with atrial fibrillation (AF). Unlike AF, discrete P waves are identifiable.

Multifocal Atrial Tachycardia

Multifocal atrial tachycardia (MAT) is characterized by a rate of *>100 per minute* with a P wave preceding each QRS complex from multiple atrial ectopic foci, as evidenced by at least *three different P-wave morphologies* on the 12-lead ECG possessing *variable P-P, PR, and R-R intervals*. The ventricular response is irregularly irregular, given the unpredictable timing of the atrial depolarization and variable AV conduction. Nonconducted atrial complexes during the ventricular absolute refractory period are also often present. Be careful not to confuse this dysrhythmia with atrial fibrillation. Unlike atrial fibrillation, discrete P waves are identifiable. (This is similar to WAP, but the atrial rate is faster.)

Atrial Fibrillation

Atrial fibrillation (AF) is characterized by a *rapid, irregular, and disorganized atrial depolarization* rate of 400 to 600 per minute *devoid of identifiable discrete P waves, instead characterized by fibrillatory waves*.

In the absence of fixed AV block, the ventricular response to AF is *irregularly irregular*. Be careful not to confuse this dysrhythmia with WAP or MAT. The key is the lack of identifiable P waves.

Atrial Flutter

Atrial flutter (AFL) is characterized by a *rapid, regular atrial depolarization* rate of *250 to 350 per minute*, representing an intra-atrial re-entrant circuit. The atrial waves are termed "flutter waves" and often demonstrate a *sawtoothed* appearance, best seen in leads V_1, II, III, and aVF.

Although the atrial rate is regular, the *ventricular response rate may be either regular or irregular*, depending on the presence of fixed versus variable AV conduction. Common AV conduction ratios are 2:1 and 4:1.

Rhythms of Atrioventricular Nodal and Junctional Origin

Atrioventricular Nodal Reentrant Tachycardia

Atrioventricular nodal reentrant tachycardia (AVNRT) is a microreentrant dysrhythmia that depends on the presence of *two separate atrioventricular nodal pathways*. Slowed conduction is present in one pathway and unidirectional conduction block is present in the second pathway. *This is a regular rhythm* with a typical *ventricular rate of 140 to 200* per minute, with abrupt onset and termination. Its onset is *often initiated by premature atrial complexes (PACs)*. Atrial activity typically consists *of inverted or retrograde P waves occurring either before, during, or after the QRS* complex, *best identified in lead* V_1. The QRS complex may be conducted normally or aberrantly.

Atrioventricular Reentrant Tachycardia

Atrioventricular reentrant tachycardia (AVRT) is a *macroreentrant circuit that consists of an atrioventricular nodal pathway and an accessory pathway*. This dysrhythmia may conduct antegrade down the AV nodal pathway with retrograde conduction through the accessory pathway (orthodromic AVRT), or antegrade down the accessory pathway with retrograde conduction up the AV nodal pathway (antidromic AVRT). As opposed to AVNRT, the *P wave is always present after the QRS* complex. With antidromic AVRT, the QRS complex, by definition, is aberrantly conducted (wide).

Junctional Premature Complexes

Junctional premature complexes are *premature* QRS complexes of AV nodal origin that may have resultant *retrograde P waves* (a negative P-wave vector in leads II, III, and aVF) occurring immediately *before (with a short PR interval), during, or after the QRS* complex.

AV Junctional Bradycardia

AV junctional bradycardia is characterized by QRS complexes of AV nodal origin that occur at a regular rate of *<60 per minute*. These represent a *subsidiary pacemaker* and may have resultant *retrograde P waves* (negative P-wave vector in leads II, III, and aVF) that occur immediately *before (with a short PR interval), during, or after the QRS* complex.

Accelerated AV Junctional Rhythm

Accelerated AV junctional rhythm is characterized by QRS complexes of AV nodal origin that occur at a regular rate of *60 to 100 per minute*. These represent a *subsidiary pacemaker* and may have resultant *retrograde P waves* (negative P-wave vector in leads II, III, and aVF) that occur immediately *before (with a short PR interval), during, or after the QRS* complex. (This dysrhythmia is similar to AV junctional bradycardia, except faster.)

AV Junctional Tachycardia

AV junctional tachycardia is characterized by QRS complexes of AV nodal origin that occur at a regular rate of *typically 100 to 200 per minute*. This dysrhythmia emanates from the AV junction and serves as a dominant cardiac pacemaker with an inappropriately rapid rate. *Retrograde P waves* may be identified (negative P-wave vector in leads II, III, and aVF) that occur immediately *before (with a short PR interval), during, or after the QRS* complex. (This dysrhythmia is similar to AV junctional rhythm, except faster.)

Rhythms of Ventricular Origin

Idioventricular Rhythm

Idioventricular rhythm is a regular escape rhythm of ventricular origin that possesses a typically *widened QRS* complex (>100 milliseconds) at a rate *of less than 60* per minute. This is often seen in cases of high-degree AV block, in which the ventricle serves as a subsidiary pacemaker.

Ventricular Parasystole

Ventricular parasystole is an independent, automatic ventricular rhythm that emanates from a single ventricular focus characterized by a *widened QRS* complex with regular discharge and ventricular depolarization. Because the rhythm is independent and not suppressible, ventricular parasystole is characterized by *varying coupling intervals and unchanged interectopic R-R intervals*. Fusion complexes can be observed when the parasystolic focus discharges simultaneously with native ventricular depolarization. When the ventricle is absolutely refractory, the parasystolic focus is not recorded on the surface electrocardiogram, but its discharge remains unabated.

Accelerated Idioventricular Rhythm

Accelerated idioventricular rhythm (AIVR) is a regular rhythm of ventricular origin that typically has a *widened QRS* complex at a *rate of 60 to 100 per minute*. It is often seen in cases of high-degree AV block, in which the ventricle serves as a subsidiary pacemaker plus in cases of coronary artery reperfusion. (AIVR is similar to idioventricular rhythm, except faster.)

Ventricular Tachycardia

Ventricular tachycardia (VT) is a sustained cardiac rhythm of ventricular origin that occurs at a typical rate of 140 to 240 per minute. In differentiating this from supraventricular tachycardia with aberrant conduction, the following features suggest VT:

- AV dissociation
- Fusion or capture complexes
- Wide QRS (≥140 milliseconds if right bundle-branch block [RBBB] morphology; ≥160 milliseconds if left bundle-branch block [LBBB] morphology)
- Left-axis QRS complex deviation
- Concordance of the precordial-lead QRS complexes
- QRS morphologies similar to those of PVCs on the current or previous ECG
- Tachyarrhythmia initiated by a PVC
- If RBBB morphology, possessing an RSr′ pattern (as opposed to an rSR′ pattern)

Polymorphic Ventricular Tachycardia

Polymorphic ventricular tachycardia is a paroxysmal form of VT with a *nonconstant R-R interval*, a ventricular rate of 200 to 300 per minute, QRS complexes of alternating polarity, and a changing QRS amplitude that often resembles a sine-wave pattern (*torsade de pointes*). It is often associated with a *prolonged QT* interval at arrhythmia initiation.

Ventricular Fibrillation

Ventricular fibrillation (VF) is a terminal cardiac rhythm with chaotic ventricular activity that lacks organized ventricular depolarization.

3. Determine the P-Wave and QRS-Complex Axes

A normal P-wave axis varies from 0 to 75 degrees, but is usually between 45 degrees and 60 degrees. P waves with a normal axis are upright in leads I, II, III, and aVF and inverted in lead aVR. An abnormal P-wave axis should prompt the interpreter to consider non–sinus nodal rhythms, dextrocardia, or limb lead reversal, among other causes.

To ascertain the frontal-plane axis of the QRS complex, the QRS-complex vector is assessed in each of the limb leads. A recommended approach is to search for the limb lead in which the QRS complex is isoelectric (i.e., the area of positivity under the R wave is equal to the area of negativity above the Q and S waves). The QRS-complex frontal-plane axis will be perpendicular to the isoelectric lead, thus narrowing down the axis to one of two possibilities (90 degrees clockwise or 90 degrees counterclockwise of the isoelectric lead's axis). Next, one examines a limb lead whose vector is close to one of the two possible axes. Based on whether the

QRS complex is grossly positive or negative in that lead, one can deduce which of the two possible axes is correct.

An alternative approach is as follows:

1. Assess the QRS-complex vector in leads I and aVF. If both are positive, the QRS complex is between 0 and +90 degrees, and is therefore normal.
2. If the QRS-complex vector is positive in lead I and negative in aVF, assess the QRS-complex vector in lead II. If it is positive in lead II, the QRS-complex axis is between –30 degrees and 0 degrees, and is leftward but still not pathologically deviated. If the QRS complex is negative in lead II, then the QRS-complex axis is between –90 degrees and –30 degrees, and therefore abnormal left-axis QRS-complex deviation is present.
3. If the QRS-complex vector is negative in lead I and positive in lead aVF, abnormal right-axis QRS-complex deviation is present.
4. If the QRS-complex vector is negative in both leads I and aVF, the QRS-complex axis is profoundly deviated to between –90 degrees and –180 degrees.

4. Measure All Cardiac Intervals

PR Interval

A normal PR interval is between 120 and 200 milliseconds. This represents the interval between P-wave onset and QRS-complex onset. The PR interval represents intra-atrial and AV nodal conduction time. A short PR interval (<120 milliseconds) is suggestive of facile intra-atrial or AV conduction, and may represent ventricular pre-excitation. A prolonged PR interval (>200 milliseconds) reflects delayed intra-atrial or AV conduction. In the setting of a varying PR interval, conduction block or AV dissociation may be present.

R-R Interval

The R-R interval is inversely proportional to the rate of ventricular depolarization. If AV conduction is normal, the ventricular rate should equal the atrial rate.

Atrioventricular Block

First-Degree AV Block

First-degree AV block occurs when the *PR interval is prolonged (>200 milliseconds)*, and *each P wave is followed by a QRS* complex. Typically, the PR interval is constant.

Second-Degree AV Block, Mobitz Type I (Wenckebach)

Second-degree AV block, Mobitz type I (Wenckebach) is characterized by *progressive prolongation of the PR interval, terminating with a P wave followed by a nonconducted QRS* complex. Normal antegrade conduction resumes with a repetitive progressive prolongation of the PR interval with each cardiac depolarization, resuming the cycle. This results in a "grouped beating" pattern. In its most common form, the R-R interval shortens from beat to beat (not including the interval in which a P wave is not conducted). This typically represents conduction block within the AV node, *superior to the bundle of His*.

Second-Degree AV Block, Mobitz Type II

Second-degree AV block, Mobitz type II is characterized by regular P waves followed by intermittent nonconducted QRS complexes in the absence of atrial premature complexes. The resulting R-R interval spanning the nonconducted complex is exactly double the conducted R-R intervals. This typically represents AV conduction block *below the bundle of His, and has a high propensity to progress* to more advanced forms of AV block.

Note that when there is AV block with a ratio of 2:1, one cannot definitively distinguish between Mobitz type I and II. Longer rhythm strips, maneuvers, and intracardiac recordings may be necessary. A widened QRS complex supports Mobitz type II but lacks certainty.

Third-Degree AV Block (Complete Heart Block)

Third-degree AV block (complete heart block) is characterized by *independent atrial and ventricular activity with an atrial rate that is faster than the ventricular rate*. PR intervals vary with dissociation of the P waves from the QRS complexes. Typically, the ventricular rhythm is either a junctional (narrow complex) or a ventricular (wide complex) rhythm. (Note this should be distinguished from AV dissociation, which is also characterized by independent atrial and ventricular activity, but the ventricular rate is faster than the atrial rate.)

QRS Complex Interval

The QRS complex interval is best measured in the limb leads from the onset of the R wave (or Q wave if present) to the offset of the S wave. A normal QRS duration is <100 milliseconds.

If the QRS duration is between 100 and <120 milliseconds, the morphology should be further inspected for features of one or more of the following.

1. *Incomplete RBBB:* QRS complex duration 100 to 120 milliseconds, with a RBBB morphology with an R′ wave duration of ≥30 milliseconds (rsR′ in V_1; terminal S-wave slowing in leads I, aVL, and V_6).
2. *Left anterior fascicular block (LAFB):*
   - QRS duration <120 milliseconds
   - Significant left-axis deviation (–45 to –90 degrees)
   - Positive QRS-complex vector in lead I, negative QRS-complex vectors in the inferior leads (II, III, aVF)
   - Absence of other causes of left-axis deviation, such as an inferior myocardial infarction or an ostium primum atrial septal defect (ASD)
3. *Left posterior fascicular block (LPFB):* Early activation along the anterior fascicles produces a small R wave in leads I and aVL, and small q waves inferiorly. Mid and late forces in the direction of the posterior fascicles produce tall R waves inferiorly, deep S waves in I and aVL, and QRS-complex right-axis deviation.
   - QRS duration <120 milliseconds
   - Right axis (>120 degrees)
   - Absence of other clinical causes of right-axis QRS-complex deviation, such as pulmonary hypertension or right ventricular hypertrophy (RVH)
   - rS QRS-complex pattern in leads I and aVL
   - qR QRS-complex pattern in the inferior leads

If the QRS complex duration is >120 milliseconds, the morphology should be further inspected for features of the following:

1. *Right bundle-branch block:* The early depolarization vectors in RBBB are similar to normal depolarization reflecting left ventricular electrical events, producing early septal Q waves in leads I, aVL, V_5, and V_6, plus an early RS pattern in leads V_1 and V_2. Given the right bundle-branch conduction block, an unopposed QRS-complex vector representing delayed and slowed right ventricular depolarization is identified. These unopposed delayed left-to right-depolarization forces produce the characteristic broad second R′ wave in leads V_1 and V_2, plus the deep broad S waves in leads I, aVL, V_5, and V_6.
   - QRS duration ≥120 milliseconds
   - rsr′, rsR′, or rSR′ in lead V_1 ± lead V_2
   - Broad (>40 milliseconds) S wave in leads I and V_6
   - T-wave inversion and down-sloping ST depression often seen in leads V_1 and V_2
2. *Left bundle-branch block*: LBBB represents an altered left ventricular depolarization sequence. The right ventricle is depolarized in a timely manner via the right bundle branch. The left ventricle is depolarized after right ventricular depolarization via slowed right-to-left interventricular septal conduction. Because left ventricular depolarization initially transpires via the terminal branches of the left-sided conduction system, left ventricular depolarization occurs via an altered sequence with a prolonged QRS-complex duration.
   - QRS-complex duration ≥120 milliseconds
   - Broad and notched and/or slurred R wave in leads aVL, V_5, and V_6
   - Absent septal Q waves in leads I, aVL, V_5, and V_6
3. *Intraventricular conduction delay:*
   - QRS complex duration >100 milliseconds
   - Indeterminate morphology not satisfying the criteria for either RBBB or LBBB

QT Interval

The QT interval demonstrates heart-rate interdependence. The QT interval is directly proportional to the R-R interval. The QT interval shortens as heart rate increases. To account for this variability with heart rate, the corrected QT interval (QT_c) is calculated, in which the QT interval is divided by the square root of the R-R interval. Normative tables for heart rate and gender are available. A normal QT_c is typically <440 milliseconds. A less cumbersome approximation involves measuring the QT interval directly (typically in lead II). If this is >50% of the R-R interval, this supports QT-interval prolongation. In this circumstance, calculating a QT_c interval is appropriate.

Differential diagnosis of a prolonged QT interval includes the following:

- Congenital (idiopathic, Jervell-Lange-Nielsen syndrome, Romano-Ward syndrome)
- Medications (psychotropics, antiarrhythmics, antimicrobials, etc.)
- Metabolic disorders (hypocalcemia, hypokalemia, hypothyroidism, hypomagnesemia, etc.)
- The morphology of QT interval prolongation in hypocalcemia deserves special mention. Typically, hypocalcemia produces prolongation and straightening of the QT interval as a result of prolongation of the ST segment, without frank widening of the T wave.
- Neurogenic, such as an intracranial hemorrhage
- Ischemia

5. Determine If Cardiac Chamber Enlargement or Hypertrophy Is Present

If a patient is in sinus rhythm, the atria can be evaluated by analyzing the P-wave morphology in leads II, V_1, and V_2. Given the superior right atrial location of the sinus node, right atrial depolarization precedes left atrial depolarization. Therefore, right atrial depolarization is best represented in the first half of the surface electrocardiogram P wave. In lead II, if a bimodal P wave is present, the first peak represents right atrial depolarization and the second peak represents left atrial depolarization. In leads V_1 and V_2, the P wave is typically biphasic. The early portion is upright, representing right atrial depolarization toward lead V_1 and V_2, with the negative latter half representing left atrial depolarization, away from these leads.

Right Atrial Abnormality

Delayed activation of the right atrium due to hypertrophy, dilation, or intrinsically slowed conduction can result in the summation of right and left atrial depolarization. This typically produces a tall peaked P wave (≥2.5–3 mm) in lead II.

Left Atrial Abnormality

Delayed activation of the left atrium due to hypertrophy, dilation, or intrinsically slowed conduction can result in a broadening (>110 milliseconds) and notching of the P wave in lead II, or a deeper inverted phase of the P wave in leads V_1 and V_2:

- Negative terminal phase of P wave in lead V_1 or V_2 ≥40 milliseconds in duration and ≥1 mm in amplitude, *or*
- Biphasic P wave in lead II with peak-to-peak interval of ≥40 milliseconds (This is not very sensitive, but is quite specific.)

Right Ventricular Hypertrophy

In RVH, there is a dominance of the right ventricular forces, which produce prominent R waves in the right precordial leads and deeper S waves in the left precordial leads. RVH is suggested by one or more of the following:

- Right-axis QRS-complex deviation (greater than +90 degrees)
- R:S ratio in lead V_1 >1
- R wave in V_1 ≥7 mm
- R:S ratio in V_6 <1
- ST–T-wave "strain" pattern in right precordial leads supported by asymmetric T-wave inversion
- Right atrial abnormality

In the absence of:

- Posterior-wall myocardial infarction
- Wolff-Parkinson-White (WPW) syndrome
- Counterclockwise rotation
- Dextrocardia
- RBBB

Left Ventricular Hypertrophy

Several criteria have been described and validated for the diagnosis of left ventricular hypertrophy (LVH) by electrocardiography.

1. Sokolow and Lyon: Amplitude of the S wave in lead V_1 + amplitude of the R wave in V_5 or V_6 (whichever is the tallest) ≥35 mm
2. Cornell: Amplitude of the R wave in aVL + amplitude of the S wave in V_3 >28 mm for men, or >20 mm for women
3. Romhilt-Estes: This is a scoring system in which a total score of 4 indicates "likely LVH," and a score of ≥5 indicates "definite LVH."
   - Voltage criteria = 3 points:
     Amplitude of limb lead R wave or S wave ≥20 mm *or*
     Amplitude of S wave in V_1 or V_2 ≥30 mm *or*
     Amplitude of R wave in V_5 or V_6 ≥30 mm
     ST–T-wave changes typical of strain (in which the ST segment and T-wave vector is shifted in a direction opposite to that of the QRS complex vector) = 3 points (only 1 point if patient is taking digitalis)
   - Left atrial abnormality = 3 points:
     Terminal portion of P wave in V_1 ≥40 milliseconds in duration and ≥1 mm in amplitude
   - Left-axis deviation = 2 points:
     Axis ≥ −30 degrees
   - QRS duration = 1 point:
     Duration ≥90 milliseconds
   - Intrinsicoid deflection = 1 point:
     Duration of interval from the beginning of the QRS complex to the peak of the R wave in V_5 or V_6 ≥50 milliseconds

Combined or Biventricular Hypertrophy

Combined ventricular hypertrophy is suggested by any of the following:

- ECG meets criteria for isolated RVH and LVH. This is the most reliable criterion.

- Precordial leads demonstrate LVH by voltage, but there is right-axis deviation (greater than +90 degrees) in the frontal plane.
- Precordial leads demonstrate LVH, with limb leads demonstrating right atrial abnormality.

6. Assess the P-Wave, QRS-Complex, and T-Wave Morphologies

Once the cardiac rate, rhythm, axes, intervals, and chambers have been assessed, one should proceed with the identification of various morphologies that suggest pathologic states. There have been virtually innumerable descriptions of various morphologic criteria for a broad spectrum of pathologic states, but here we discuss those that are most common and/or most important.

ECG Abnormalities and Corresponding Differential Diagnoses

Incorrect Lead Placement

Incorrect lead placement is most commonly identified in the limb leads, with a negative P-wave vector in leads I and aVL and normal precordial R-wave progression.

Low Voltage

Low voltage in limb leads is defined as a QRS-complex amplitude of <5 mm in each of the standard limb leads (I, II, and III). Low voltage of all leads is defined as low voltage in the limb leads plus a QRS-complex amplitude of <10 mm in each of the precordial leads.

Low voltage on the ECG may be of primary myocardial origin or secondary to high-impedance tissue conduction. Differential diagnosis possibilities include:

- Cardiomyopathy (infiltrative or restrictive)
- Pericardial effusion
- Pleural effusion
- Anasarca
- Obesity
- Myxedema
- Chronic obstructive pulmonary disease

Q Waves

Q waves represent an initial negative QRS-complex vector. Pathologic Q waves are present if they are ≥1 mm (0.1 mV) in depth and ≥40 milliseconds in duration. Q waves are most commonly associated with a myocardial infarction. To diagnose a myocardial infarction, Q waves must be identified in two contiguous leads:

- Inferior leads—II, III, and aVF
- Anteroseptal leads—V_2 and V_3
- Anterior leads—V_2, V_3, and V_4
- Lateral leads—V_5 and V_6
- High lateral leads—I and aVL
- Posterior leads V_1 and V_2 (R-wave amplitude > S-wave amplitude)

Contiguous regions on an electrocardiogram include the following:

- Inferior, posterior, and lateral
- Anteroseptal, anterior, and lateral
- Lateral and high lateral

Other etiologies of Q waves include:

- "Septal" Q waves (small Q waves as a result of the septal left-to-right depolarization vector)—leads I, aVL, V_5, and V_6
- Hypertrophic cardiomyopathy—any lead
- Left anterior fascicular block—leads I and aVL
- Wolfe-Parkinson-White syndrome—any lead

ST-Segment Elevation

ST-segment elevation refers to elevation of the segment between the terminal aspect of the QRS complex and the T-wave onset. This elevation is relative to the isoelectric comparative TP segment located between the end of the T wave and the start of the P wave.

Causes of ST-segment elevation include the following:

- *Acute myocardial injury:* convex upward ST-segment elevation in at least two contiguous ECG leads
- *Coronary spasm (Prinzmetal angina):* similar morphology to acute myocardial injury, with the distinction that the ST-segment elevation is typically transient
- *Pericarditis:* diffuse concave upward ST-segment elevation not confined to contiguous ECG leads
- *Left ventricular aneurysm:* most often seen in the right precordial leads, with convex upward ST-segment elevation overlying an infarct zone, with ST-segment elevation persisting for months to years after the initial myocardial infarction

- *LBBB:* typically discordant from the QRS-complex vector
- *Early repolarization:* manifest as J-point elevation with normal ST segments, best seen in the lateral precordial leads
- *Brugada syndrome:* ST-segment elevation in the right precordial leads with a pattern of right ventricular conduction delay
- *Hypothermia:* Osborne waves

ST-Segment Depression

The most common causes of ST-segment depression are the following:

- *Myocardial ischemia or non–ST-segment-elevation myocardial infarction (NSTEMI):* Horizontal or down-sloping ST-segment depression demonstrates the greatest specificity for myocardial ischemia. Positive cardiac biomarkers distinguish ischemia versus infarction.
- *Ventricular hypertrophy:* Down-sloping asymmetric ST-segment depression and T-wave inversion is often present in both LVH and RVH.

Peaked T Waves

The most common causes of peaked, positive T waves are the following:

- Hyperkalemia
- Hyperacute phase of myocardial infarction
- Acute transient ischemia (Prinzmetal angina)

U Waves

U waves are seen immediately following the T wave. They are best observed in leads V_2, V_3, and V_4 and are typically up to one quarter the amplitude of the T wave. Prominent U waves are ≥1.5 mm (≥0.15 mV) in amplitude.

Prominent U waves are commonly observed in the presence of:

- Hypokalemia
- Bradyarrhythmias
- Certain medications

Pathologic States and Corresponding ECG Abnormalities

Myocardial Injury and Infarction

- *Acute myocardial infarction:* Q waves and ST-segment elevation. Reciprocal ST-segment depression is often observed but is not necessary.
- *Recent myocardial infarction:* Q waves with ischemic T-wave changes, often inverted; the ST segments are typically no longer elevated.
- *Age-indeterminate myocardial infarction:* persistent Q waves devoid of ST-segment elevation or ischemic T-wave changes.
- *Acute myocardial injury:* regional ST-segment elevation without Q waves.

Acute Pericarditis

Acute pericarditis is characterized by diffuse ST-segment elevation and/or PR-segment depression. Lead aVR classically demonstrates PR-segment elevation and is highly specific.

- Diffuse ST-segment elevation.
- Diffuse PR-segment depression with PR-segment elevation in lead aVR.
- T-wave inversions typically do not appear until ST-segment elevations have resolved.

Pericardial Effusion

The ECG manifestations of pericardial effusions are a result of the increased impedance of the electrical signal through the pericardial fluid collection coupled with translational cardiac motion within the pericardium. These include:

- Electrical alternans
- Low-voltage QRS complexes

Digitalis Effect

- Most commonly manifests as ST-segment and T-wave changes
- Concave depression/sagging of the ST segment (usually without frank J-point depression) seen best in leads V_5 and V_6
- PR-interval prolongation
- T-wave flattening with QT-interval shortening

Digitalis Toxicity

Digitalis toxicity exerts its effects via a combination of an increase in myocardial automaticity plus suppression of sinus nodal and AV nodal pacemaker function. This manifests as a combination of conduction defects and arrhythmias including but not limited to:

- Atrial tachycardia
- Accelerated junctional rhythm

- First-, second-, or third-degree AV block
- Bidirectional ventricular tachycardia (VT with alternating right and LBBB morphology)
- Ventricular fibrillation

Hyperkalemia

- Tall, peaked, narrow-based T waves
- PR-interval prolongation
- Advanced conduction block
- Atrial standstill or arrest
- Widening of the QRS complex, which can progress to a "sine wave" pattern
- Ventricular tachycardia or fibrillation

Hypokalemia

- Prominent U waves, especially in leads V_2, V_3, and V_4
- ST-segment depression
- Decreased T-wave amplitude
- Increase in P-wave amplitude and duration

Hypercalcemia

- Shortened QT_c, predominantly via decreased ST-segment duration

Hypocalcemia

- Prolonged QT_c, predominantly via increased ST-segment duration and straightening without a significant increase in the T-wave duration

Sick Sinus Syndrome

Sick sinus syndrome is characterized by combinations of the following:

- Marked sinus bradycardia
- Sinus arrest
- Prolonged recovery time of the sinus node following PACs or atrial tachyarrhythmias
- Alternating bradycardia and tachycardia

Acute Cor Pulmonale

The following suggest acute cor pulmonale:

- Sinus tachycardia
- Anterior precordial T-wave inversion (leads V_1 to V_3)
- Right atrial abnormality
- Right-axis QRS-complex deviation
- An S1, Q3, T3 QRS complex limb lead pattern
- RBBB (may be transient)

Atrial Septal Defect, Secundum

The following ECG findings are suggestive of a secundum ASD:

- Right-axis QRS-complex deviation
- Incomplete RBBB
- RVH
- Right atrial abnormality
- PR-interval prolongation

Atrial Septal Defect, Primum

The following ECG findings are suggestive of a primum ASD:

- Left-axis QRS-complex deviation
- PR-interval prolongation
- Incomplete RBBB

Dextrocardia

The following ECG findings suggest dextrocardia:

- Precordial R-wave regression (R-wave amplitude decreases from V_1 to V_6)
- Negative P-wave vector in leads I and aVL

Wolff-Parkinson-White Syndrome

WPW syndrome is suggested by the following ECG findings:

- Shortened PR interval (<120 milliseconds)
- Delta wave representing ventricular preexcitation (slurring of the initial portion of the QRS complex)
- QRS complex may be wide, representing altered ventricular depolarization

Hypertrophic Cardiomyopathy

The following ECG criteria are suggestive of hypertrophic cardiomyopathy:

- High-voltage QRS complex
- Deep Q waves not ascribable to a specific coronary artery territory
- ST–T-wave changes including deep T-wave inversions

Hypothermia

The following ECG criteria are suggestive of hypothermia:

- Osborne waves (elevated J point that is proportional to the degree of hypothermia)
- Bradycardia
- PR-interval, QRS-complex interval, and QT-interval prolongation

Myxedema

The following ECG criteria are suggestive of myxedema:

- Sinus bradycardia
- PR-interval prolongation
- Low-voltage QRS complexes

7. Draw Conclusions and Correlate Clinically

Electrocardiography has its largest clinical impact when interpreted in the context of the patient's presenting symptoms and available past medical and surgical history. It is within this context that an overall diagnostic and treatment plan can be developed with the electrocardiogram interpretation fulfilling an important role.

Electrocardiography Review

A CASE-BASED APPROACH

Electrocardiogram Case Study **#1**

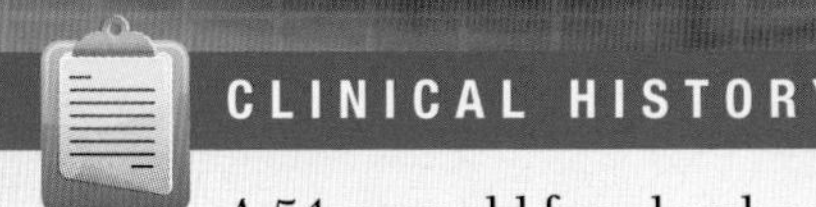

CLINICAL HISTORY

A 54-year-old female who presents for a routine physical examination.

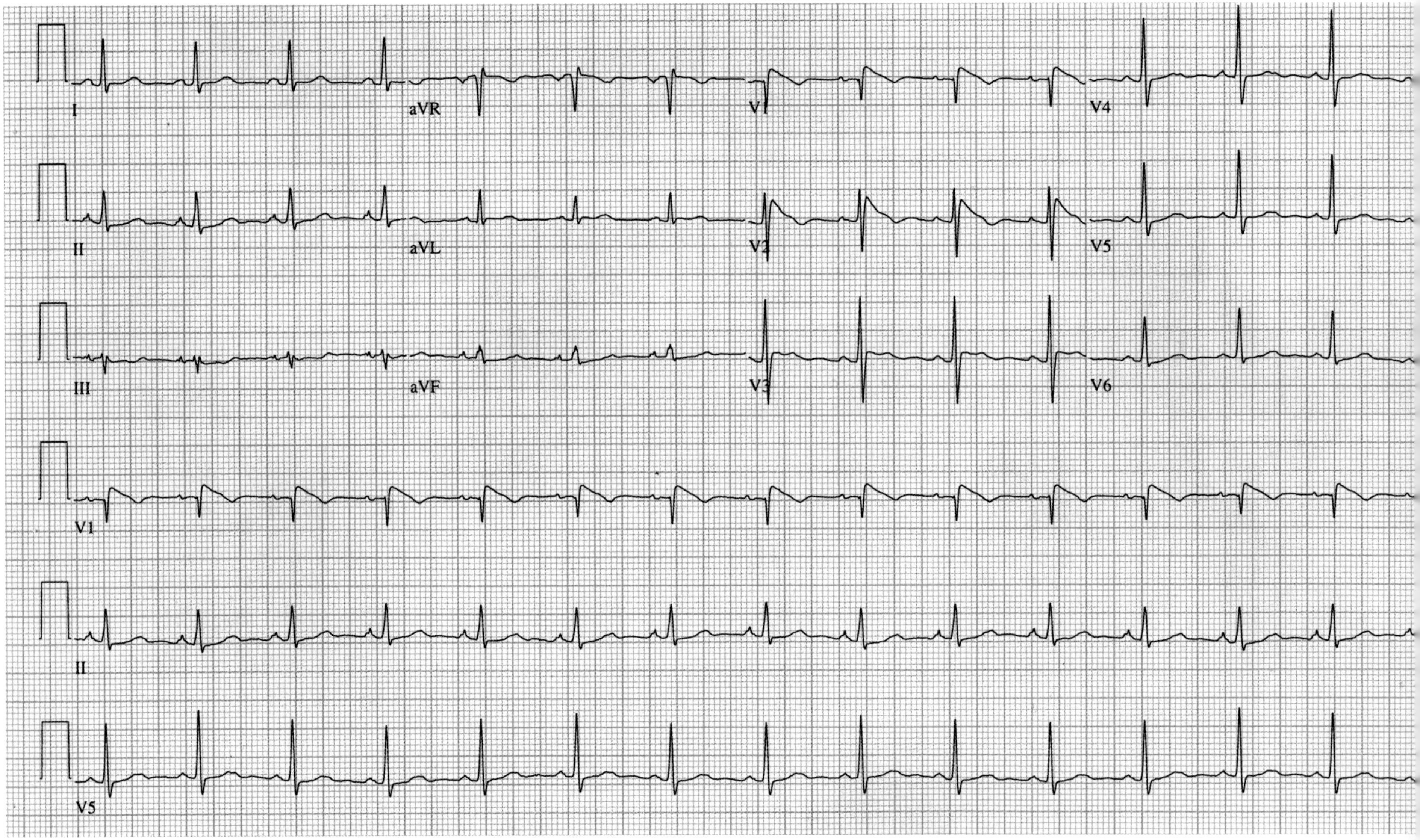

Interpretation Notes:

Electrocardiogram Case Study #1

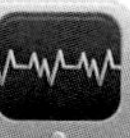

ELECTROCARDIOGRAM INTERPRETATION

This electrocardiogram demonstrates normal sinus rhythm at an atrial rate of approximately 80 per minute. J-point and ST-segment elevation is seen in leads V1 and V2. This morphology suggests terminal right ventricular conduction delay. Note the absence of a terminally prolonged S wave in leads 1, aVL, V5, and V6 as would normally be seen in the presence of a right ventricular conduction delay. This pattern of abnormality, particularly as seen in the right precordial leads, is consistent with Brugada syndrome.

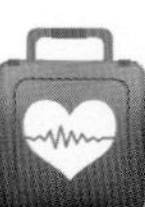

KEY DIAGNOSES

- Normal sinus rhythm
- Brugada syndrome

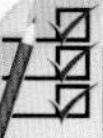

KEY TEACHING POINTS

- Brugada syndrome is electrocardiographically reflected by a characteristic pattern in leads V1 and V2 as depicted on this electrocardiogram.
- This is an important pattern to recognize as Brugada syndrome patients are at a heightened risk for unexpected sudden cardiac death in the setting of fatal ventricular arrhythmias.

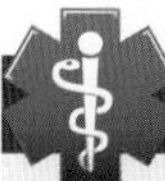

BOARD EXAMINATION ESSENTIALS

Brugada syndrome is an important board exam example. Brugada syndrome may also occur as a question incorporating a patient care scenario, an electrocardiogram example, and asking for the best form of patient management. Consideration should be given for implantable cardiac defibrillator placement.

Electrocardiogram Case Study #2

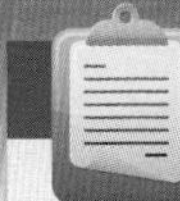

CLINICAL HISTORY

A 46-year-old male with a severe episode of anterior chest pain 2 weeks previously who presents to his physician with persistent shortness of breath.

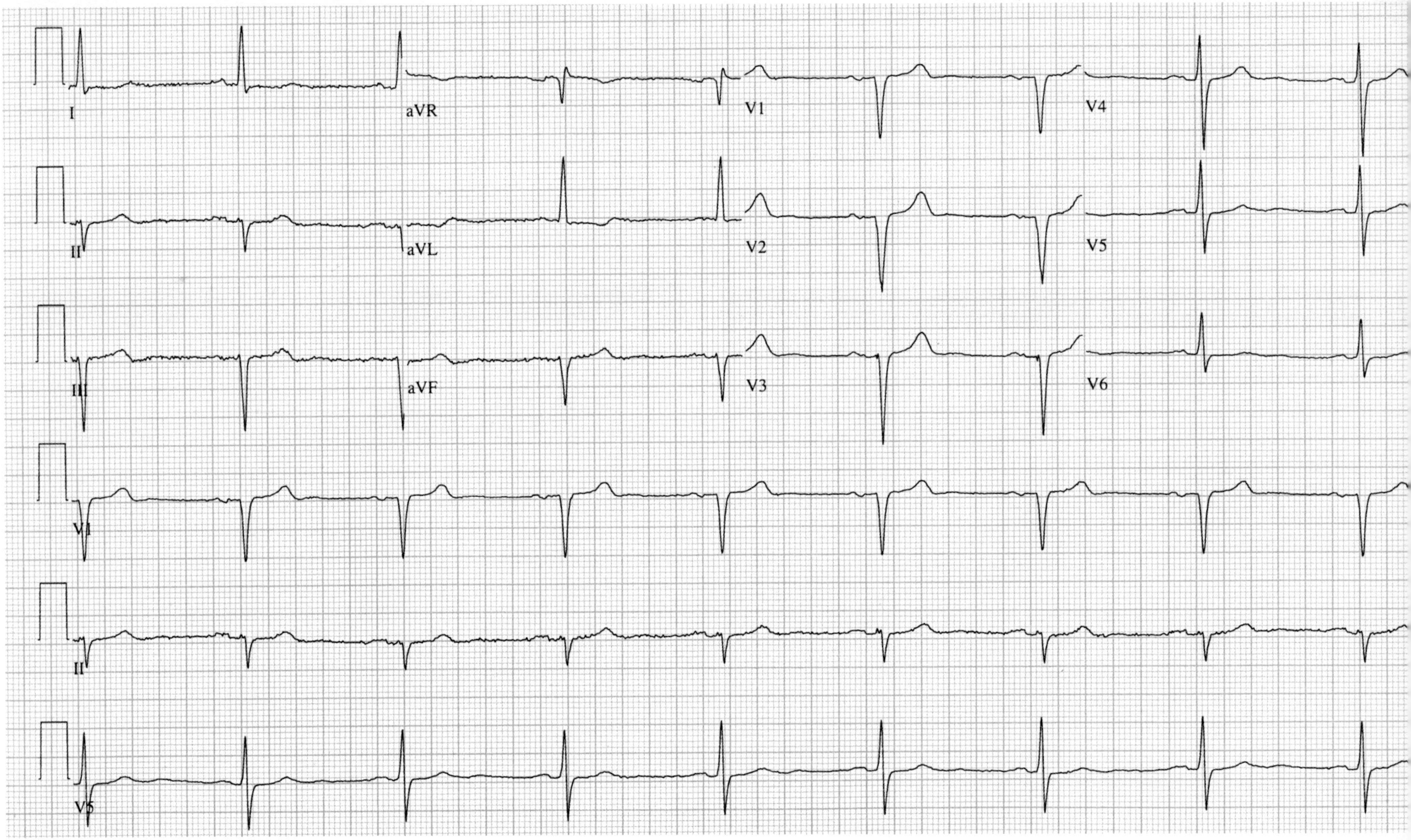

I aVR V1 V4
II aVL V2 V5
III aVF V3 V6
V1
II
V5

Interpretation Notes:

Electrocardiogram Case Study #2

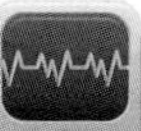

ELECTROCARDIOGRAM INTERPRETATION

This electrocardiogram demonstrates sinus bradycardia at an atrial rate of approximately 55 per minute. Left atrial abnormality is suspected as there is a bifid and prolonged P wave in lead II. Left anterior fascicular block is also present given the positive QRS complex vector in lead I and negative QRS complex vectors in leads II, III and aVF with a preserved R wave. Q waves are seen in leads V1, V2, and V3. In lead V3, a very small or "splinter" Q wave is seen that is highly specific for an anteroseptal myocardial infarction of indeterminate age.

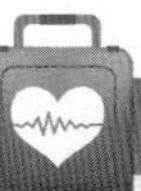

KEY DIAGNOSES

- Sinus bradycardia
- Left atrial abnormality
- Left anterior fascicular block
- Anteroseptal myocardial infarction age indeterminate

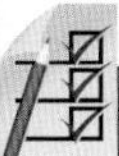

KEY TEACHING POINTS

- In lead II, the P wave appears bifid with initial right atrial depolarization and subsequently left atrial depolarization. This reflects slowed atrial conduction.
- Q waves are seen in leads V1, V2, and V3 confirming an anteroseptal myocardial infarction of indeterminate age. In lead V3, the QRS complex demonstrates an initial brief negative deflection followed by a slight R wave followed by a dominant S wave. This is termed a splinter Q wave and lends greater specificity to the diagnosis of a myocardial infarction. At times, this may be the only finding supporting the presence of ischemic heart disease.

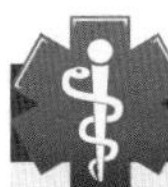

BOARD EXAMINATION ESSENTIALS

When coding for left anterior fascicular block, make sure the QRS complex duration is ≤100 milliseconds and the QRS complex frontal plane vector is ≥ negative 45 degrees. This is easily determined if the predominantly positive QRS complex vector is in lead AVL and the QRS complex vector in lead II is significantly negative. If Q waves are isolated to leads V1 and V2, do not code an anteroseptal myocardial infarction as this is not diagnostic. A definite Q wave must be present in lead V3, even more important in the presence of left anterior fascicular block given the initial posterior and inferior QRS complex depolarization vector. This electrocardiogram depicts a classic splinter Q wave where the initial QRS complex vector is negative with a Q-wave duration typically not diagnostic of a Q-wave myocardial infarction (≤25 milliseconds) in the precordial leads. The splinter Q wave is an exception to this rule where a Q-wave myocardial infarction diagnosis can be made with confidence with a short duration Q wave. In summary, diagnostic board exam codes include sinus bradycardia, left atrial abnormality/enlargement, left anterior fascicular block, and anteroseptal myocardial infarction, age indeterminate.

Electrocardiogram Case Study **#3**

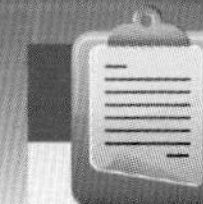

CLINICAL HISTORY

A 72-year-old male with known coronary artery disease and two past myocardial infarctions, last in the left anterior descending coronary artery distribution approximately 3 years prior to this electrocardiogram.

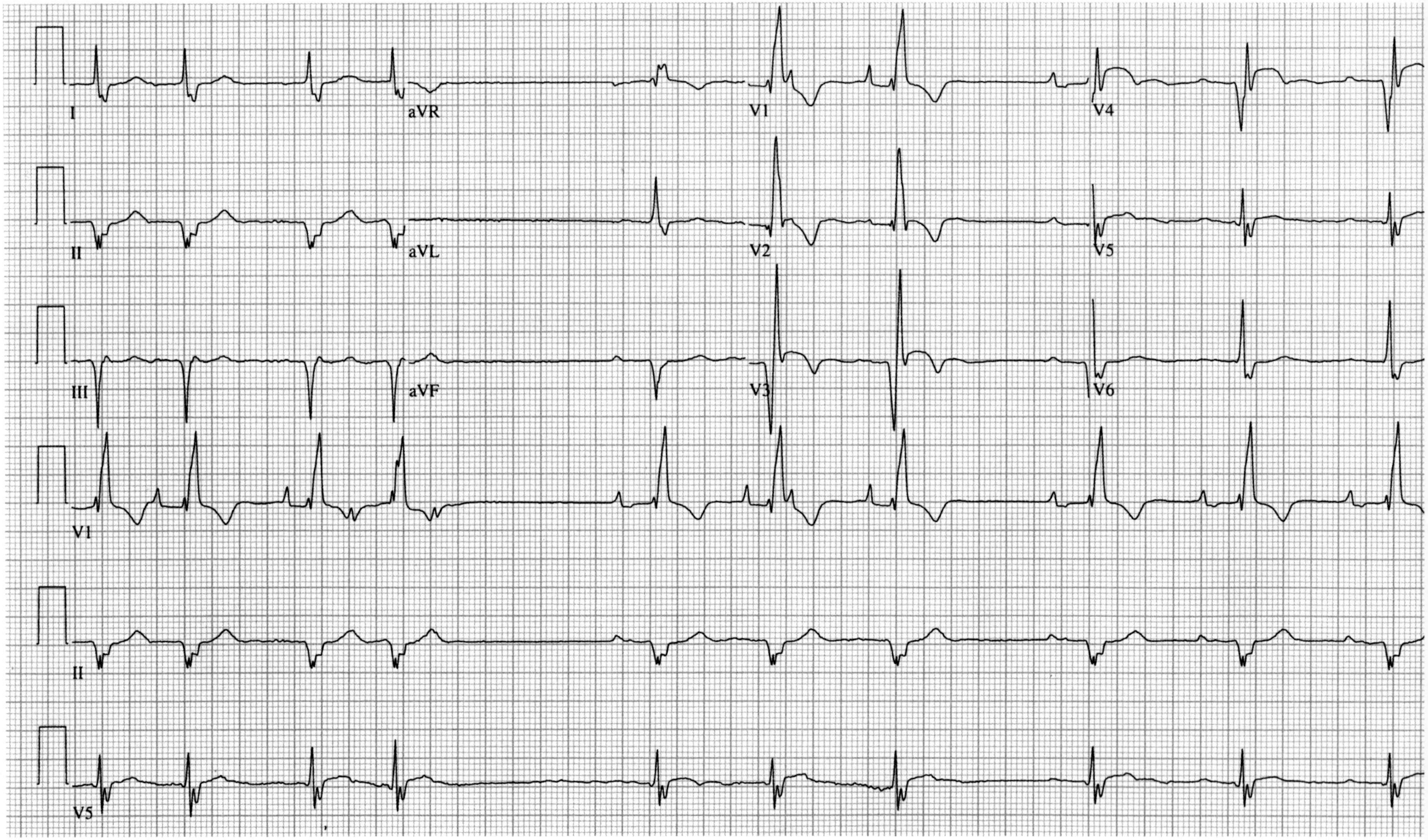

Interpretation Notes:___

Electrocardiogram Case Study #3

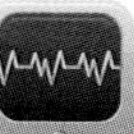

ELECTROCARDIOGRAM INTERPRETATION

This electrocardiogram demonstrates sinus bradycardia at a rate of approximately 55 per minute. The native P waves are best seen on the right-hand portion of the electrocardiogram in the lead V1 rhythm strip. The P wave appears prolonged and is somewhat peaked in lead V1 suggesting right atrial abnormality. There is a prolonged, terminally negative component to the P wave in lead V1 suggesting left atrial abnormality. Both conducted and nonconducted premature atrial complexes with a differing P-wave morphology are seen toward the left-hand portion of the electrocardiogram in the lead V1 rhythm strip. Q waves are seen in leads II, III, and AVF consistent with an age-indeterminate inferior myocardial infarction. The PR interval is also prolonged consistent with first-degree atrioventricular block. Complete right bundle branch block is seen as there is a RSR′ complex in leads V1 and V2 with terminal S-wave conduction delay seen in leads I, aVL, V5, and V6 and a QRS complex duration of >120 milliseconds. Q waves of diagnostic duration are seen in leads V3 and V4 consistent with an age-indeterminate anterior myocardial infarction. Persistent and unchanged based on prior electrocardiograms, ST-segment elevation is seen consistent with the patient's known history of a left ventricular aneurysm.

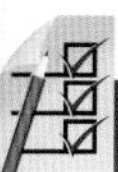

KEY TEACHING POINTS

- The findings on this electrocardiogram suggest multivessel coronary artery disease, in the least involving both the right coronary artery and left anterior descending coronary artery distributions.
- Clues to the presence of a left ventricular aneurysm include the patient's asymptomatic status, history of a prior myocardial infarction, prominent Q waves, and upwardly coved ST segments with associated J-point elevation in the absence of a clinical history or biochemical evidence of acute myocardial injury.
- A posterior myocardial infarction is not demonstrated on this electrocardiogram. The initial R wave is diminutive. Avoid the potential trap of suspecting a posterior myocardial infarction in the presence of complete right bundle branch block with a prominent R′ deflection. It is the R wave or initial ventricular vector that reflects left ventricular depolarization.

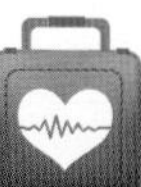

KEY DIAGNOSES

- Sinus bradycardia
- Right atrial abnormality
- Left atrial abnormality
- Premature atrial complexes
- Nonconducted premature atrial complexes
- Inferior myocardial infarction age indeterminate
- First-degree atrioventricular block
- Complete right bundle branch block
- Anterior myocardial infarction age indeterminate
- Left ventricular aneurysm

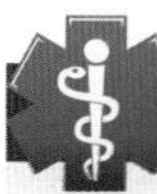

BOARD EXAMINATION ESSENTIALS

Note the lack of an R wave in leads II, III, and aVF. This finding precludes the diagnosis of left anterior fascicular block, instead supporting an inferior myocardial infarction age indeterminate. It is important to locate the native P wave if at all possible. On most electrocardiograms, the native P wave will reflect a sinus node origin but not always. Once the native P wave is identified, it is easier to identify ectopic P waves and to characterize them as premature, as in this case, versus escape complexes. For the board exam, thoroughly evaluating the heart rhythm is essential including ectopic complexes, both conducted and nonconducted. Note the lack of a code for a left ventricular aneurysm on the board exam coding sheet. Without a supporting clinical history of a remote myocardial infarction and continued clinical stability, this electrocardiogram could alternatively be coded for an anterior myocardial infarction acute and possibly anterolateral if you believed the Q wave in lead V5 was of diagnostic duration. Board exam diagnostic codes include sinus bradycardia; right atrial abnormality/enlargement; left atrial abnormality/enlargement; atrial premature complexes; inferior myocardial infarction, age indeterminate; AV block, first degree; right bundle branch block, complete; and anterior myocardial infarction, age indeterminate.

Electrocardiogram Case Study #4

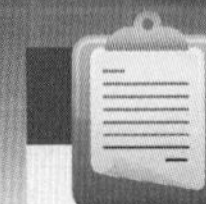

CLINICAL HISTORY

A 34-year-old male with congenital bicuspid aortic valve disease and severe aortic valve insufficiency.

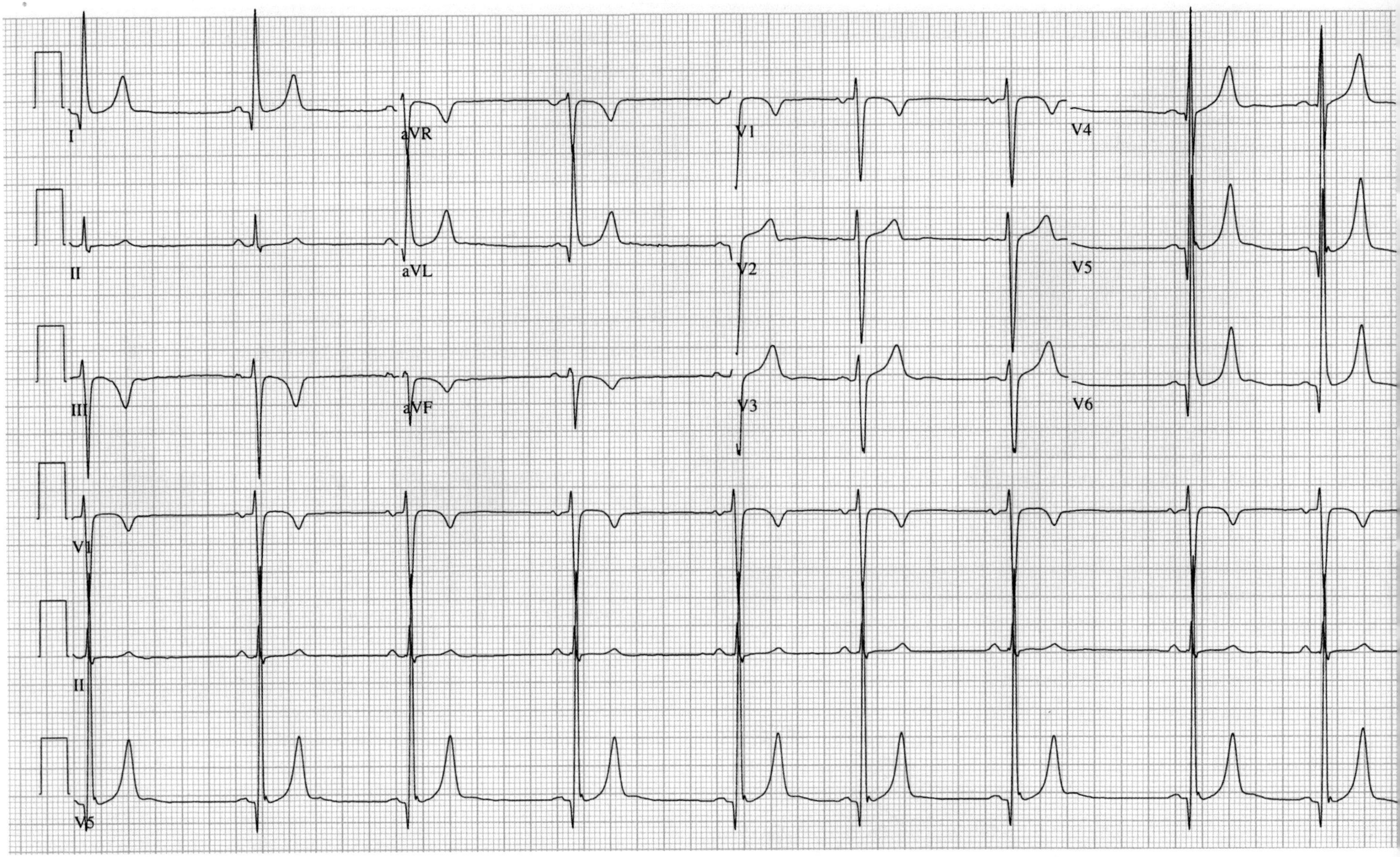

I aVR V1 V4

II aVL V2 V5

III aVF V3 V6

V1

II

V5

Interpretation Notes:

Electrocardiogram Case Study #4

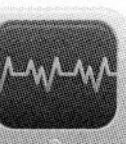

ELECTROCARDIOGRAM INTERPRETATION

This electrocardiogram demonstrates sinus bradycardia at an approximate rate of 50 per minute with coexisting sinus arrhythmia. Prominent QRS complex voltage is seen with overlapping QRS complexes in leads V4, V5, and V6. Prominent narrow Q waves are evident in leads V5 and V6 and also leads I and aVL. This is an example of a younger patient with severe bicuspid aortic valve insufficiency and the volume overload pattern of left ventricular hypertrophy. In this circumstance, while prominent voltage is seen typically over the left precordial leads, there is a lack of asymmetric T-wave inversion, better known as repolarization changes or a strain pattern. This is very typical of a volume overload pattern of left ventricular hypertrophy that one might see in the presence of severe aortic or mitral insufficiency.

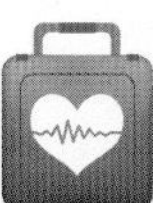

KEY DIAGNOSES

- Sinus bradycardia
- Sinus arrhythmia
- Left ventricular hypertrophy

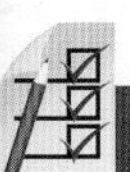

KEY TEACHING POINTS

- Distinguishing the more common pressure overload pattern of left ventricular hypertrophy from the volume overload pattern is important and can provide insight as to the pathophysiology of the increased left ventricular mass.
- As demonstrated on this electrocardiogram, in the volume overload pattern of left ventricular hypertrophy, prominent, narrow and deep septal Q waves are seen in the lateral precordial leads. Additionally, the lack of asymmetric T-wave inversion and significant repolarization changes favors a left ventricular volume overload pattern.

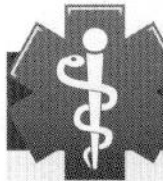

BOARD EXAMINATION ESSENTIALS

Not all ventricular hypertrophy patterns possess abnormal ST segments. For the board examination, keep in mind that coding for hypertrophy patterns is a separate selection from the ST and/or T-wave changes secondary to hypertrophy. When the latter is present, make sure it is coded for in addition to the hypertrophy pattern. Also, whenever hypertrophy is present, pay close attention to the QRS complex frontal plane axis and also to the P-wave morphology, especially atrial enlargement patterns. Diagnostic board exam codes include sinus bradycardia, sinus arrhythmia, and left ventricular hypertrophy.

Electrocardiogram Case Study #5

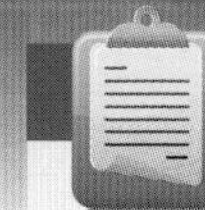

CLINICAL HISTORY

A 54-year-old female with intermittent palpitations and light-headedness for the past 6 months.

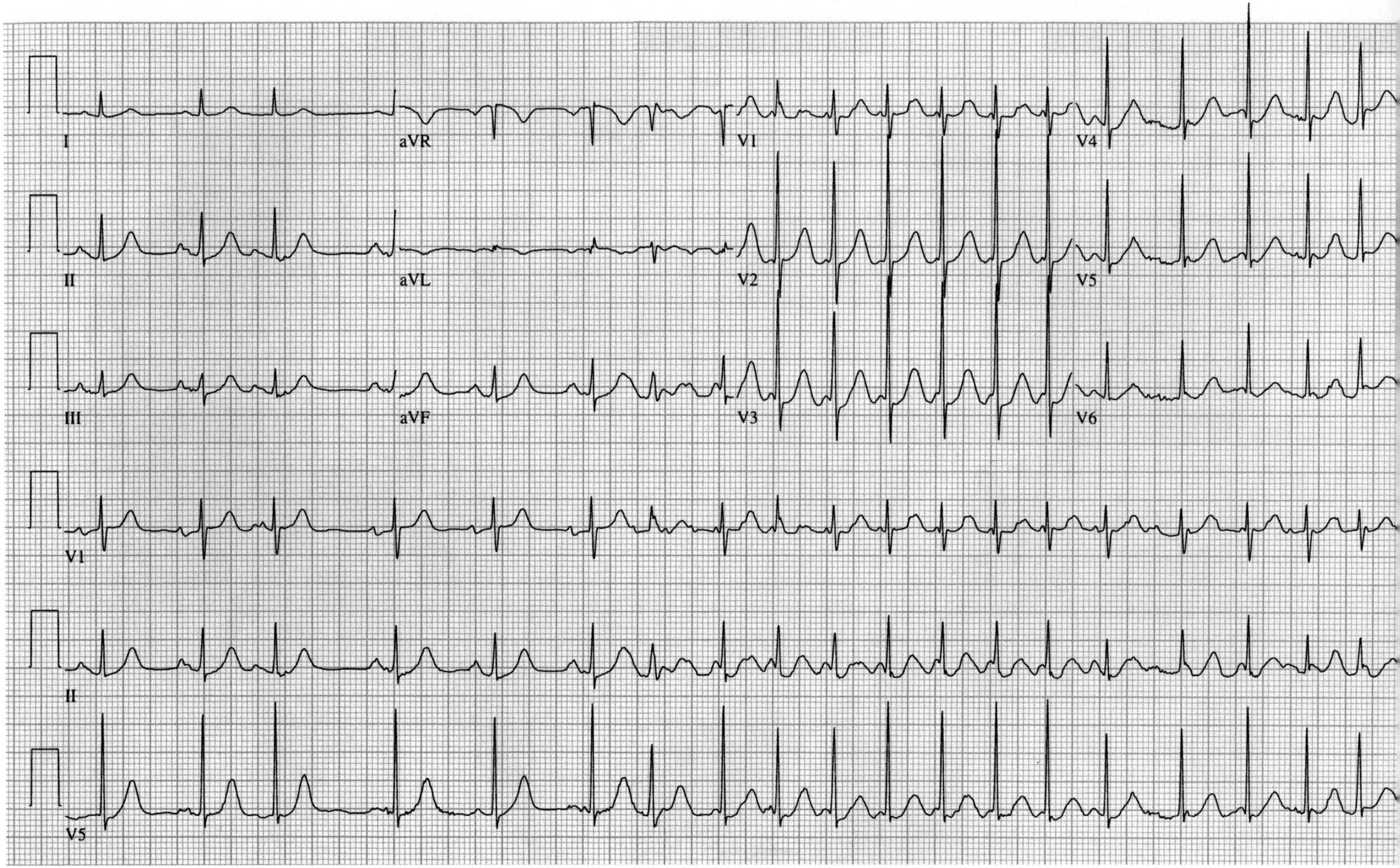

I aVR V1 V4
II aVL V2 V5
III aVF V3 V6
V1
II
V5

Interpretation Notes:______________________________

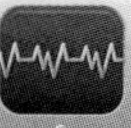

ELECTROCARDIOGRAM INTERPRETATION

On the left-hand portion best seen in the limb leads I, II, and III, this electrocardiogram demonstrates normal sinus rhythm at a rate of approximately 80 per minute. The third P wave followed by a QRS complex represents a premature atrial complex. Similarly, this is seen in the seventh P wave followed by a premature QRS complex that conducts aberrantly. This begins a paroxysm of a supraventricular tachycardic rhythm at a rate of about 150 per minute composed of atrial flutter waves best identified in the lead II rhythm strip. Approximately half way across the electrocardiogram, best identified in the lead V1 and lead II rhythm strips, an ectopic atrial focus is seen that appears dissimilar to the native P wave. A subsequent paroxysm of atrial flutter ensues. Of note, in lead II the native P wave is best seen and the second P-wave component lends a bifid appearance, suggesting slowed intra-atrial conduction and likely the substrate for atrial arrhythmia initiation.

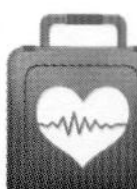

KEY DIAGNOSES

- Normal sinus rhythm
- Atrial flutter
- Premature atrial complex
- Aberrant conduction

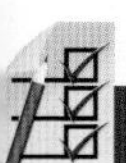

KEY TEACHING POINTS

- Atrial arrhythmias such as atrial flutter and atrial fibrillation are often initiated by premature atrial complexes, as demonstrated on this electrocardiogram.
- Be careful not to interpret the widened QRS complex as a premature ventricular complex. As on this electrocardiogram, instead, this represents a supraventricular complex conducted to the ventricle with aberrant and thus slowed intraventricular conduction. The most important clue is the fact that the widened QRS complex is preceded by a premature atrial depolarization.

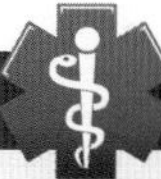

BOARD EXAMINATION ESSENTIALS

Make certain to code functional (rate-related) aberrancy when present. In this case, this is due to the rapid increase in heart rate and partial conduction system refractoriness. While the ST segments appear normal on this electrocardiogram, ST-segment and T-wave changes may be seen during tachycardic heart rhythms. These should be coded as nonspecific ST and/or T-wave abnormalities unless another specific cause is readily identifiable. Board exam diagnostic codes include normal sinus rhythm, atrial flutter, atrial premature complex, and aberrant conduction.

Electrocardiogram Case Study #6

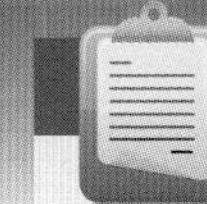

CLINICAL HISTORY

A 61-year-old male seen preoperatively prior to a planned lung mass resection.

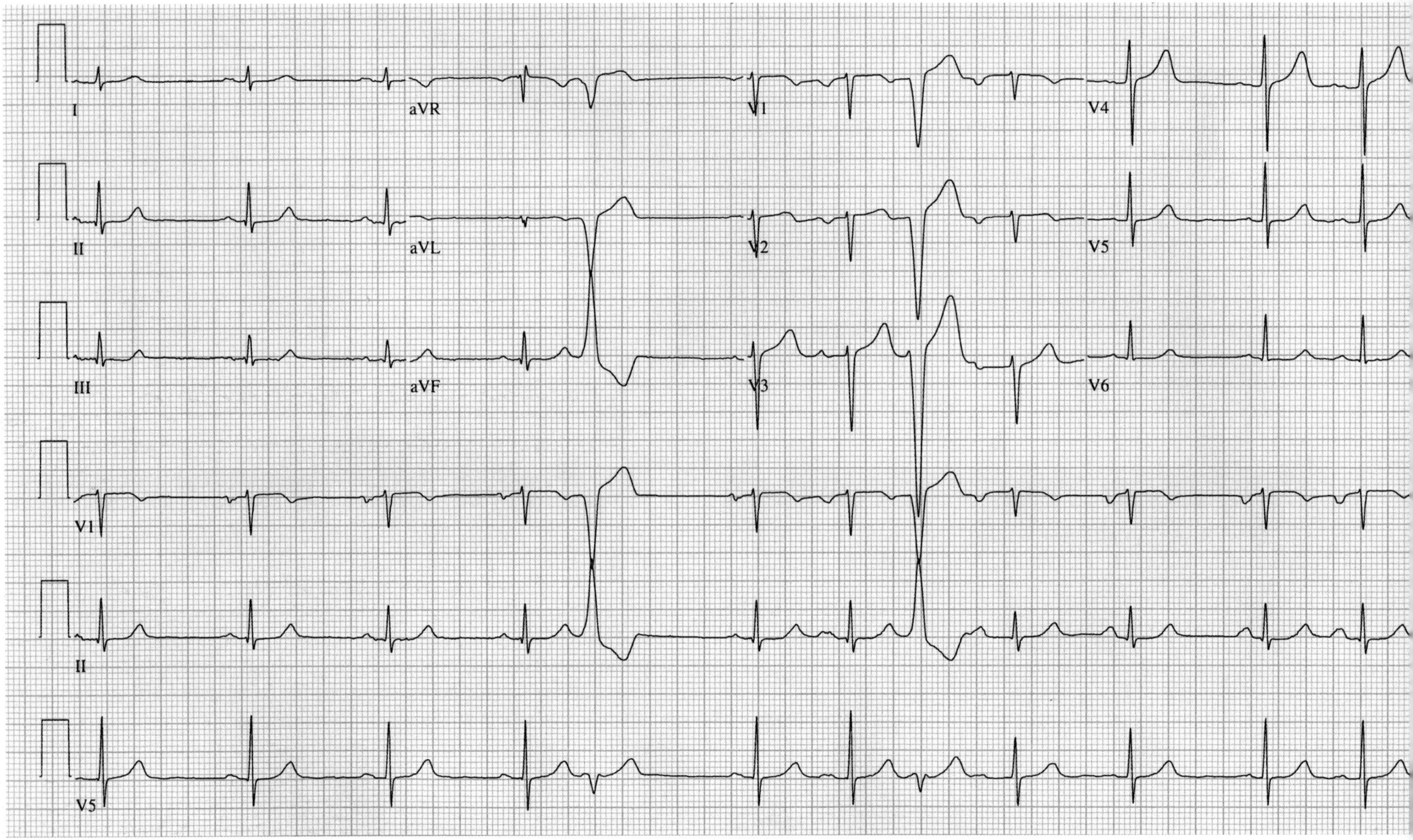

I aVR V1 V4
II aVL V2 V5
III aVF V3 V6
V1
II
V5

Interpretation Notes:

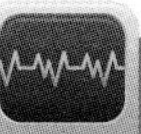

ELECTROCARDIOGRAM INTERPRETATION

On the left-hand side of the electrocardiogram, normal sinus rhythm is present. Two premature ventricular complexes are seen. Both conduct with a complete left bundle branch block morphology and therefore are right ventricular in origin. The first premature ventricular complex demonstrates a tighter coupling interval in relation to the previous QRS complex. What follows is a compensatory pause and resetting of the sinus node. In the middle of the electrocardiogram, the P-wave morphology changes just prior to the second premature ventricular complex and an ectopic atrial rhythm commences. During this ectopic atrial rhythm paroxysm, a subsequent premature ventricular complex of similar morphology is seen. This is slightly less tightly coupled to the proceeding QRS complex, and the subsequent ectopic atrial P wave demonstrates a prolonged PR interval suggesting retrograde ventriculoatrial concealed conduction at least into the AV node and perhaps beyond into the atrial conduction system.

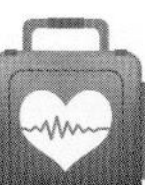

KEY DIAGNOSES

- Normal sinus rhythm
- Ectopic atrial rhythm
- Premature ventricular complex
- Concealed conduction

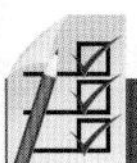

KEY TEACHING POINTS

- In the presence of a premature ventricular complex, prolongation of the subsequent PR interval is frequently seen and is the most common 12-lead electrocardiogram example of concealed conduction.
- It is important to assess the P-wave morphology and P-wave electrical axis. An abnormal and variable P-wave morphology is an important diagnostic finding as it may be a precursor to future atrial arrhythmias such as atrial flutter and atrial fibrillation.

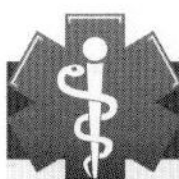

BOARD EXAMINATION ESSENTIALS

This electrocardiogram requires coding for two atrial rhythms, normal sinus rhythm and an ectopic atrial rhythm. Interestingly, ectopic atrial rhythm is not a coding option on the present scoring sheet. A more likely electrocardiogram possibility might include a paroxysm of atrial tachycardia with a P-wave axis differing from the sinus P wave. The main point here is that premature complexes, in this case ventricular in origin, can influence both ventricular and atrial refractoriness, the latter with intact ventriculoatrial conduction, influencing a subsidiary pacemaker to assume dominance. Additionally, while left atrial abnormality may be present when assessed echocardiographically, the sinus P wave at best approximates a terminally negative area of 1 cm^2. Avoid making this diagnosis on the basis of an ectopic atrial complex as only a sinus P wave should be assessed. Board exam diagnostic codes include normal sinus rhythm and ventricular premature complexes.

Electrocardiogram Case Study #7

CLINICAL HISTORY

A 78-year-old male with recent symptoms of light-headedness and one episode of syncope.

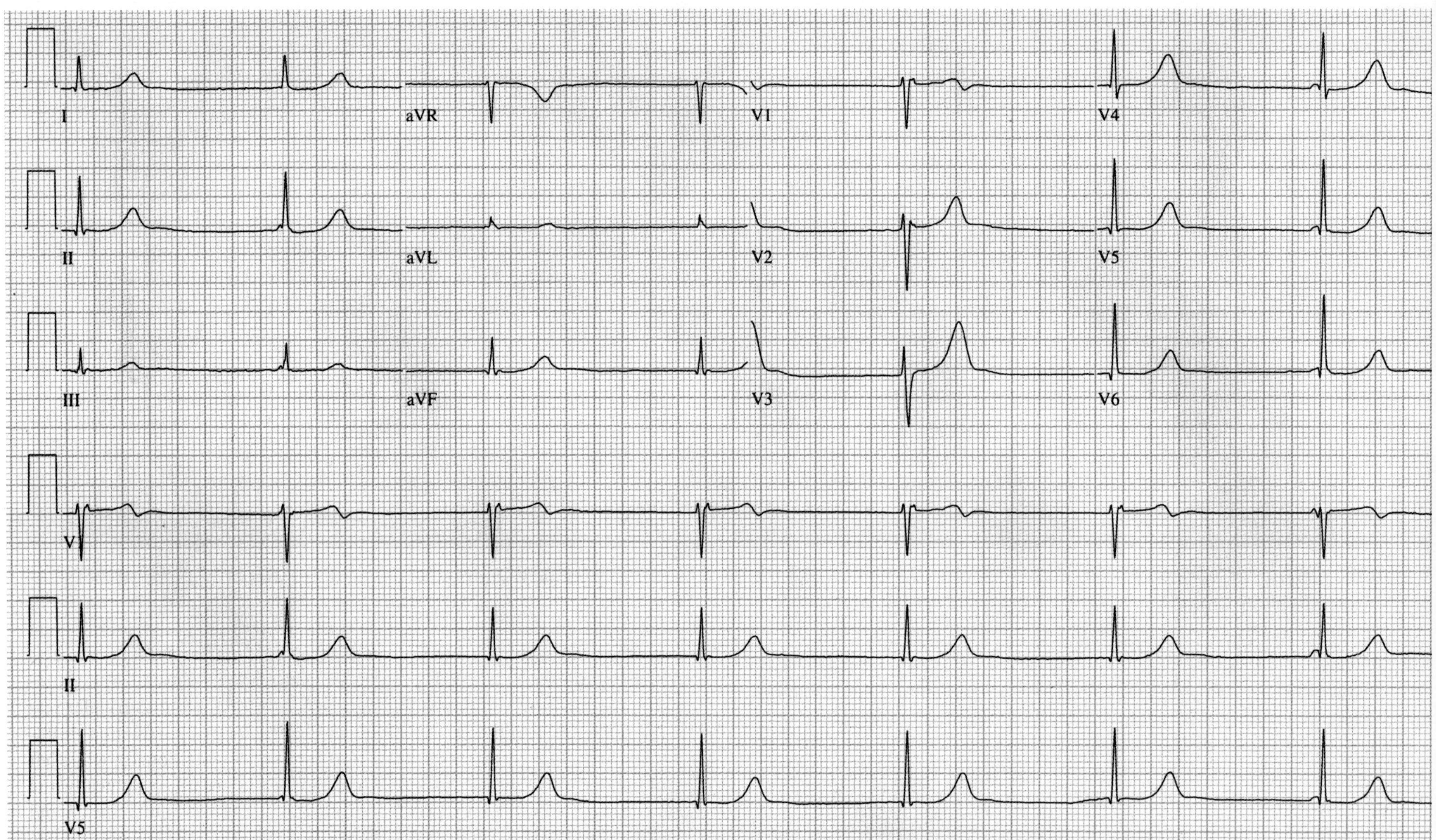

Interpretation Notes:

Electrocardiogram Case Study #7

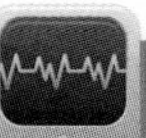

ELECTROCARDIOGRAM INTERPRETATION

This electrocardiogram demonstrates QRS complexes with a constant R-to-R interval at a ventricular rate <40 per minute consistent with junctional bradycardia. In the lead V1 rhythm strip, the QRS complex morphology varies slightly, leading one to believe there may be an intermittent incomplete right bundle branch block. Instead, immediately preceding the last QRS complex, a P wave is identified. This represents an atrial rhythm most likely reflecting sinus bradycardia coexisting with junctional bradycardia. Atrioventricular dissociation is present, and a longer rhythm strip would be necessary to see if in fact this represents complete heart block. A favorable PR interval for antegrade atrioventricular conduction does not exist. This could also represent retrograde P waves with variable junctional to atrial conduction times therefore occurring before, within, and slightly after the widened QRS complex. Subtle ST-T changes are also seen with slight ST segment sagging in leads I, II, V5, and V6.

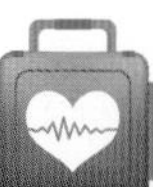

KEY DIAGNOSES

- Junctional bradycardia
- Sinus bradycardia
- Nonspecific ST-T changes
- Atrioventricular dissociation

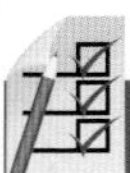

KEY TEACHING POINTS

- In the presence of a junctional rhythm, it is important to investigate for a coexisting atrial rhythm.
- Since a favorable PR interval to assess for antegrade atrioventricular conduction does not exist, it is important to obtain a longer rhythm strip or even a prolonged recording such as a Holter monitor before concluding complete heart block is present.
- The biggest clue on this electrocardiogram for the presence of two underlying heart rhythms is the variable QRS complex morphology. While incomplete right bundle branch conduction delay is suggested, a more careful assessment readily identifies atrial activity.

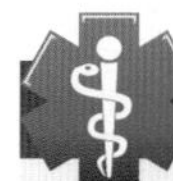

BOARD EXAMINATION ESSENTIALS

This is another example where coding for two coexisting heart rhythms is important. In the presence of a junctional rhythm, carefully inspect all aspects of the electrocardiogram for identifiable P waves. If located, assess if they are retrograde, and if so, they will possess a negative P-wave vector in the inferior leads and will possess a constant coupling interval to the prior QRS complex. If atrioventricular (AV) dissociation is present, the ventriculoatrial coupling interval will vary and a separate atrial rhythm should be coded. For this electrocardiogram, a cursory review suggests incomplete right bundle branch block. This is incorrect as the apparent terminal QRS complex conduction delay varies and is in fact a superimposed P wave, most evident as it occurs just prior to the last QRS complex on this electrocardiogram. Diagnostic codes for the board exam include AV junctional rhythm, sinus bradycardia, nonspecific ST and/or T-wave abnormalities, and AV dissociation.

Electrocardiogram Case Study #8

CLINICAL HISTORY

A 78-year-old male with known coronary artery disease who suffered a myocardial infarction 2 years prior to this electrocardiogram.

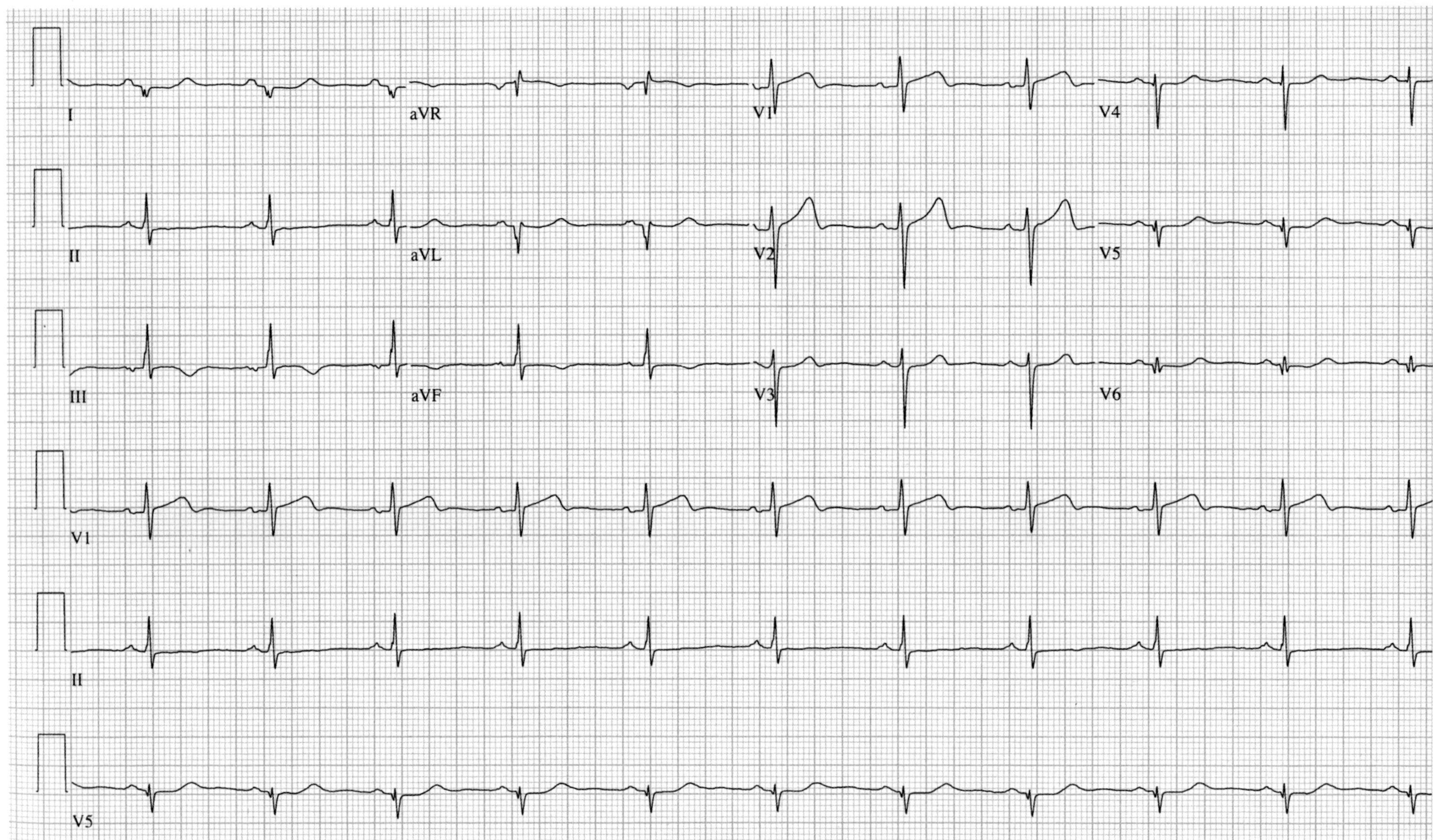

Interpretation Notes:

Electrocardiogram Case Study #8

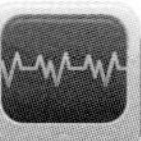

ELECTROCARDIOGRAM INTERPRETATION

This electrocardiogram demonstrates normal sinus rhythm at a rate of 68 per minute. Nonspecific ST-T changes are seen in leads II, III, and aVF. A prominent R wave is seen in lead V1. The R wave regresses across the precordial leads from V2, V3, V4, V5 to V6. Q waves are seen in leads I and aVL as well as in leads V5 and V6. This group of findings is consistent with an age-indeterminate posterolateral and high lateral myocardial infarction. When evaluating an electrocardiogram for a prominent R wave in lead V1, diagnostic considerations include a posterior myocardial infarction, right ventricular conduction delay, counterclockwise rotation, and right ventricular hypertrophy. In this circumstance, Q waves are seen in both the high lateral and lateral leads. Even though they are at a distance on the electrocardiogram, anatomically they reflect contiguous myocardial territories. Therefore, the largest hint on this electrocardiogram of underlying obstructive coronary artery disease is the tall R wave in lead V1. Lastly, Wolff-Parkinson-White Syndrome merits consideration. However, in the presence of Wolff-Parkinson-White Syndrome, the PR interval is typically shortened and most importantly ventricular preexcitation in the form of a delta wave is present. Neither of these findings is demonstrated on this electrocardiogram.

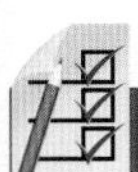

KEY TEACHING POINTS

- Electrocardiogram R-wave regression is an abnormal finding and always merits explanation.
- It is important to be familiar with contiguous myocardial territories on the electrocardiogram. In this circumstance, the high lateral leads I and aVL are contiguous with lead V1 and also with the lateral leads V5 and V6.

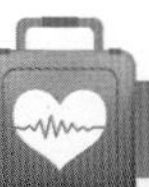

KEY DIAGNOSES

- Normal sinus rhythm
- Nonspecific ST-T changes
- Posterolateral myocardial infarction age indeterminate
- High lateral myocardial infarction age indeterminate

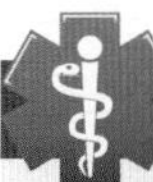

BOARD EXAMINATION ESSENTIALS

For the purposes of the board exam, separate codes for an age-indeterminate posterior and lateral myocardial infarction are required. Note the presence of the R wave in lead V4, negating the possibility of an anterolateral myocardial infarction. Cardiac catheterization demonstrated a complete occlusion of the left circumflex coronary artery. The posterior and lateral myocardial infarction patterns actually represented one myocardial infarction and two contiguous myocardial territories. For the board exam, they are coded separately. There is no evidence of ST-segment elevation to suggest acute myocardial injury. The fact that prominent R waves are present in leads II, III, and aVF supports the lack of right coronary artery involvement. Should you discover a posterior or lateral myocardial infarction pattern, be sure to assess the inferior leads as an infarction pattern will frequently be present as the inferior wall can also represent a contiguous myocardial territory. Diagnostic codes for the board exam include normal sinus rhythm; posterior myocardial infarction, age indeterminate; and lateral myocardial infarction, age indeterminate.

Electrocardiogram Case Study #9

CLINICAL HISTORY

A 69-year-old male with recent symptoms of light-headedness.

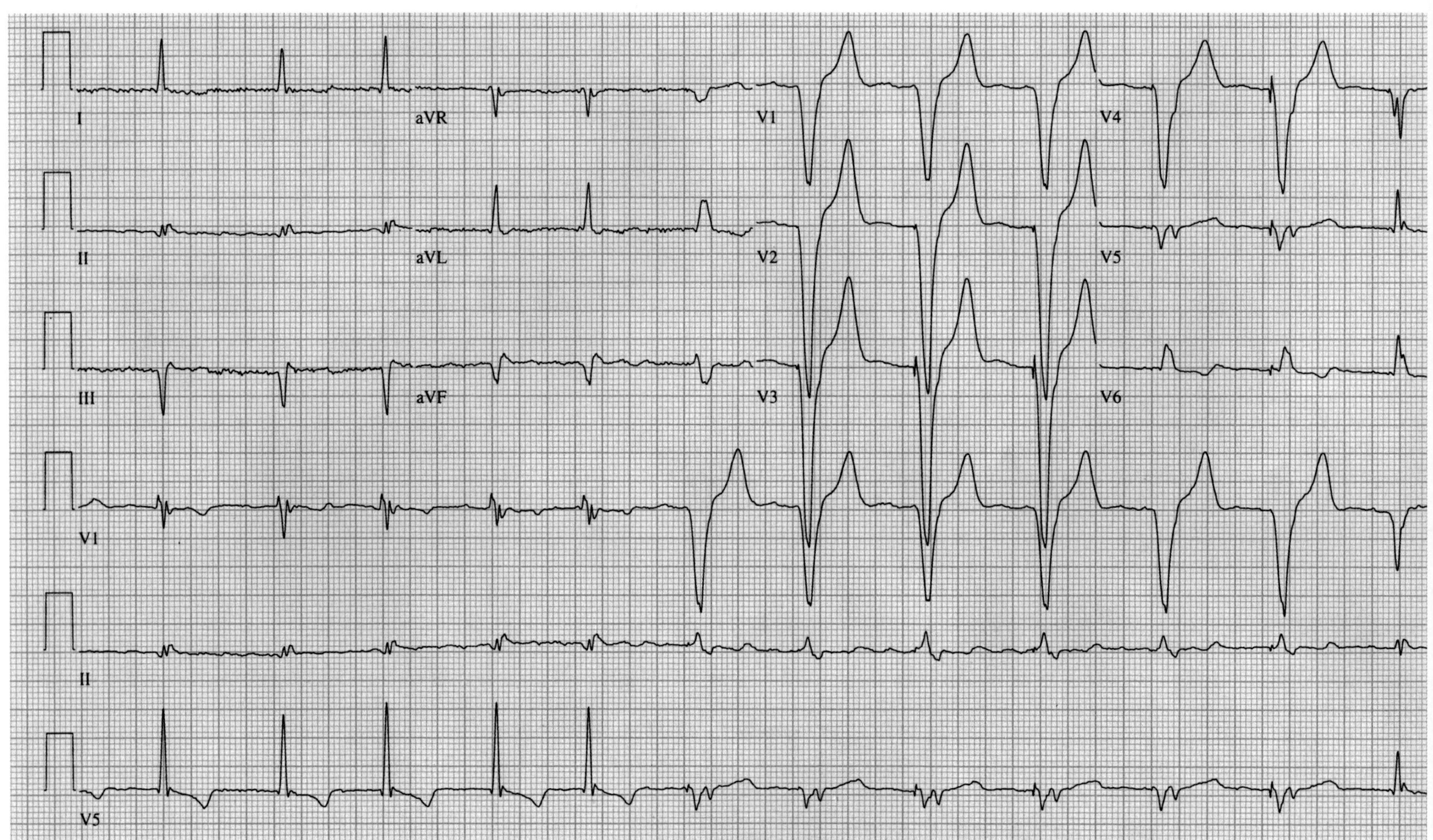

Interpretation Notes:

Electrocardiogram Case Study #9

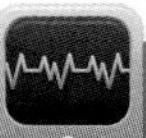

ELECTROCARDIOGRAM INTERPRETATION

On the left-hand portion of the electrocardiogram, atrial fibrillation is present. Additionally, Q waves of diagnostic duration are present in leads II, III, and aVF consistent with an age-indeterminate myocardial infarction. The QRS complex demonstrates terminal conduction delay particularly in leads II, III, and aVF consistent with peri-infarction block or delayed conduction toward the infarct zone. Approximately 50% across the electrocardiogram, a wide QRS complex ensues. In leads V3, V4, and V5, pacemaker deflections are seen. The QRS complex demonstrates a complete left bundle black morphology given the right ventricular apical location of the ventricular pacemaker lead. This is consistent with a paroxysm of ventricular pacing. The last QRS complex represents a pacemaker fusion complex as simultaneous ventricular depolarization transpires via the native conduction system and also via the pacemaker. During this period of ventricular pacing, atrial fibrillation continues. This is seen as an undulating baseline particularly in the lead V2 rhythm strip without evidence of discrete atrial depolarizations. In lead aVF, one notes the prominent diagnostic Q waves. In the paced QRS complex, the diagnostic Q wave is no longer seen. Additionally, due to the ventricular pacing, posterior or lateral extension of the inferior myocardial infarction, representing contiguous myocardial territories, cannot be assessed.

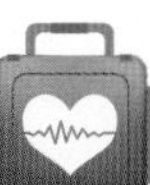

KEY DIAGNOSES

- Atrial fibrillation
- Inferior myocardial infarction age indeterminate
- Peri-infarction block
- Ventricular pacemaker

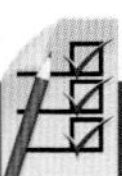

KEY TEACHING POINTS

- Ventricular pacing precludes the diagnosis of an age-indeterminate myocardial infarction.
- Acute myocardial injury in the form of ST-segment elevation can still be discerned during ventricular pacing.
- It is of importance to accurately diagnose the underlying atrial rhythm, if possible, in the presence of a ventricular pacemaker.
- Intermittent ventricular pacing provides an opportunity to assess the QRS complex morphology and cardiac intervals, otherwise obscured during ventricular pacing.

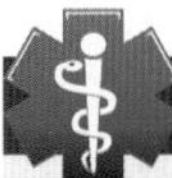

BOARD EXAMINATION ESSENTIALS

This is an excellent example of a potential board exam electrocardiogram. It possesses two heart rhythms, atrial fibrillation and a ventricular pacemaker. The ventricular pacemaker deflections may be overlooked with some examinees falling into a trap coding complete left bundle branch block. Others may not identify the inferior myocardial infarction of indeterminate age or the intraventricular conduction disturbance, nonspecific type. In leads I and aVL, nonspecific ST and/or T-wave abnormalities are present. These are not essential to code, but at the same time you are unlikely to be penalized for doing so. Board exam diagnostic codes include atrial fibrillation; inferior myocardial infarction, age indeterminate; intraventricular conduction disturbance, nonspecific type; and ventricular demand pacemaker (VVI), normally functioning.

Electrocardiogram Case Study #10

CLINICAL HISTORY

A 74-year-old female with recent pacemaker placement and post-procedure persistent shortness of breath.

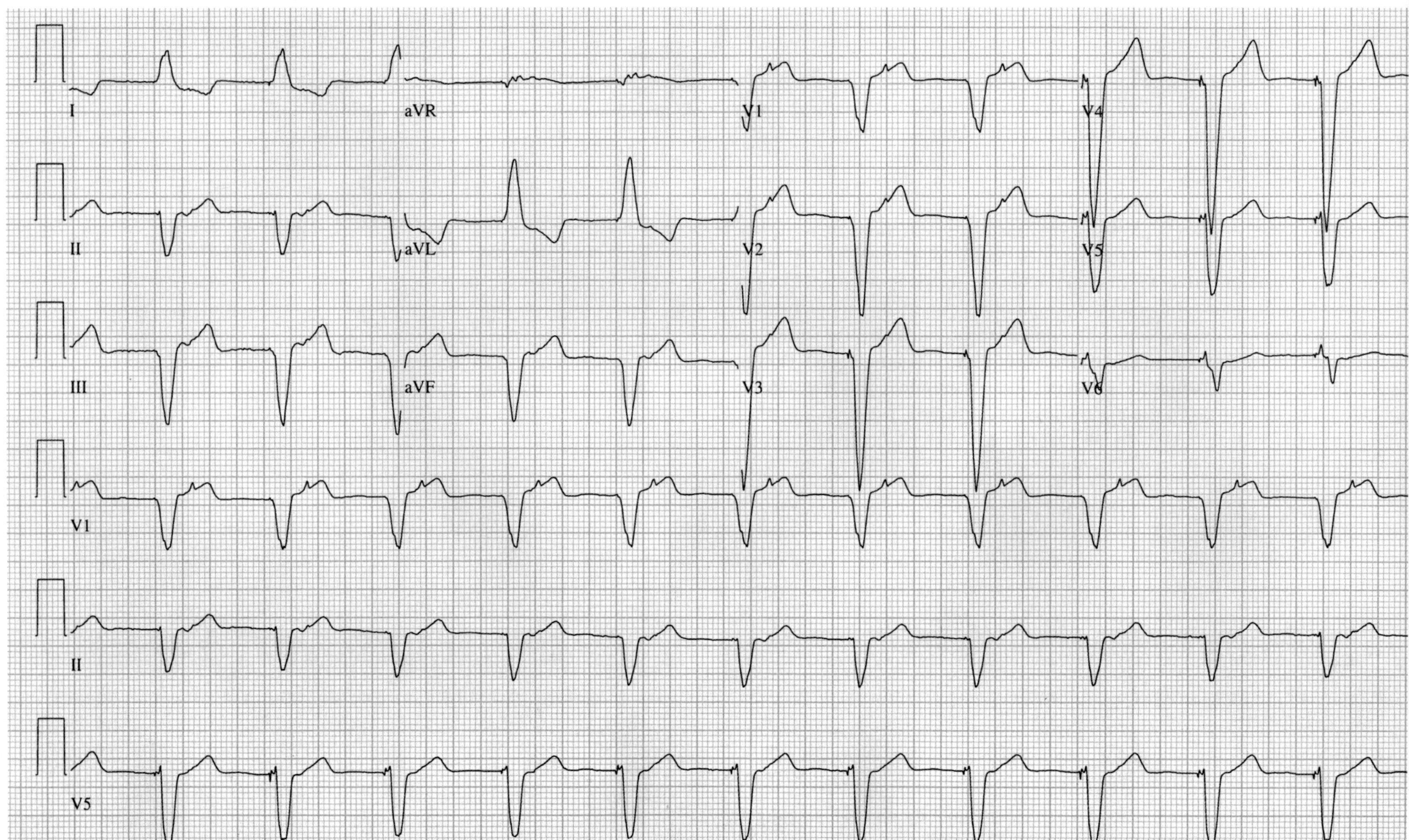

Interpretation Notes:

Electrocardiogram Case Study #10

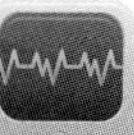

ELECTROCARDIOGRAM INTERPRETATION

This electrocardiogram demonstrates a regular wide QRS complex rhythm at a rate slightly less than 75 per minute. Pacemaker deflections are identified immediately preceding each QRS complex best seen in leads V3, V4, V5, and V6. This is consistent with ventricular pacing. P waves are also identified within the mid-ST segment best seen in leads V1 and V2 and also demonstrated in leads II, III, and aVF. These represent retrograde ventriculoatrial conduction. This is clinically important and relevant to assess, particularly in a symptomatic patient who continues with fatigue and/or shortness of breath post–pacemaker implantation. This may in fact be the first clinical evidence of the pacemaker syndrome where atrial contraction transpires simultaneously against a closed mitral and tricuspid valve.

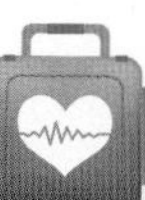

KEY DIAGNOSES

- Ventricular pacemaker
- Retrograde ventriculoatrial conduction

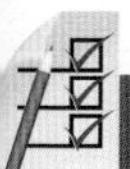

KEY TEACHING POINTS

- Pacemaker deflections may be seen in some but not all leads. Be sure to review each lead carefully and avoid misinterpreting the electrocardiogram as complete left bundle branch block.
- Note the QRS complex axis of the ventricular paced complexes. It demonstrates left axis deviation with greatest positivity toward lead aVL. This is due to the right ventricular apical location of the ventricular pacemaker lead depolarizing the heart from the apex to base in a direction opposite normal antegrade atrioventricular conduction.

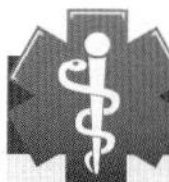

BOARD EXAMINATION ESSENTIALS

This is another example of a ventricular pacemaker that could potentially be confused with complete left bundle branch block and QRS complex left axis deviation. For the board exam, whenever you suspect complete left bundle branch block, make sure that you carefully search for pacemaker deflections. They can be subtle. No code exists for retrograde atrial activation. Should a clinical history of exertional intolerance and fatigue accompany this type of electrocardiogram, pacemaker reprogramming is indicated. Board exam diagnostic codes include ventricular demand pacemaker (VVI), normally functioning.

Electrocardiogram Case Study #11

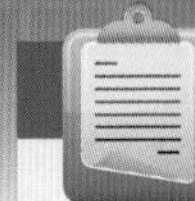

CLINICAL HISTORY

A 57-year-old male with the acute onset of severe anterior chest discomfort of 45-minute duration.

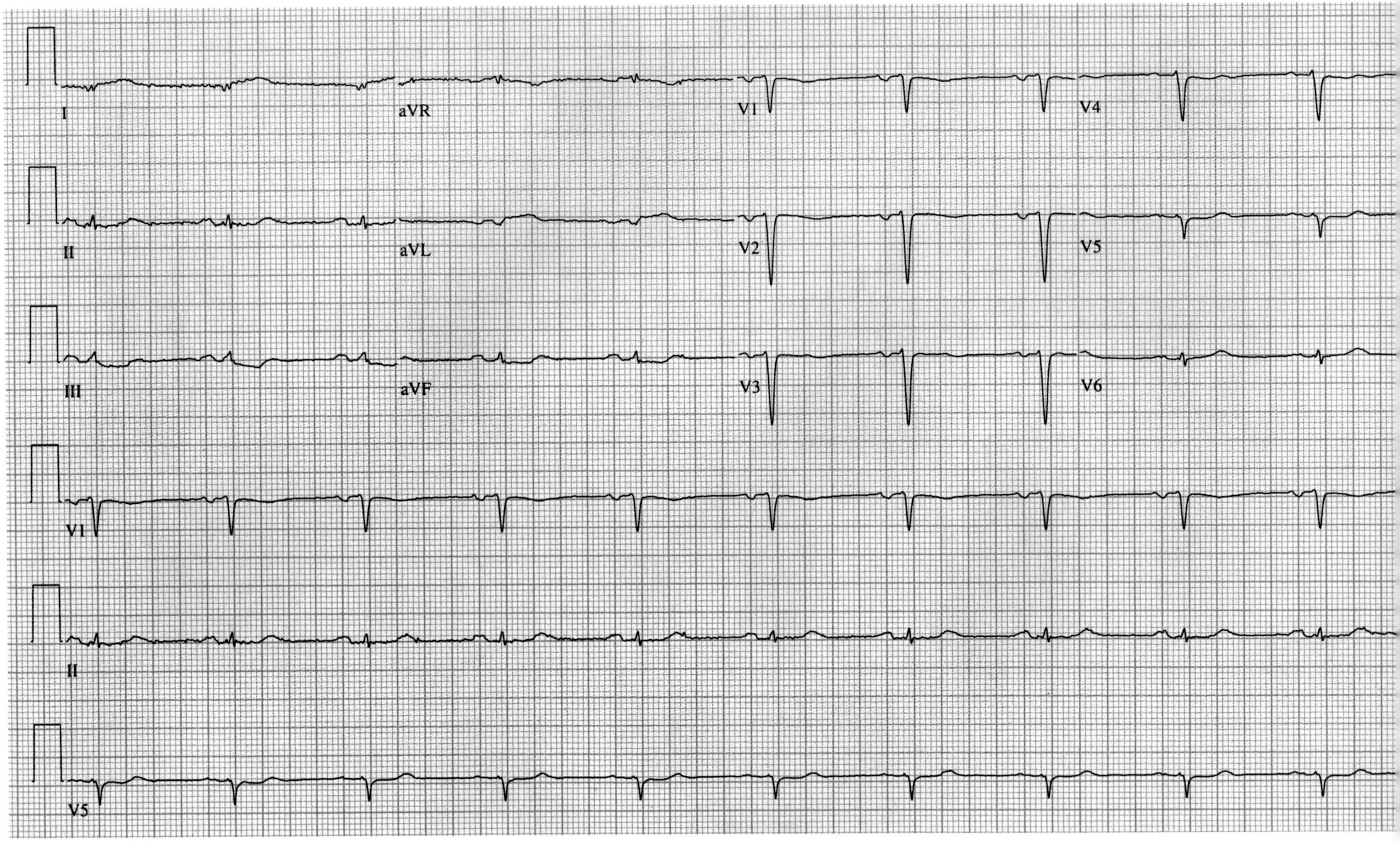

I aVR V1 V4

II aVL V2 V5

III aVF V3 V6

V1

II

V5

Interpretation Notes: ______________________________

____

Electrocardiogram Case Study #11

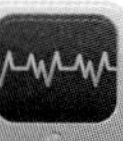

ELECTROCARDIOGRAM INTERPRETATION

This electrocardiogram demonstrates normal sinus rhythm at an atrial rate of approximately 60 per minute. Baseline artifact is present. A bifid P wave is seen in lead II and P-wave terminal negativity is demonstrated in lead V1 consistent with slowed left atrial conduction best termed left atrial abnormality. R-wave progression is delayed across the precordium as one proceeds from leads V2 to V6. Q waves are seen in leads 1 and aVL with associated ST-segment elevation. Reciprocal down sloping ST-segment depression is identified in leads III and aVF. This is consistent with an acute high lateral myocardial infarction and reciprocal inferior ST-T changes. Both injury and infarction are transpiring given the associated ST-segment elevation and diagnostic Q waves in leads I and aVL. Low-voltage QRS complexes are present in the limb leads as no QRS complex exceeds 0.5 millivolts in amplitude.

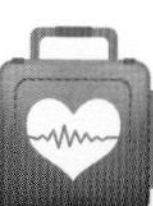

KEY DIAGNOSES

- Normal sinus rhythm
- Left atrial abnormality
- High lateral myocardial infarction acute
- Reciprocal ST-T changes
- Low-voltage QRS complexes—limb leads
- Artifact

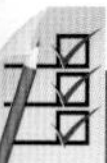

KEY TEACHING POINTS

- Note that the QRS complexes do not have to be extremely high in amplitude to render the diagnosis of acute myocardial infarction. Instead, the diagnostic duration of the Q wave is most important and in this case is clearly greater than 40 milliseconds.
- The high lateral leads, leads I and aVL, are the most often overlooked electrocardiogram leads. An isolated high lateral myocardial infarction may reflect the left circumflex coronary artery, ramus intermedius coronary artery, or a large branching diagonal system derived from the left anterior descending coronary artery.

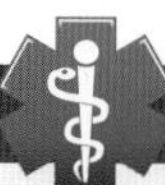

BOARD EXAMINATION ESSENTIALS

This electrocardiogram reflects a lateral myocardial infarction acute. Additionally, it is appropriate to code for ST and/or T-wave changes suggesting acute myocardial injury. Note the lack of significant R-wave progression from lead V1 to lead V6. Despite this finding, R waves are present negating the presence of a left anterior descending coronary artery territory myocardial infarction. Other board exam diagnostic codes include normal sinus rhythm, left atrial abnormality and/enlargement, low voltage, limb leads, and artifact.

Electrocardiogram Case Study **#12**

CLINICAL HISTORY

An 84-year-old male postoperative day #1 partial colon resection with acute onset severe shortness of breath and chest discomfort.

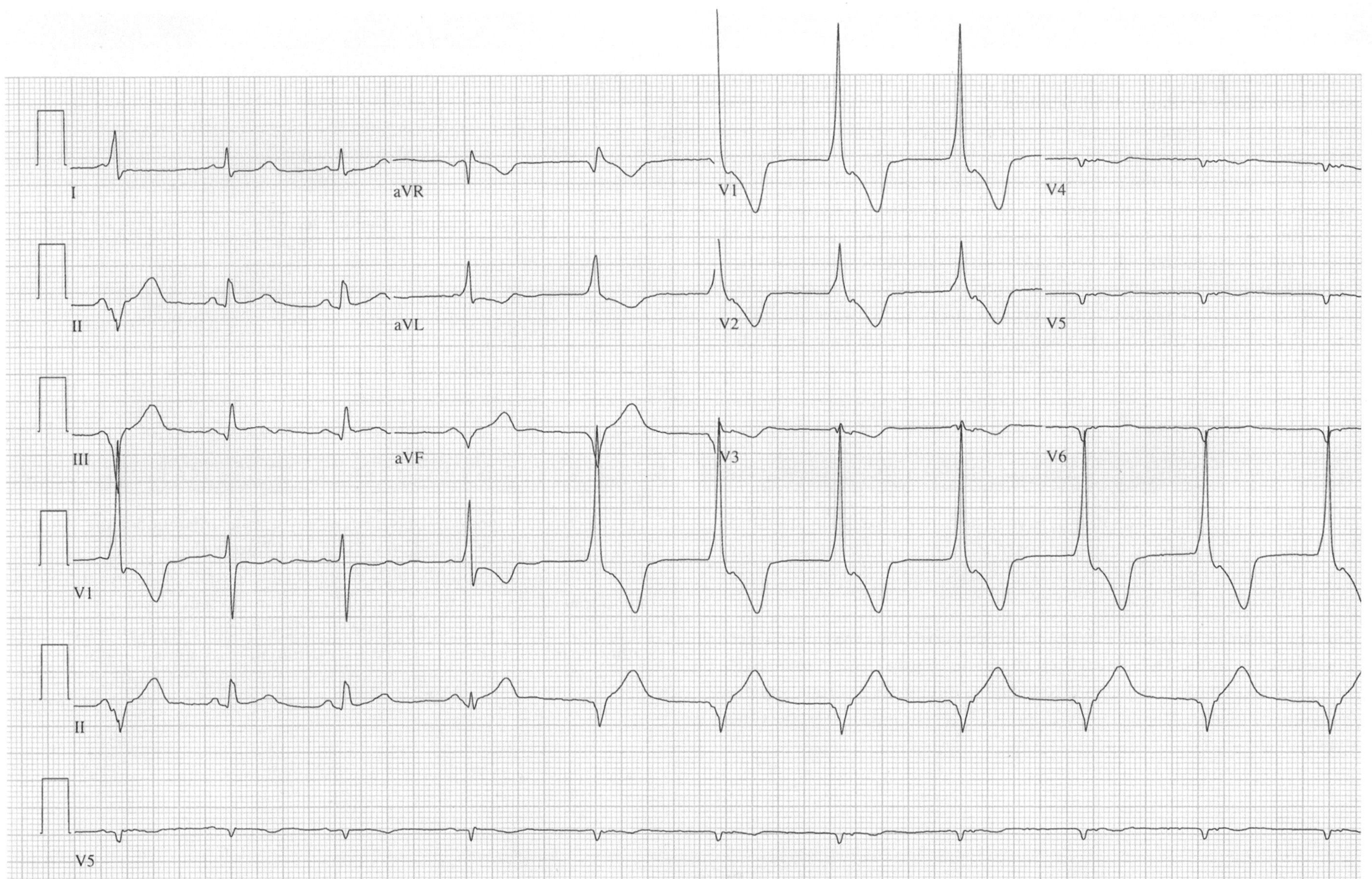

Interpretation Notes:

Electrocardiogram Case Study #12

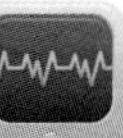

ELECTROCARDIOGRAM INTERPRETATION

This electrocardiogram toward the left-hand portion of the tracing demonstrates two narrow QRS complexes each preceded by a P wave with a normal P-wave axis indicative of normal sinus rhythm at a rate of about 70 per minute. ST-segment elevation as well as J-point elevation is seen in leads II and III, highly suggestive of acute myocardial injury. The Q wave in lead III is not of diagnostic duration to confidently render the diagnosis of an acute myocardial infarction. Following the second narrow QRS complex, slowing of sinus node discharge ensues and a wide QRS complex rhythm with constant R to R intervals is identified at a ventricular rate of about 65 per minute. The fourth QRS complex represents a fusion or hybrid complex that morphologically is reflective of superimposed native antegrade ventricular depolarization and pure ventricular depolarization from an ectopic focus as seen in the presence of this accelerated idioventricular rhythm. P waves are seen in the proximal ST segment of the accelerated idioventricular rhythm complexes suggesting retrograde ventriculoatrial conduction. Additionally, the accelerated idioventricular focus demonstrates a complete right bundle branch block morphology consistent with a left ventricular origin.

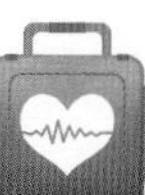

KEY DIAGNOSES

- Normal sinus rhythm
- Acute myocardial injury
- Fusion complex
- Accelerated idioventricular rhythm
- Retrograde ventriculoatrial conduction

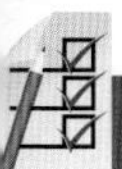

KEY TEACHING POINTS

- A Q wave is seen in lead aVF highly suggesting both myocardial injury and infarction. Due to the fact that the idioventricular focus is from the left ventricle, initial depolarization of the ventricle should solely represent left ventricular events.
- Utilizing the strictest criteria for the diagnosis of an inferior myocardial infarction, a Q wave 40-millisecond duration or greater should be present in lead aVF. For this electrocardiogram, the accelerated idioventricular rhythm obscures the native QRS complex morphology in lead aVF. Repeating the electrocardiogram once the accelerated idioventricular rhythm abates would be appropriate.
- An accelerated idioventricular rhythm has been identified as a reperfusion arrhythmia, often indicating a restoration of coronary artery blood flow to a previously 100% obstructed coronary artery.

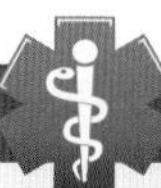

BOARD EXAMINATION ESSENTIALS

This electrocardiogram demonstrates a regular wide complex rhythm including the board exam diagnostic codes of normal sinus rhythm, an inferior myocardial infarction acute and ST and/or T-wave abnormalities suggesting acute myocardial injury. The wide complex rhythm is best coded as an accelerated idioventricular rhythm. During the accelerated idioventricular rhythm, the P waves appear retrograde with a constant coupling interval to the QRS complex. Thus, atrioventricular dissociation is not coded.

Electrocardiogram Case Study #13

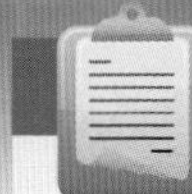

CLINICAL HISTORY

A 66-year-old male with known coronary artery disease and a prior coronary artery bypass operation. He has been experiencing 2 hours of severe chest pain and hypotension.

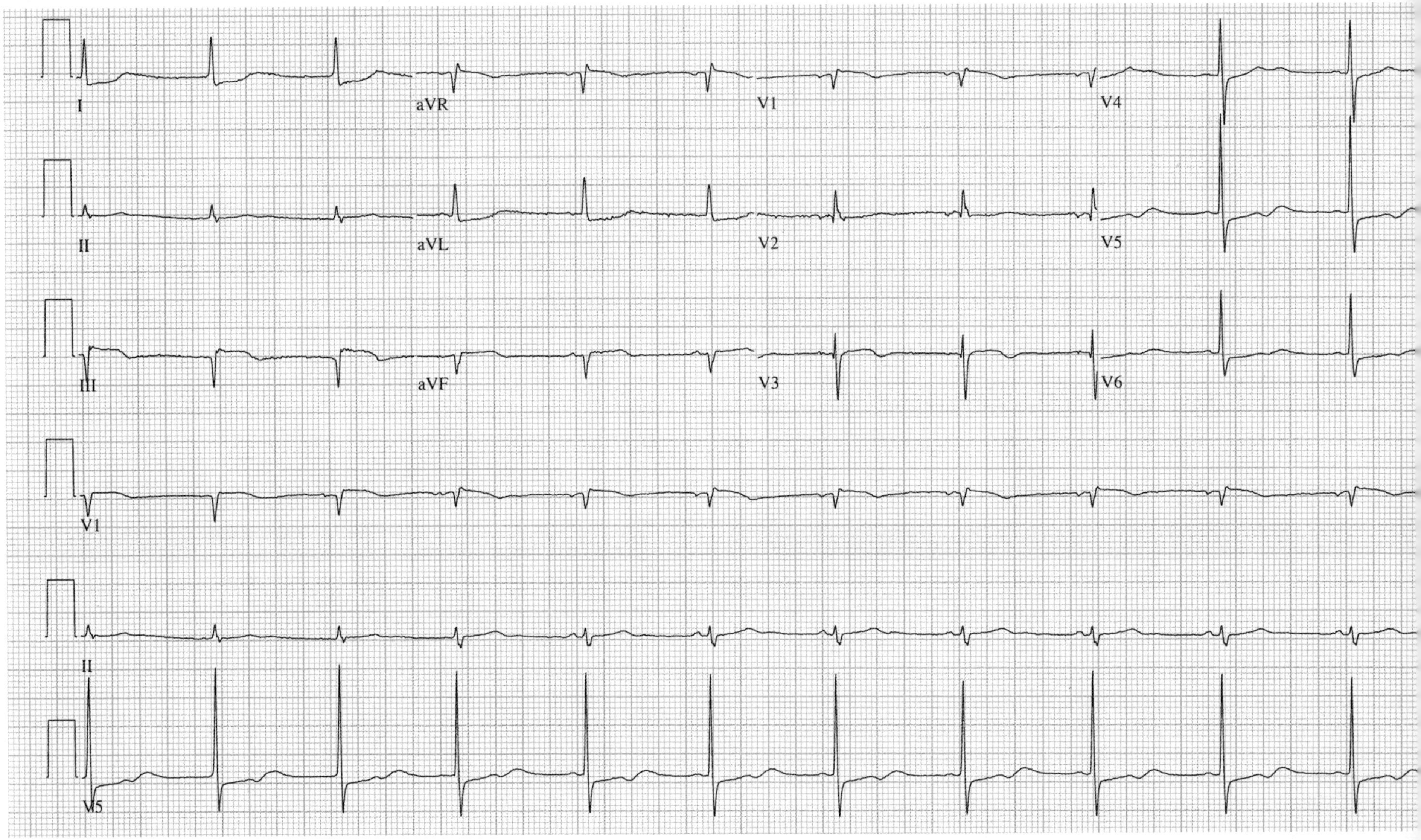

I aVR V1 V4

II aVL V2 V5

III aVF V3 V6

V1

II

V5

Interpretation Notes:

Electrocardiogram Case Study #13

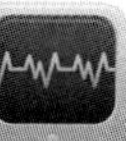

ELECTROCARDIOGRAM INTERPRETATION

This electrocardiogram demonstrates an abnormal P-wave axis with a nearly isoelectric baseline in leads I, II, and III. A diminutive P wave is seen in lead aVF and also in lead V1 with a short PR interval. This is consistent with an ectopic atrial rhythm at a rate approximating 65 per minute. Diagnostic inferior Q waves are seen consistent with an inferior myocardial infarction. Associated ST-segment elevation is demonstrated in leads III and aVF consistent with acute myocardial injury and in conjunction with the Q wave reflects an acute inferior myocardial infarction. ST-segment elevation is also seen in lead V1. Otherwise, lead V1 is diminutive. In the setting of an acute inferior myocardial infarction, this represents an acute right ventricular myocardial injury pattern. This supports the presence of a right coronary artery occlusion proximal to the right ventricular marginal branch. Lateral and high lateral ST-T changes are seen as is a prolonged QT-U interval. A prominent positive U wave is seen in leads V4, V5, and V6.

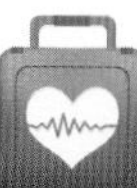

KEY DIAGNOSES

- Ectopic atrial rhythm
- Inferior myocardial infarction acute
- Right ventricular myocardial injury
- Prolonged QT-U interval
- Acute myocardial injury
- Prominent U waves

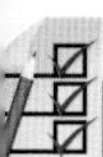

KEY TEACHING POINTS

- When making the electrocardiogram diagnosis of an acute inferior myocardial injury/infarction pattern, it is important to carefully review contiguous myocardial territories
  - Posterior myocardial infarction—R wave greater than or equal to the S wave with reciprocal ST-segment depression in leads V1 and V2 (not identified on this electrocardiogram).
  - Lateral myocardial infarction—Q wave of diagnostic duration in lead V6 (not identified on this electrocardiogram).
  - Acute right ventricular myocardial injury—ST-segment elevation in leads V1 and V2 with right-sided precordial leads assisting with confirmation of acute right ventricular myocardial injury.

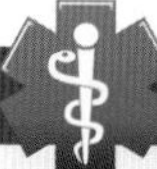

BOARD EXAMINATION ESSENTIALS

The P-wave axis is abnormal, most consistent with an ectopic atrial rhythm. Unless the coding sheet is modified, the diagnosis of an ectopic atrial rhythm will not appear on the board examination. Inferior Q waves of diagnostic duration with associated ST-segment elevation support an inferior myocardial infarction acute. Right ventricular myocardial injury/acute myocardial infarction is also not found on the coding sheet. Instead, anticipate at least one question on patient management with a corresponding electrocardiogram. The most important point here is to avoid preload reducing agents, instead emphasizing volume replacement in the form of intravenous fluid administration. Do not forget to also code for ST- and/or T-wave abnormalities suggesting myocardial injury and prominent U waves.

Electrocardiogram Case Study #14

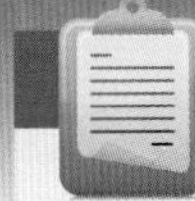

CLINICAL HISTORY

A 54-year-old female who had this electrocardiogram performed as part of a physical examination. She presently feels well without cardiovascular symptoms.

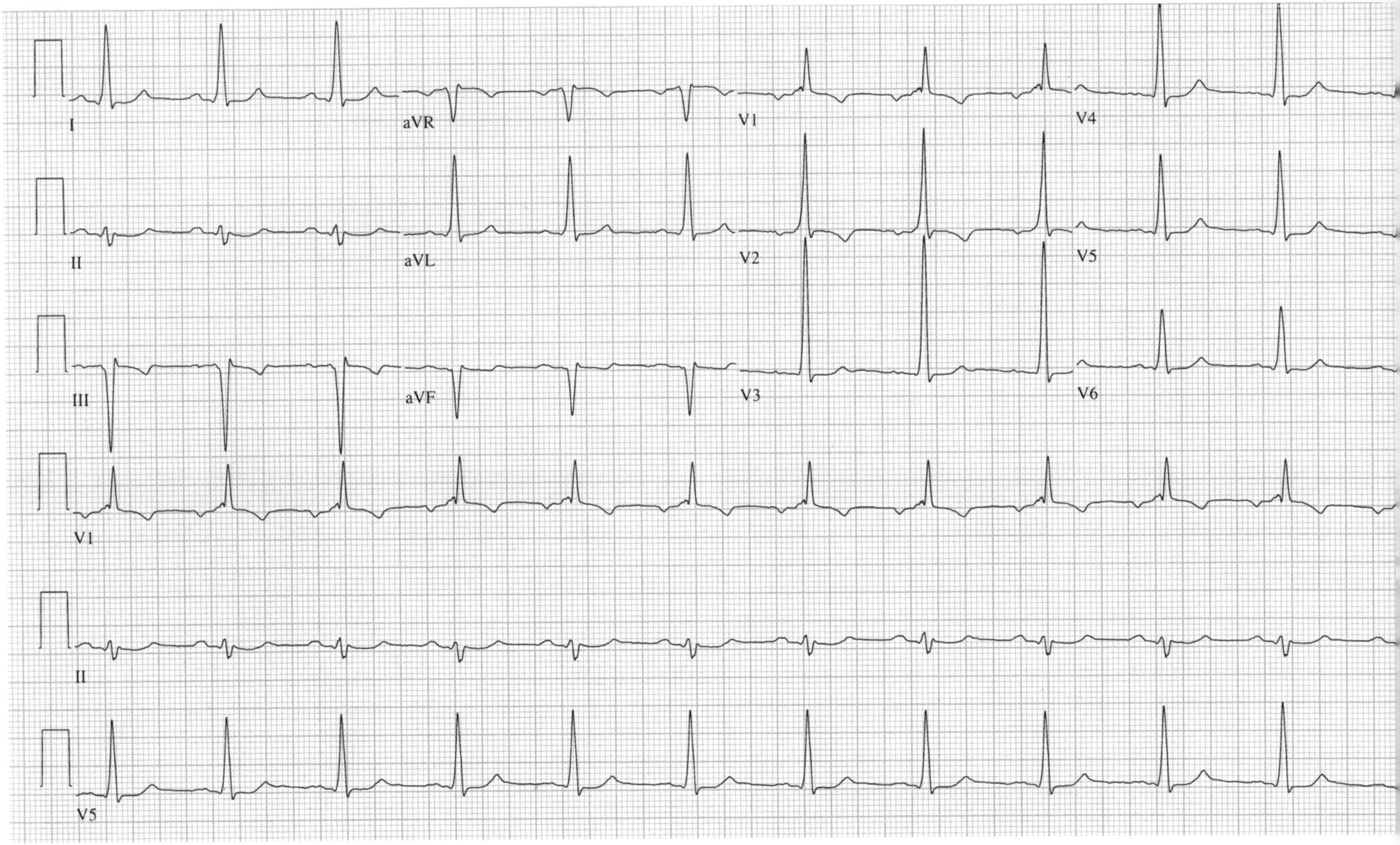

I aVR V1 V4

II aVL V2 V5

III aVF V3 V6

V1

II

V5

Interpretation Notes:

Electrocardiogram Case Study #14

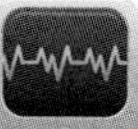

ELECTROCARDIOGRAM INTERPRETATION

This electrocardiogram demonstrates normal sinus rhythm with a normal P-wave axis and an atrial rate of approximately 70 per minute. Terminal P-wave negativity in lead V1 supports left atrial abnormality. A prominent R wave is present in lead V1. The differential diagnosis includes ventricular pre-excitation, a posterior myocardial infarction, right ventricular hypertrophy, right ventricular conduction delay, and counter clockwise rotation. This electrocardiogram is most consistent with ventricular pre-excitation. A delta wave is seen in leads I, V2, V3, V4, V5, and V6. Additionally, a delta wave is seen in lead aVL. What makes this more challenging is that inferior Q waves are present in leads III and aVF. In the presence of ventricular pre-excitation, this precludes ascribing the diagnosis of an age-indeterminate inferior myocardial infarction and instead, initial ventricular depolarization through the accessory pathway is away from leads III and aVF thus generating a Q wave in the form of a delta wave as the initial QRS complex vector.

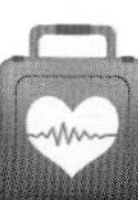

KEY DIAGNOSES

- Normal sinus rhythm
- Wolff-Parkinson-White Syndrome
- Pseudoinfarction pattern
- First-degree atrioventricular block
- Left atrial abnormality

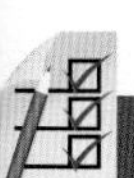

KEY TEACHING POINTS

- It is incorrect to ascribe the diagnosis of an age-indeterminate inferior posterior myocardial infarction in this circumstance. Initial left ventricular depolarization transpires through the accessory pathway, precluding accurate interpretation of initial left ventricular forces.
- The inferior Q waves and prominent R wave in lead V1 is best collectively termed a pseudoinfarction pattern. If possible, repeating the electrocardiogram in the absence of ventricular pre-excitation to best assess the native QRS complex morphology is recommended.
- Note the slightly prolonged PR interval. This coupled with the positive QRS complex vector in lead V1 suggests a left lateral accessory pathway with a prolonged atrioventricular conduction time and thus the slightly prolonged PR interval length.

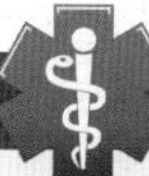

BOARD EXAMINATION ESSENTIALS

For this electrocardiogram, coding less than more is best. Normal sinus rhythm; Wolff-Parkinson-White Pattern; and AV block, first degree, represents a complete interpretation. Left atrial abnormality/enlargement is also likely given the P-wave terminal negativity seen in lead V1. Do not code for an infarction pattern in the presence of Wolff-Parkinson-White Pattern.

Electrocardiogram Case Study #15

CLINICAL HISTORY

A 63-year-old male with intermittent exertional lightheadedness and chest pressure.

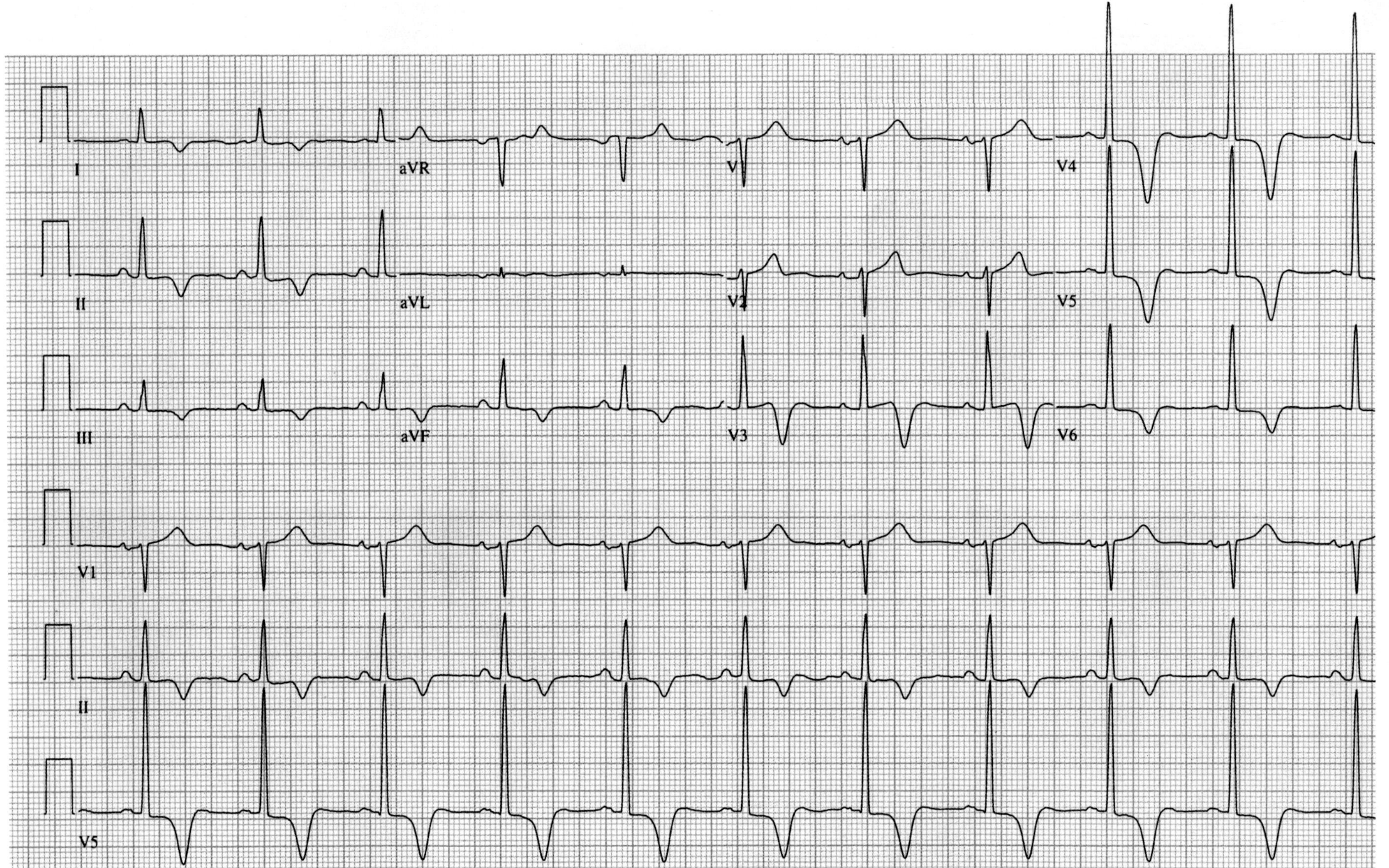

Interpretation Notes:

Electrocardiogram Case Study #15

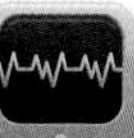

ELECTROCARDIOGRAM INTERPRETATION

This electrocardiogram demonstrates normal sinus rhythm at an atrial rate of approximately 65 per minute. T-wave inversion is seen inferiorly, apically and laterally. Prominent voltage criteria for left ventricular hypertrophy is present and the T-wave inversion, unlike the typical strain pattern as seen in the pressure overload pattern of left ventricular hypertrophy, is symmetric. This is a patient who was diagnosed with the apical form of hypertrophic cardiomyopathy, also known as Yamaguchi disease. Lead V3 is felt to represent the cardiac apex and when symmetric T-wave inversion is seen beginning in lead V3 and extending to leads V4, V5, and V6 with heightened QRS complex voltage, Yamaguchi disease should be suspected. Inferior T-wave symmetric inversion reflects the apical portion of the inferior wall and the apical hypertrophic cardiomyopathy involvement.

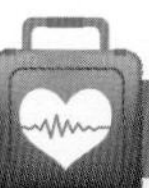

KEY DIAGNOSES

- Normal sinus rhythm
- Yamaguchi disease
- Hypertrophic cardiomyopathy

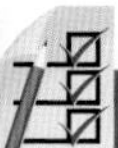

KEY TEACHING POINTS

- Lead V3 can be exceedingly helpful as it reflects the anteroseptal and the apical myocardial regions.
- Note the lack of prominent septal Q waves in a Yamaguchi disease patient as compared to asymmetric septal hypertrophy and the more common forms of hypertrophic cardiomyopathy.

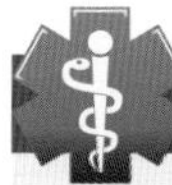

BOARD EXAMINATION ESSENTIALS

This is a form of hypertrophic cardiomyopathy and with the appropriate clinical history perhaps including exertional lightheadedness or presyncope, it would be appropriately coded for under the Clinical Disorders section. In addition to normal sinus rhythm, code left ventricular hypertrophy and ST- and/or T-wave abnormalities secondary to hypertrophy. While not present on this electrocardiogram, make sure to assess for left and /or right atrial abnormality/enlargement as these findings are commonly found together with ventricular hypertrophy patterns and hypertrophic cardiomyopathy. Lastly, hypertrophic cardiomyopathy may also demonstrate right ventricular hypertrophy, less often seen in the apical hypertrophy Yamaguchi variant.

Electrocardiogram Case Study **#16**

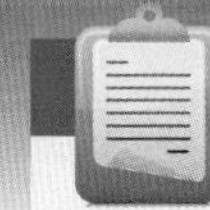

CLINICAL HISTORY

A 68-year-old male with longstanding hypertension and known coronary artery disease.

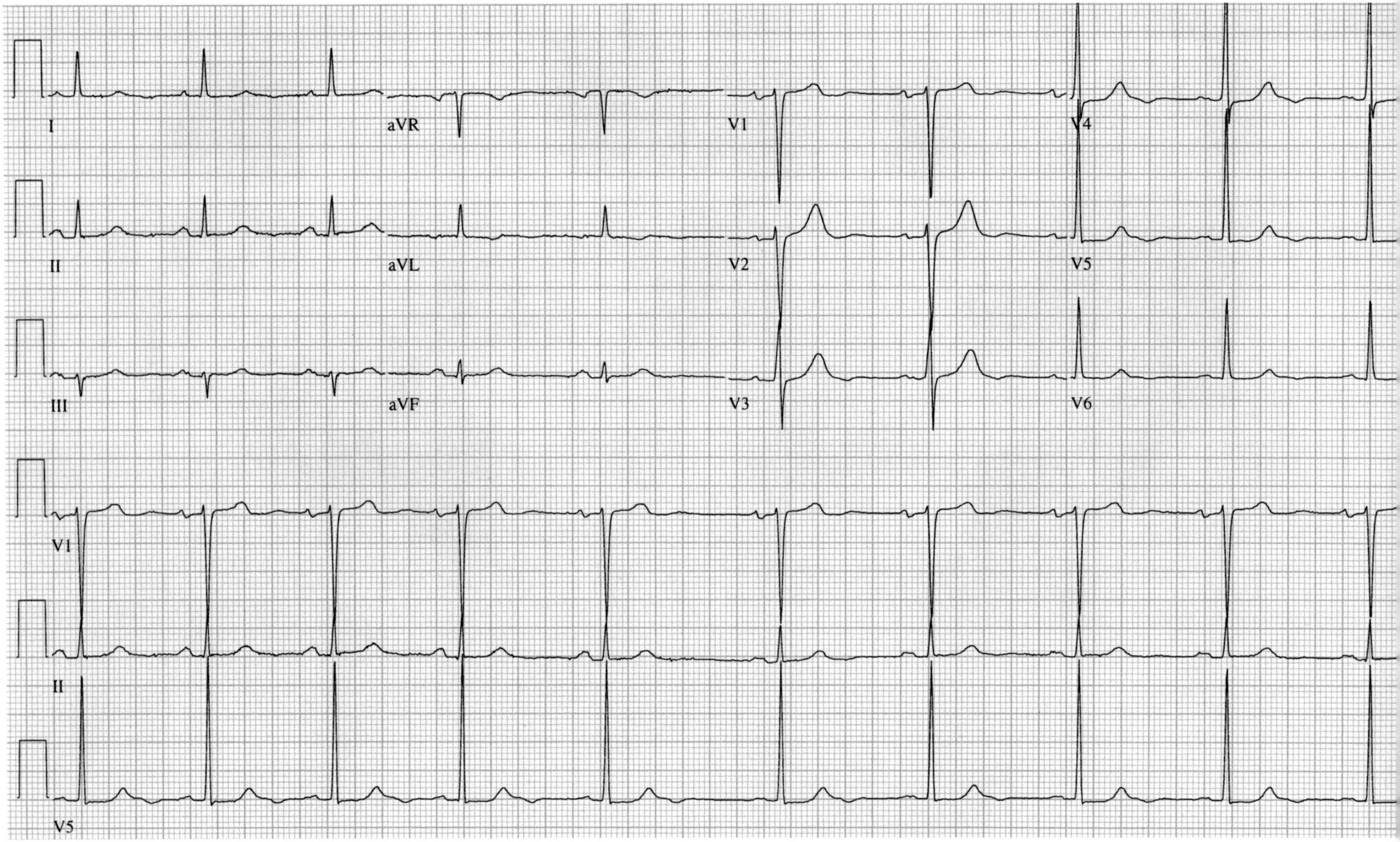

I aVR V1 V4

II aVL V2 V5

III aVF V3 V6

V1

II

V5

Interpretation Notes:

Electrocardiogram Case Study #16

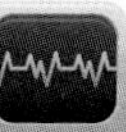

ELECTROCARDIOGRAM INTERPRETATION

This electrocardiogram demonstrates normal sinus rhythm with sinus arrhythmia at an average atrial rate approximating 60 per minute. Initial interpretation would render this to be a normal electrocardiogram. However, negative U waves are present in leads V4, V5, and V6. After the positive T-wave deflection, there is a negative or a scooped deflection of the electrocardiogram baseline indicative of the negative U wave.

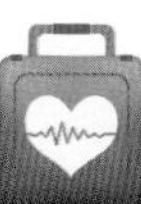

KEY DIAGNOSES

- Normal sinus rhythm
- Sinus arrhythmia
- Negative U waves

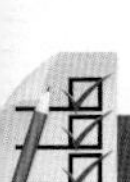

KEY TEACHING POINTS

- Negative U waves can be seen in the presence of left ventricular hypertrophy/increased left ventricular mass and coronary artery disease. There is no significant voltage on this electrocardiogram to satisfy the criteria for left ventricular hypertrophy. Therefore, coronary artery disease merits consideration.
- In the presence of coronary artery disease, negative U waves can be a transient finding, present in the setting of a flow-limiting obstruction. Once the obstruction is relieved, the negative U waves disappear soon thereafter.
- Negative U waves can also be transient finding during exercise stress testing, appearing during periods of transient myocardial ischemia.

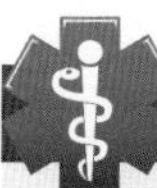

BOARD EXAMINATION ESSENTIALS

Sinus arrhythmia, when present, is easily overlooked. Make sure to code for both the underlying atrial rhythm in addition to sinus arrhythmia. It is unlikely negative U waves will appear on the board exam. They certainly are helpful clinically and can also be helpful on the board exam when considering the possibilities of coronary artery disease and left ventricular hypertrophy. The QRS complex voltage does not quite satisfy the criteria for left ventricular hypertrophy and should not be coded for the board exam. Left atrial abnormality/enlargement may also be present, but the criteria of a terminally negative P wave in lead V1 possessing an area of 1 cm^2 are not met and the P-wave duration in lead II is <110 milliseconds. In summary, for the board exam code normal sinus rhythm, sinus arrhythmia and consider coding normal electrocardiogram understanding negative U waves are an abnormal finding.

Electrocardiogram Case Study #17

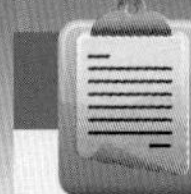

CLINICAL HISTORY

A 54-year-old male who presents for a follow-up cardiovascular medicine evaluation in the context of known coronary artery disease. He is feeling well at the present time.

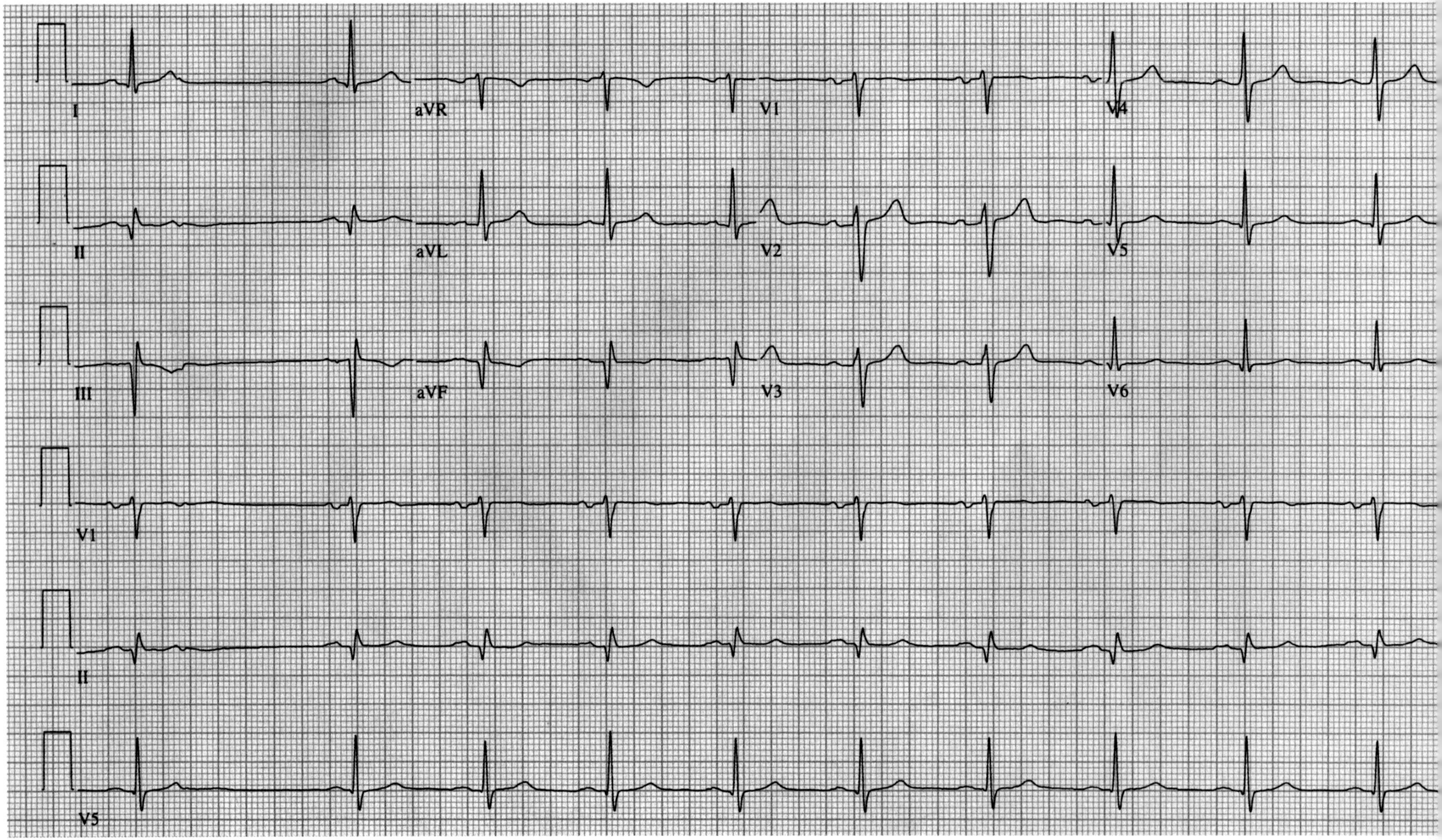

Interpretation Notes:

Electrocardiogram Case Study #17

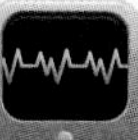

ELECTROCARDIOGRAM INTERPRETATION

This electrocardiogram demonstrates normal sinus rhythm at a rate of about 65 per minute. The P waves demonstrate a terminal negativity in lead V1 and a broadened appearance in lead II consistent with left atrial abnormality. Q waves of diagnostic duration are seen in leads II, III, and aVF consistent with an age-indeterminate inferior myocardial infarction. Terminal conduction delay best classified as peri-infarction block is also present. Additionally, R-wave regression is seen from leads V4 to V5 to V6. A small, likely diagnostic Q wave is seen in lead V6 that represents the lateral wall and contiguous territory to the inferior myocardial region. Therefore, although the Q wave is present in only one isolated lead in V6, this is considered a contiguous lead and together with R-wave regression supports the diagnosis of an age-indeterminate inferolateral myocardial infarction. At the beginning of the electrocardiogram, an apparent pause is seen. There is deformation of the T wave following the initial QRS complex consistent with a nonconducted premature atrial complex and thus the apparent prolonged R to R interval.

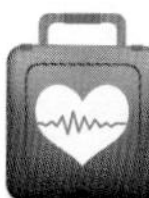

KEY DIAGNOSES

- Normal sinus rhythm
- Left atrial abnormality
- Inferolateral myocardial infarction, age indeterminate
- Peri-infarction block
- Nonconducted premature atrial complex

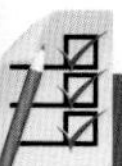

KEY TEACHING POINTS

- It is important not only to assess QRS complex morphology but also amplitude. Should R-wave regression be identified in the precordial leads, the presence of a Q wave should be sought. Another diagnostic possibility is misplaced precordial leads. That is not the case for this electrocardiogram.
- Normally, two contiguous leads with diagnostic Q waves are necessary to conclude an age-indeterminate myocardial infarction. This electrocardiogram is an exception to that rule as a diagnostic lateral Q wave is confined to lead V6. This is because of lead V6 being contiguous with the inferior leads and the age-indeterminate inferior myocardial infarction.
- Additionally, lead V1 should be carefully inspected for evidence of posterior involvement. On this electrocardiogram, the R-wave amplitude is less than the S wave and, therefore, a posterior myocardial infarction is not suspected.

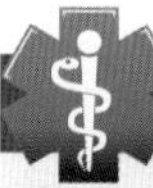

BOARD EXAMINATION ESSENTIALS

The appropriate codes for this electrocardiogram include normal sinus rhythm; atrial premature complex; inferior myocardial infarction, age indeterminate; lateral myocardial infarction, age indeterminate; intraventricular conduction disturbance, nonspecific type. The apparent pause is due to a nonconducted premature atrial complex and not a more advanced form of heart block. In the setting of an inferior myocardial infarction, R-wave regression and a Q wave in a single contiguous lead such as lead V6 supports a lateral myocardial infarction of indeterminate age.

Electrocardiogram Case Study #18

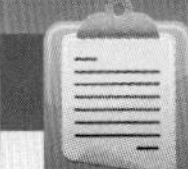

CLINICAL HISTORY

A 73-year-old male who returns for an outpatient cardiovascular medicine follow-up evaluation. He feels well at the present time. He has known coronary artery disease and ischemic left ventricular systolic dysfunction.

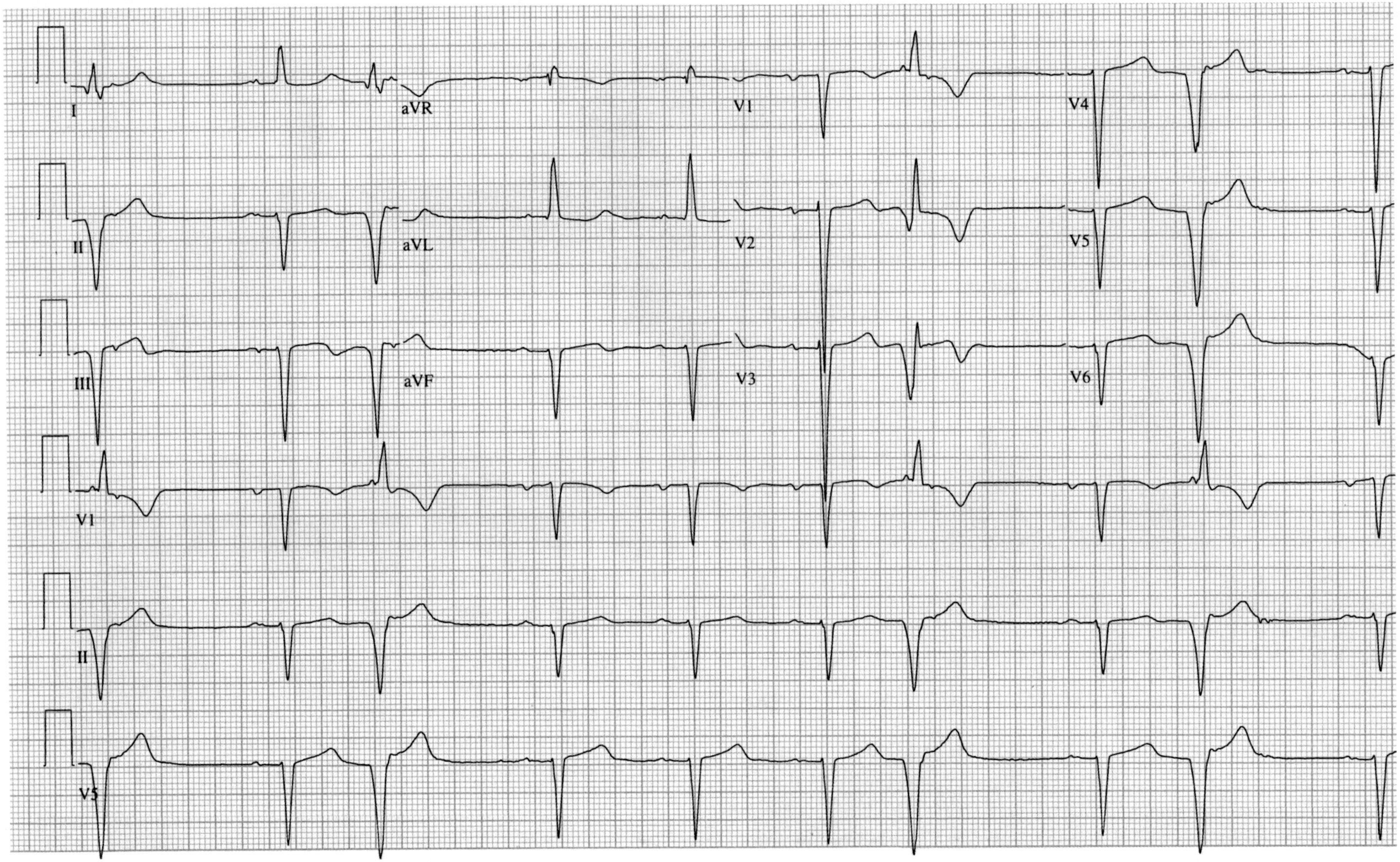

Interpretation Notes:

Electrocardiogram Case Study #18

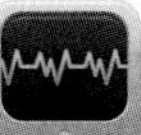

ELECTROCARDIOGRAM INTERPRETATION

Normal sinus rhythm is present. The atrial rate is approximately 60 per minute. The PR interval is >200 millisecconds confirming first-degree atrioventricular block. Frequent premature ventricular complexes are seen and demonstrate a similar QRS complex morphology including an RSR' conduction pattern in lead V1. This is consistent with right ventricular conduction delay and left ventricular premature ventricular complex origin. The atrial rate is approximately 60 per minute. Left anterior fascicular block is seen as the QRS complex is positive in lead I and negative in leads II, III, and aVF. A small R wave is seen in leads II, III, and aVF not supporting the diagnosis of an inferior myocardial infarction. The R-wave spanning leads V2 to V6 demonstrates poor progression. Small R waves are present in each lead. The premature ventricular complex of left ventricular origin, which is timed with the right and the left precordial leads, demonstrates prominent Q waves. This likely solidifies the diagnosis of an anterolateral myocardial infarction of indeterminate age. The PVC also demonstrates Q waves in leads II and III raising the high likelihood of an age-indeterminate inferior myocardial infarction. Both myocardial territory infarctions are unmasked by the premature ventricular complexes of left ventricular origin.

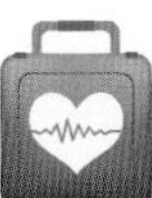

KEY DIAGNOSES

- Normal sinus rhythm
- First-degree atrioventricular block
- Premature ventricular complexes
- Left ventricular fascicular block
- Anterolateral myocardial infarction, age indeterminate
- Inferior myocardial infarction, age indeterminate.

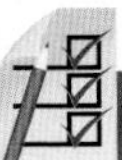

KEY TEACHING POINTS

- Premature ventricular complexes of left ventricular origin permit an initial accounting of pure left-sided electrical events. For this electrocardiogram, the premature ventricular complexes clearly delineate myocardial infarctions in both the left anterior descending and the right coronary artery distributions.
- Within the premature ventricular complexes, prominent ST-T changes in the form of ST-segment elevation are noted in lead V3, raising the possibility of a left ventricular aneurysm.

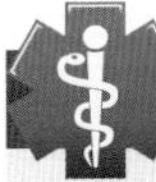

BOARD EXAMINATION ESSENTIALS

For the board exam, diagnostic codes include normal sinus rhythm; left anterior fascicular block; AV block, first degree; ventricular premature complexes; and nonspecific ST- and/or T-wave abnormalities. Since small R waves are present in each lead, it is not recommended to code an infarction pattern for the board exam. Stay with the criteria of a Q wave of diagnostic duration in at least two contiguous leads before coding a myocardial infarction pattern. While interesting and of clinical utility, the ventricular premature complex finding suggesting an anterolateral and inferior myocardial infarction should not be used to code a myocardial infarction pattern on the board exam.

Electrocardiogram Case Study #19

CLINICAL HISTORY

A 74-year-old male having undergone coronary artery bypass grafting surgery earlier the same day.

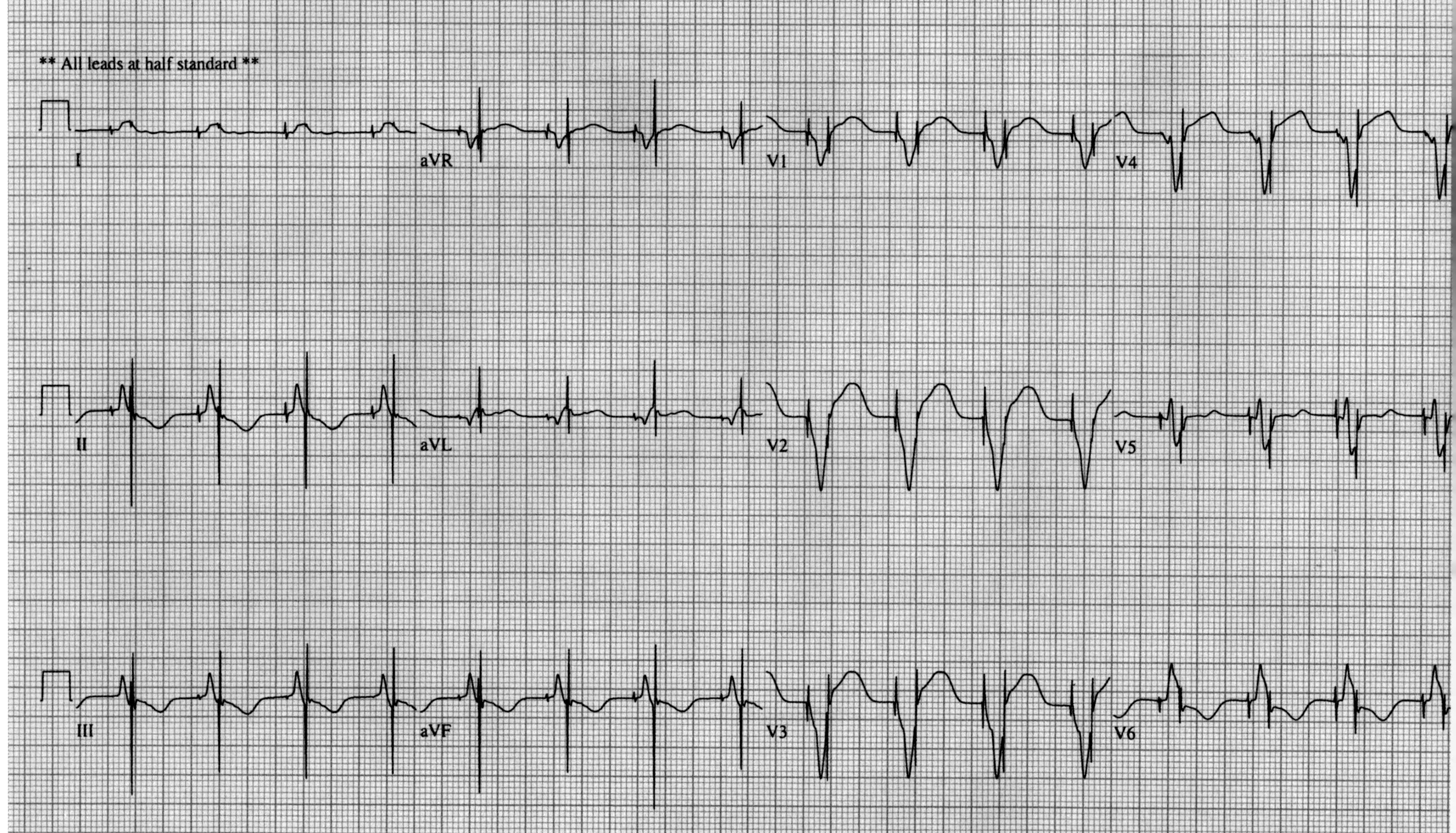

Interpretation Notes:

Electrocardiogram Case Study #19

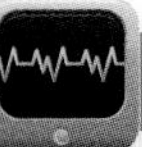

ELECTROCARDIOGRAM INTERPRETATION

This electrocardiogram demonstrates two discrete deflections representing atrial and ventricular pacemaker output. The initial pacemaker deflection is seen immediately preceding the QRS complex and the subsequent pacemaker discharge is present after the QRS complex within the proximal ST segment. This is an example of an epicardial atrioventricular pacemaker placed intraoperatively at the time of open heart surgery. This is a temporary system and the atrial and the ventricular leads were switched at the pulse generator. Thus, the atrial lead is attached to the ventricular output and the ventricular lead is attached to the atrial output of the pulse generator. This explains the altered sequence of pacemaker discharge and depolarization.

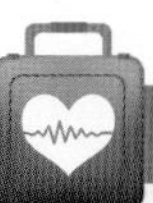

KEY DIAGNOSES

- Atrioventricular pacemaker
- Pacemaker malfunction

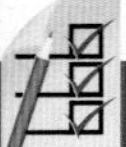

KEY TEACHING POINTS

- In this situation, this is quickly reversed by switching the lead wires at the temporary pulse generator.
- This patient was not harmed as an adequate cardiac output was maintained via ventricular pacing. This error was quickly recognized and immediately rectified.

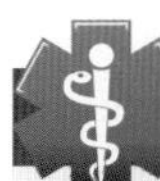

BOARD EXAMINATION ESSENTIALS

The best code for this electrocardiogram is pacemaker malfunction, not constantly sensing (atrium or ventricle). Pacemaker rhythms on the cardiovascular medicine board exam are typically straightforward and will potentially include normal function, abnormalities of capture and sensing. It should not be too complex and, in this case, a single code suffices.

Electrocardiogram Case Study #20

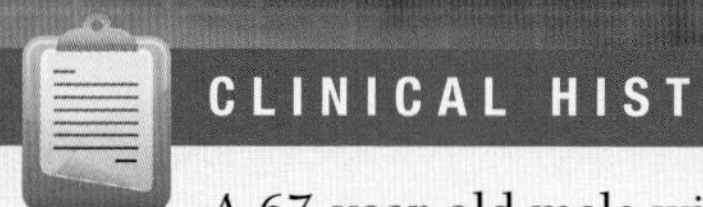

CLINICAL HISTORY

A 67-year-old male with acute onset chest pain of 2-hour duration.

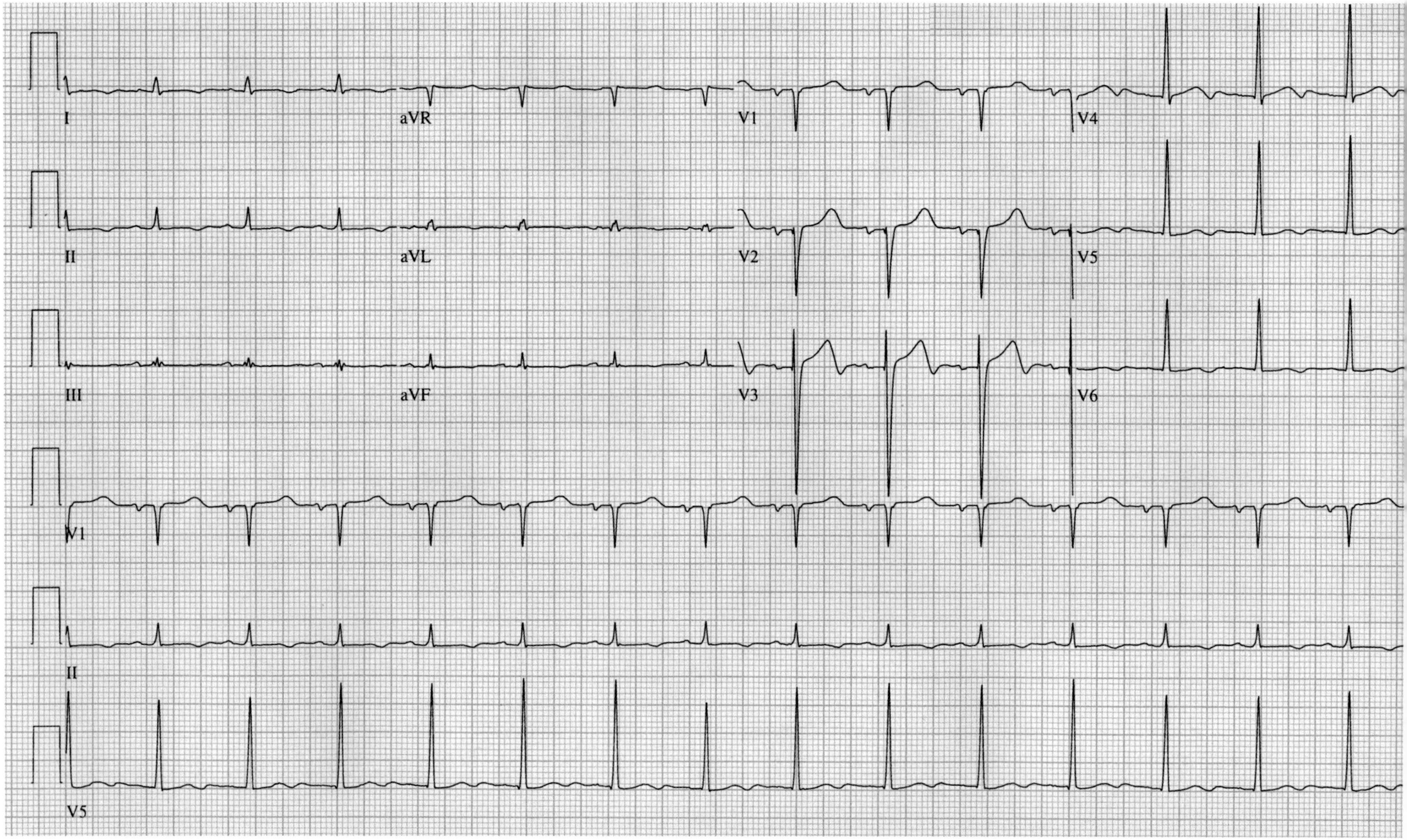

I aVR V1 V4
II aVL V2 V5
III aVF V3 V6
V1
II
V5

Interpretation Notes:

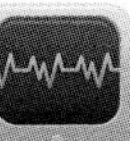

ELECTROCARDIOGRAM INTERPRETATION

This electrocardiogram demonstrates normal sinus rhythm at a rate of approximately 90 per minute. Low-voltage QRS complexes are seen over the limb leads as none are >0.5 milliVolt in amplitude. Anterolateral ST-T changes are also seen. In lead V3, the T wave is biphasic and terminally negative. The J-point is slightly elevated as is the ST segment. In lead V4, there is ST-segment straightening. This is a subtle example of an anterior ST-segment elevation myocardial infarction. Splinter Q waves are best identified in lead V3 supporting the diagnosis of a myocardial infarction. The most important clue on this electrocardiogram is the biphasic T-wave inversion seen in lead V3. Recognizing this abnormality allows the interpreter to focus on other potential abnormalities, likewise subtle in appearance.

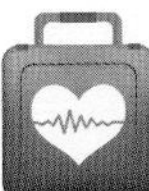

KEY DIAGNOSES

- Normal sinus rhythm
- Acute myocardial injury
- Anterior myocardial infarction acute
- Low-voltage QRS complexes

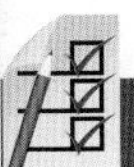

KEY TEACHING POINTS

- Subtle J-point elevation and ST-T changes are seen in leads I and aVL. While not diagnostic, this raises the possibility of acute myocardial infarction high lateral myocardial involvement.
- The initial small q wave seen in leads V2 and V3 is termed a splinter q wave given its extremely short duration. This finding is highly specific for a myocardial infarction, especially when located in leads V2 and V3.

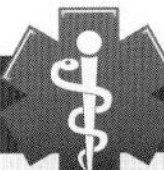

BOARD EXAMINATION ESSENTIALS

When coding for the board exam, normal sinus rhythm, and low voltage, limb leads are both correct codes as are ST- and/or T-wave abnormalities suggesting acute myocardial injury. While Q waves are present in leads V2 and V3, in the context of the board exam they are not of diagnostic duration. In this circumstance, do not code for a myocardial infarction but instead solely focus on the ST- and the T-wave abnormalities of acute myocardial injury. Clinically, this patient demonstrated positive serum biomarkers for acute myocardial injury and the splinter Q waves in hindsight reflected an acute myocardial infarction.

Electrocardiogram Case Study #21

CLINICAL HISTORY

A 42-year-old male with known coronary artery disease and a myocardial infarction 2 years previously at which time urgent stenting of his left circumflex coronary artery was successfully undertaken.

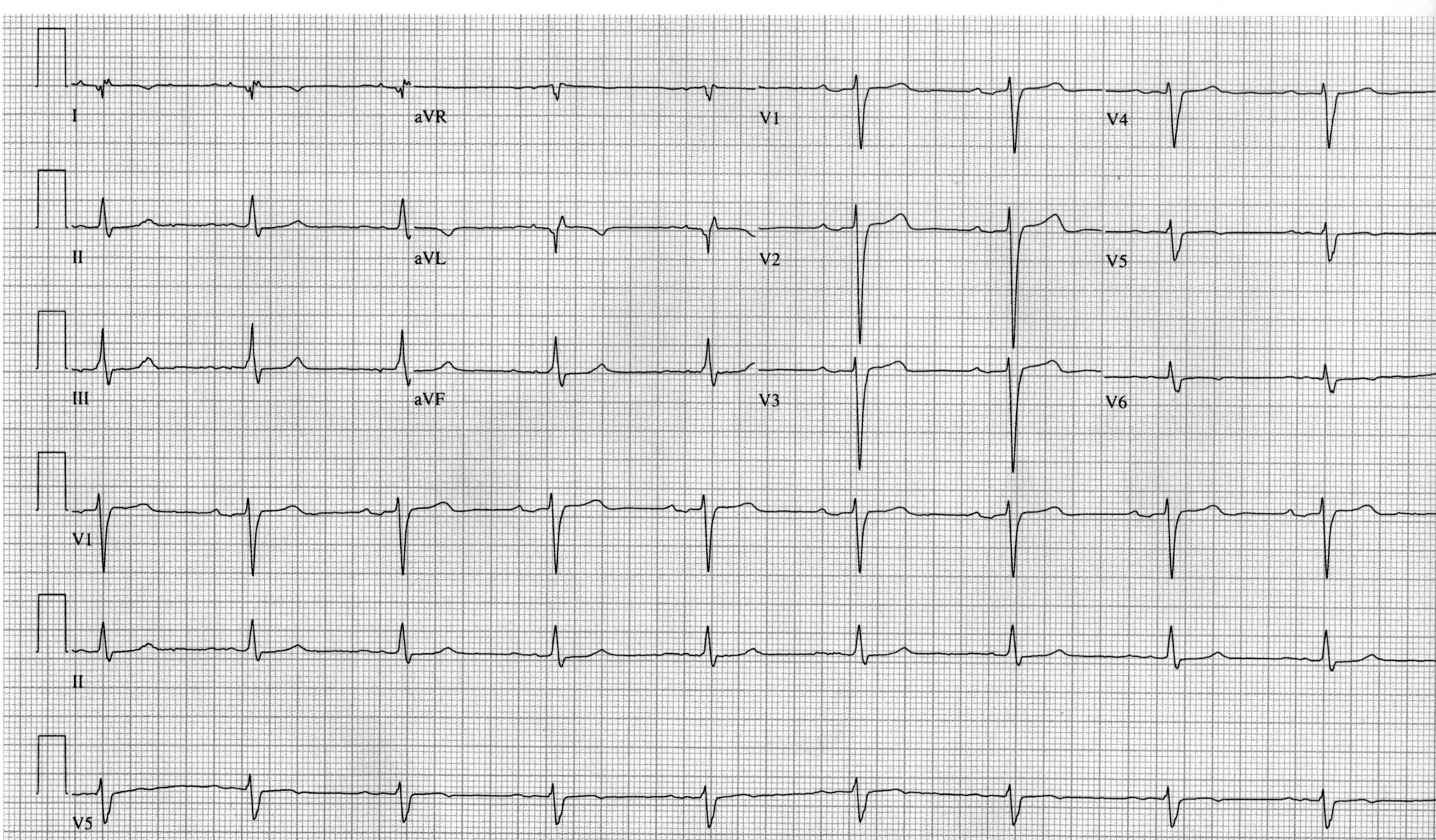

Interpretation Notes:

Electrocardiogram Case Study #21

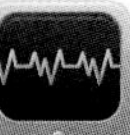

ELECTROCARDIOGRAM INTERPRETATION

This electrocardiogram demonstrates sinus bradycardia at a rate of approximately 55 per minute. Left atrial abnormality is seen given the prolonged terminal aspect of the P-wave best observed in lead V1 and the bifid P wave, which is also prolonged in lead II. In leads V5 and V6, T-wave flattening is identified with subtle T-wave inversion. The high lateral leads demonstrate diminutive QRS complexes and Q waves of diagnostic duration with terminal T-wave inversion and terminal QRS complex conduction delay in the form of peri-infarction block. These abnormal findings are best assessed as a high lateral myocardial infarction of indeterminate age, easily overlooked in the setting of the small- or low-amplitude QRS complexes in leads I and aVL. The most important clue is the terminal conduction delay best seen in lead aVL and the terminal T-wave inversion. This allows the interpreter to focus more carefully on the initial component of the QRS complex where a diagnostic Q wave is identified.

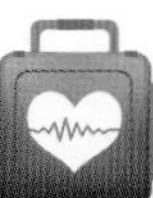

KEY DIAGNOSES

- Sinus bradycardia
- Left atrial abnormality
- High lateral myocardial infarction, age indeterminate
- Peri-infarction block

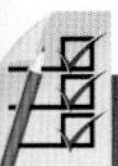

KEY TEACHING POINTS

- An important clue to the presence of a myocardial infarction is the terminal conduction delay best seen in lead aVL and the associated terminal T-wave inversion. This allows the interpreter to focus more carefully on the initial component of the QRS complex where a diagnostic Q wave is identified.
- In the setting of recent chest discomfort, the findings on this electrocardiogram support a recent myocardial event. That was not the case in this circumstance.
- Findings in the high lateral leads I and aVL are often overlooked on the electrocardiogram. These leads may be the only electrocardiogram indication of underlying coronary artery disease.

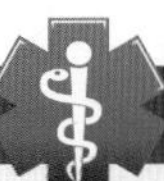

BOARD EXAMINATION ESSENTIALS

Diagnostic codes for the board exam include sinus bradycardia as the sinus rate is slightly <60 per minute. The QRS complex is prolonged >100 milliseconds supporting an intraventricular conduction disturbance, nonspecific type. Since a high lateral myocardial infarction, age indeterminate, is not a coding choice, code lateral myocardial infarction even when leads I and aVL are the leads solely reflecting a myocardial infarction. Lastly, left atrial abnormality/enlargement should be coded for, particularly based on the significantly prolonged P-wave duration >110 milliseconds as evidenced in lead II.

Electrocardiogram Case Study #22

CLINICAL HISTORY

A 66-year-old female with anterior precordial crushing pain of 45-minute duration. She has known coronary artery disease.

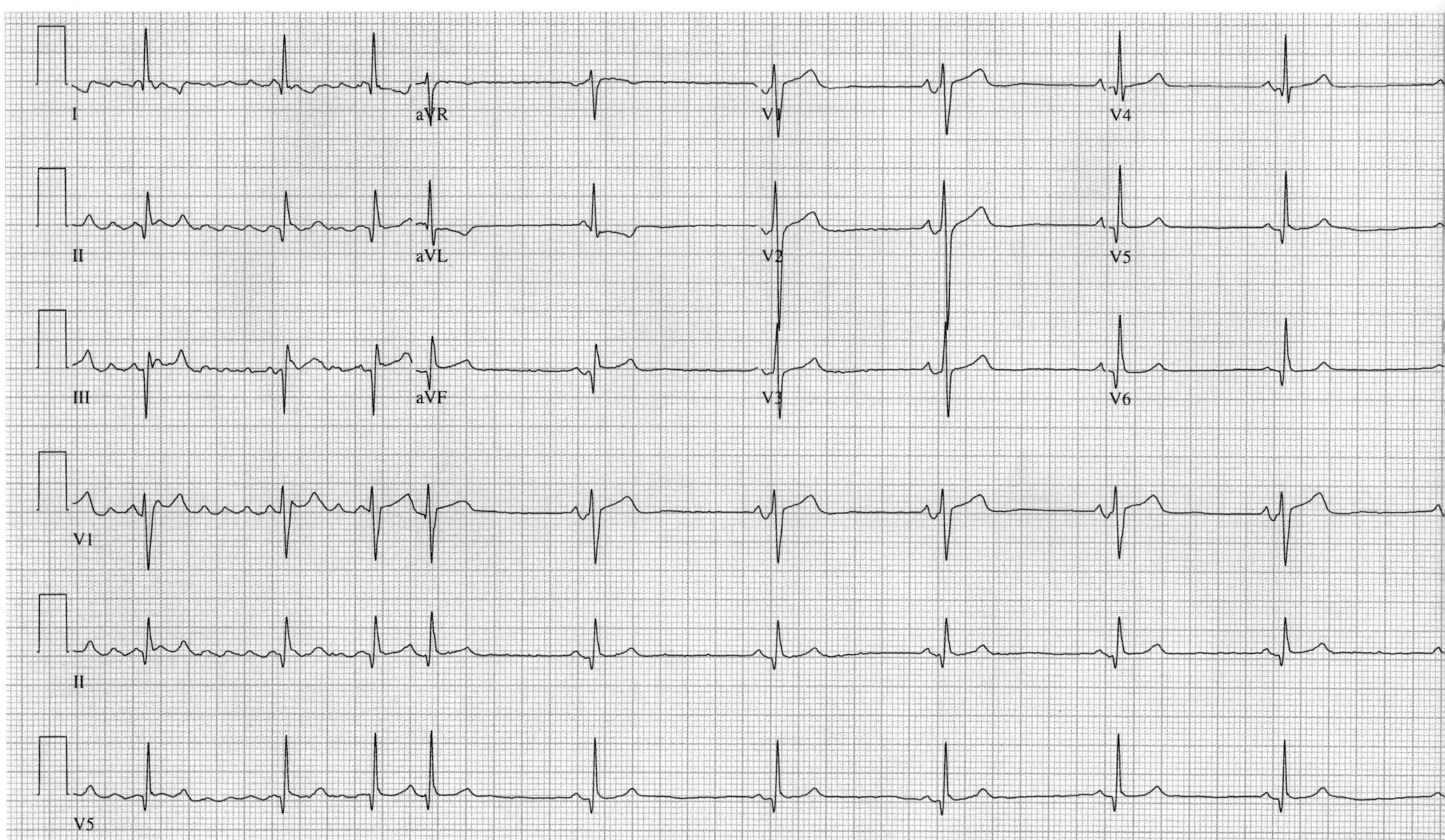

Interpretation Notes:

Electrocardiogram Case Study #22

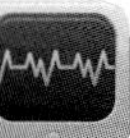

ELECTROCARDIOGRAM INTERPRETATION

On the right hand portion of this electrocardiogram, a supraventricular bradycardic rhythm is demonstrated with eight discrete atrial depolarizations identified with a short PR interval. This most likely represents either an ectopic atrial bradycardia or a sinus bradycardia. If sinus bradycardia, terminal P-wave inversion is noted in lead V1 consistent with left atrial abnormality. On the left hand side of the electrocardiogram, atrial flutter waves are identified, best observed in lead II. The fourth QRS complex is premature and interrupts the paroxysm of atrial flutter converting to ectopic atrial bradycardia versus normal sinus rhythm. Inferior Q waves of borderline diagnostic duration are seen in leads II, III, and aVF with J-point elevation seen in leads III and aVF suspicious for an acute inferior myocardial infarction. Q waves are also seen in leads V5 and V6 without associated J-point and ST-segment elevation. These are not of diagnostic duration to assure the diagnosis of a lateral myocardial infarction.

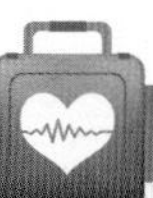

KEY DIAGNOSES

- Ectopic atrial bradycardia
- Atrial flutter
- Inferior myocardial infarction acute

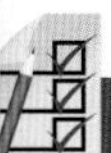

KEY TEACHING POINTS

- Atrial arrhythmias are commonly present in the setting of acute myocardial injury and infarction.
- The atrial flutter sequence terminates with a premature complex that interrupts the atrial flutter macro re-entrant circuit.
- The duration of the Q waves is of borderline diagnostic significance. The J-point and ST-segment elevation lends greater confidence to the diagnosis of an acute inferior myocardial infarction. The lateral precordial Q waves, while of similar appearance, are devoid of associated J-point elevation or ST-segment change.

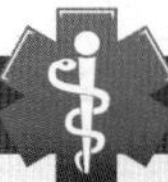

BOARD EXAMINATION ESSENTIALS

Since ectopic atrial bradycardia is not a coding choice for the board exam, sinus bradycardia is the most closely available coding option. Atrial flutter is also present and should be coded. Inferior and lateral Q waves are present but they are not of diagnostic duration (40 milliseconds) to confidently code a myocardial infarction. For the board exam, apply strict criteria when coding for an infarction pattern. In this case, instead code for ST-and/or T-wave abnormalities suggesting acute myocardial injury given the J-point and ST-segment elevation seen in leads III and aVF in the context of the supporting clinical history.

Electrocardiogram Case Study #23

CLINICAL HISTORY

A 68-year-old male with a history of coronary artery disease who experienced a myocardial infarction 3 years previously. The patient returns for outpatient cardiovascular medicine follow-up.

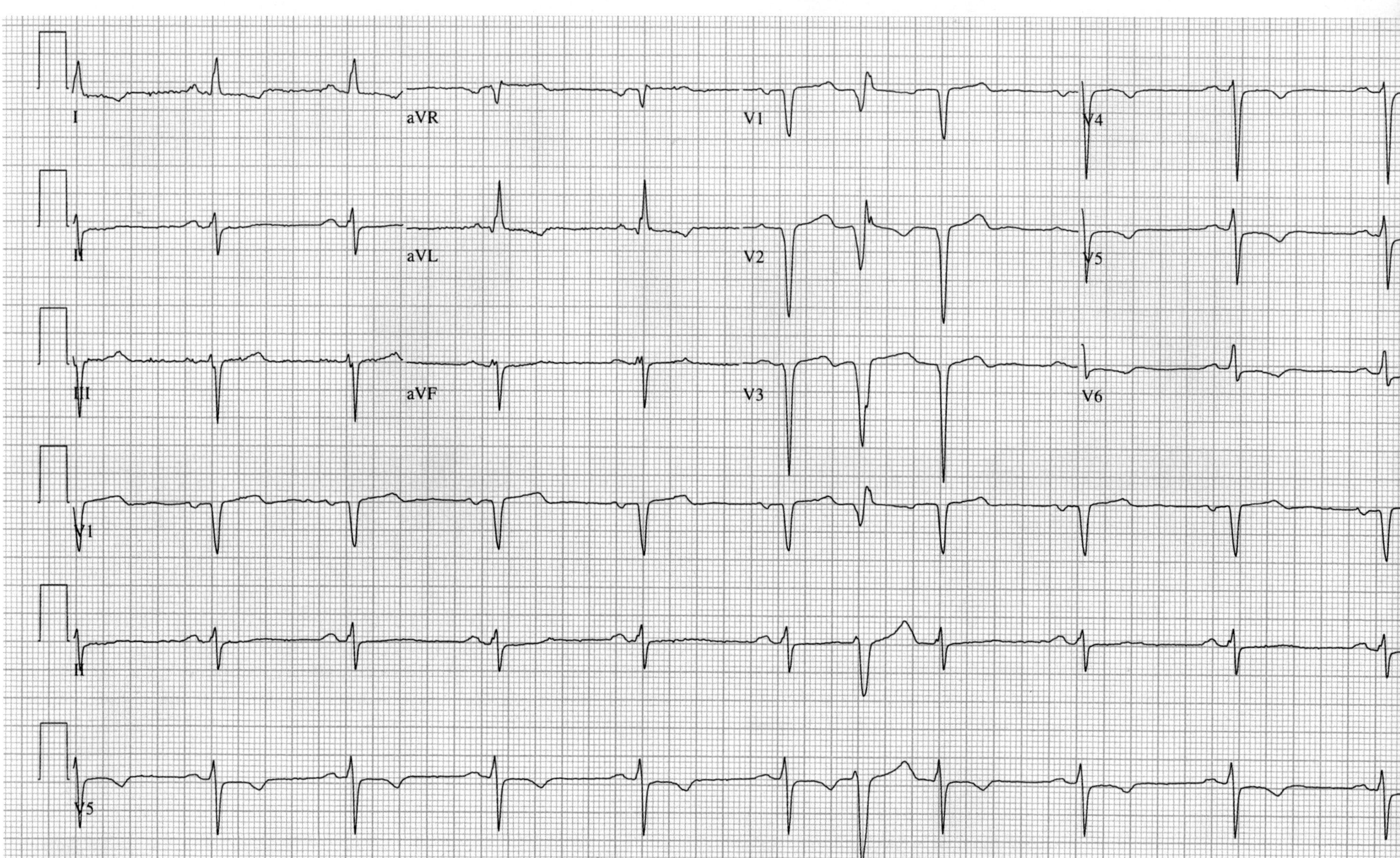

Interpretation Notes:

Electrocardiogram Case Study #23

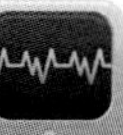

ELECTROCARDIOGRAM INTERPRETATION

This electrocardiogram demonstrates sinus bradycardia at an atrial rate slightly <60 per minute. Left anterior fascicular block is present given the positive QRS complex vector in lead I and negative QRS complex vectors in leads II, III, and aVF. Q waves are present in leads V1, V2, and V3 consistent with an anteroseptal myocardial infarction of indeterminate age. An interpolated premature ventricular complex is identified with subsequent prolongation of the ensuing PR interval. The interpolated premature ventricular complex has a QRS complex morphology best identified in lead V1, indicating right ventricular conduction delay and therefore left ventricular in origin. Of note, within the QRS complex, deep Q waves are seen further substantiating the presence of an age-indeterminate anteroseptal myocardial infarction. Anterolateral ST-T wave changes best characterized as T-wave inversion are also identified.

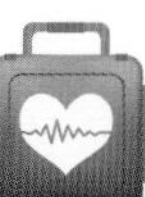

KEY DIAGNOSES

- Sinus bradycardia
- Left anterior fascicular block
- Anteroseptal myocardial infarction age indeterminate
- Premature ventricular complex interpolated
- Nonspecific ST-T changes

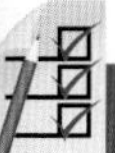

KEY TEACHING POINTS

- Premature ventricular complexes of right ventricular origin result in initial left ventricular depolarization. The early most portion of the premature ventricular complex reflects left ventricular forces, permitting the interpreter to gain additional insight to the presence of pathologic Q waves and age-indeterminate myocardial infarction patterns.
- In the presence of left anterior fascicular block, initial left ventricular forces are directed posteriorly and inferiorly away from the left anterior fascicle. This can result in Q waves in leads V1, V2, and sometimes lead V3 complicating the accurate diagnosis of an age-indeterminate anteroseptal myocardial infarction. On this electrocardiogram, the premature ventricular complex of left ventricular origin lends greater support to the myocardial infarction diagnosis.

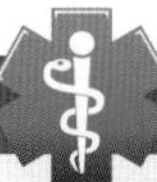

BOARD EXAMINATION ESSENTIALS

This is an example of sinus bradycardia as the sinus rate is slightly less than 60 per minute. Left anterior fascicular block should also be coded as the QRS complex is of normal duration and the QRS complex vector is positive in lead I and significantly negative in lead II. Q waves are present in leads V1, V2 and V3. The Q wave in lead V3 is key and supports coding an anteroseptal myocardial infarction, age indeterminate. Also, make sure to code the ventricular premature complex. The PR interval prolongation seen after the premature ventricular complex does not qualify as first-degree atrioventricular block and should not be coded. The ST-T changes are likely related to the ischemic heart disease. Coding for this finding is equivocal as they are not truly nonspecific.

Electrocardiogram Case Study **#24**

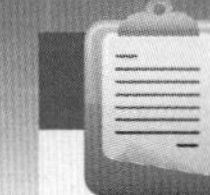

CLINICAL HISTORY

A 78-year-old female who presented 24 hours earlier with severe anterior chest discomfort consistent with an acute myocardial infarction.

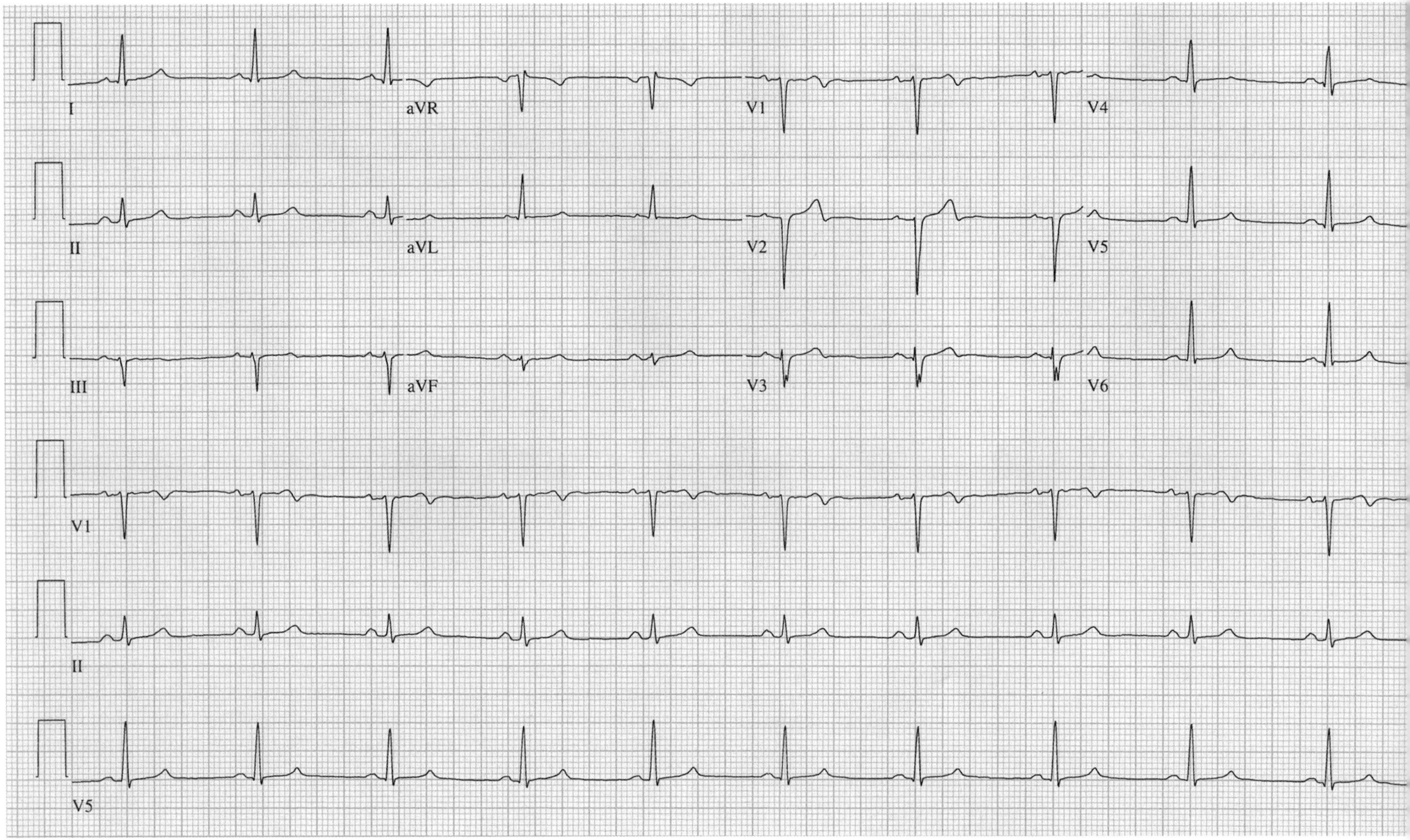

I aVR V1 V4

II aVL V2 V5

III aVF V3 V6

V1

II

V5

Interpretation Notes:

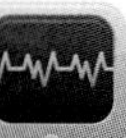

ELECTROCARDIOGRAM INTERPRETATION

This electrocardiogram demonstrates normal sinus rhythm at an atrial rate slightly >60 per minute. On first glance, this appears to be a normal electrocardiogram. However, a biphasic T wave with terminal T-wave inversion is seen best in leads V1 and V2. This is abnormal and, in fact, this patient was known to experience a recent left anterior descending coronary artery occlusion and acute myocardial injury based on serial cardiac enzymes. In the appropriate clinical context, terminal biphasic T-wave inversion can be extremely helpful as an indicator for obstructive coronary artery disease.

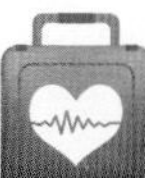

KEY DIAGNOSES

- Sinus bradycardia
- T-wave changes

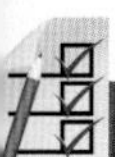

KEY TEACHING POINTS

- This electrocardiogram reinforces the premise to approach each interpretation opportunity in a logical and sequential manner. For unclear reasons, despite the left anterior descending coronary artery occlusion, this electrocardiogram presents minimal abnormal findings in the form of subtle biphasic terminal T-wave inversion.
- In the clinical context of an acute chest discomfort syndrome, this finding helps localize the infarction-related artery to the left anterior descending coronary artery territory.
- Since the biphasic T-wave inversion is noted both in leads V1 and V2, this further localizes the left anterior descending coronary artery obstruction within the proximal vessel, before the first septal perforator branch.

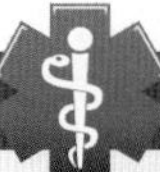

BOARD EXAMINATION ESSENTIALS

Subtle T-wave findings as found on this electrocardiogram may appear on the board exam. In the context of an appropriate clinical history supporting an acute coronary syndrome, acute myocardial injury should be suspected. For the board exam, coding selections should include sinus bradycardia and nonspecific ST- and/or T-wave changes. Myocardial injury, while supported by the clinical history, is not definitively demonstrated on the electrocardiogram.

Electrocardiogram Case Study **#25**

CLINICAL HISTORY

A 46-year-old male with hypertension who presents for blood pressure follow-up.

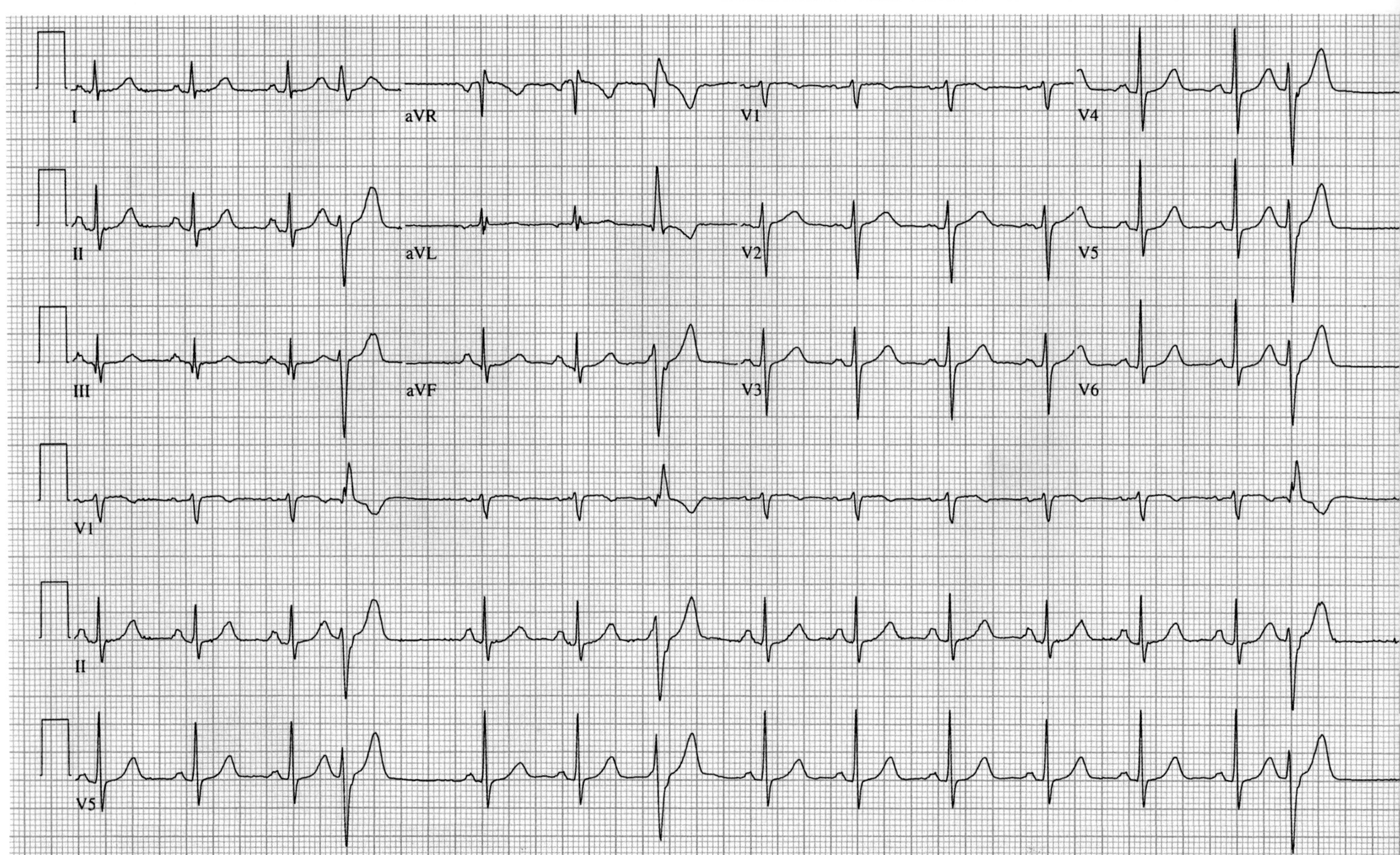

Interpretation Notes:____

____

Electrocardiogram Case Study #25

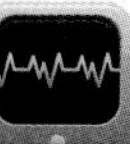

ELECTROCARDIOGRAM INTERPRETATION

This electrocardiogram demonstrates normal sinus rhythm at a rate of approximately 85 per minute. Widened QRS complexes are seen with a QR pattern in the lead V1 rhythm strip suggesting premature ventricular complexes of left ventricular origin. These premature ventricular complexes demonstrate a varying coupling interval, a similar QRS complex morphology, and a constant R to R interval as assessed by caliper measurement. This is also termed a constant interectopic interval. One of the premature ventricular complexes appears to be missing or nonconducted. The ventricle is absolutely refractory at that instant due to the native atrioventricular conduction and ventricular depolarization. This is an example of ventricular parasystole. The electrocardiogram is otherwise normal.

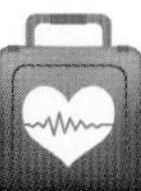

KEY DIAGNOSES

- Normal sinus rhythm
- Ventricular parasystole

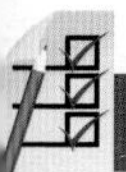

KEY TEACHING POINTS

- Ventricular parasystole is a relatively uncommon finding without a known adverse prognosis. It is easily overlooked and more often than not is interpreted as frequent premature ventricular complexes.
- The criteria of a constant interectopic interval, varying coupling intervals and a similar QRS complex morphology satisfy the criteria for ventricular parasystole. Even less commonly recognized is atrial parasystole.
- Fusion complexes can be seen when the ventricular parasystolic focus depolarizes the ventricles simultaneously with intact native antegrade ventricular depolarization.

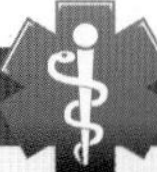

BOARD EXAMINATION ESSENTIALS

For the board examination, coding normal sinus rhythm and ventricular parasystole are appropriate. It is not necessary to code ventricular premature complexes.

Electrocardiogram Case Study #26

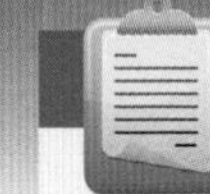

CLINICAL HISTORY

A 66-year-old female with known mitral regurgitation and a history of atrial arrhythmias who is presently postoperative day 1, status post colorectal surgery.

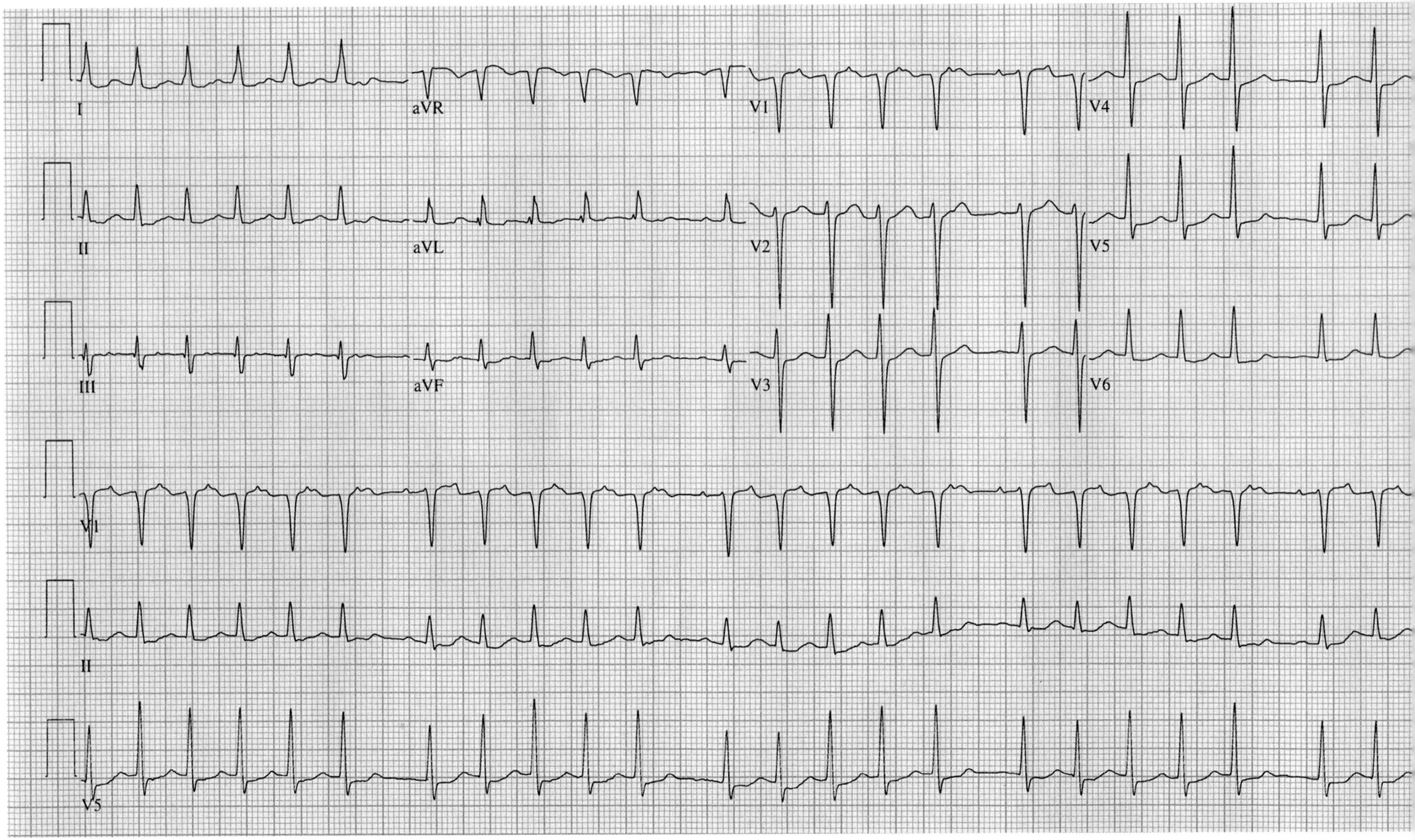

I aVR V1 V4
II aVL V2 V5
III aVF V3 V6
V1
II
V5

Interpretation Notes:

Electrocardiogram Case Study #26

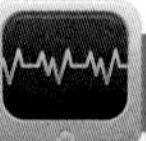

ELECTROCARDIOGRAM INTERPRETATION

This electrocardiogram demonstrates discrete atrial activity best seen in the lead V1 rhythm strip at an atrial rate slightly >150 per minute with an abnormal P-wave axis including isoelectric P waves in lead III consistent with ectopic atrial tachycardia. The QRS complexes are grouped with an ectopic atrial depolarization preceding each QRS complex with a successively prolonging atrial depolarization to QRS complex interval consistent with Wenckebach periodicity and varying conduction ratios. Diffuse nonspecific ST-T changes are also present.

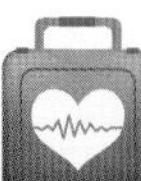

KEY DIAGNOSES

- Ectopic atrial tachycardia
- Mobitz I Wenckebach atrioventricular block
- Nonspecific ST-T changes

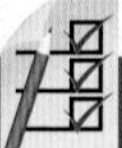

KEY TEACHING POINTS

- The initial approach to electrocardiogram interpretation should be determination of the heart rhythm. Oftentimes, the heart rhythm is best elucidated in a rhythm strip, in this case the lead V1 rhythm strip.
- After identifying the P waves, it is important to determine the P-wave axis.
- Once the P waves are identified and the P-wave axis is determined, it is best to assess if the P waves are associated with the QRS complexes.
- In this case, P waves are readily identified, the P-wave axis is abnormal, and a P wave precedes each QRS complex.
- Wenckebach periodicity not only occurs in the presence of normal sinus rhythm but can also be seen in the presence of ectopic atrial rhythms such as demonstrated on this electrocardiogram.

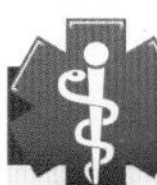

BOARD EXAMINATION ESSENTIALS

For the board examination, appropriate codes include atrial tachycardia; AV block, second degree—Mobitz type I (Wenckebach); and nonspecific ST- and/or T-wave abnormalities. Be careful not to code atrial fibrillation because of the apparent irregularly irregular ventricular response. In fact, the ventricular response demonstrates periodicity in the form of grouped complexes. This is the most important clue to investigate further for the presence of discrete P waves and progressive PR interval prolongation in the form of Wenckebach atrioventricular block.

Electrocardiogram Case Study #27

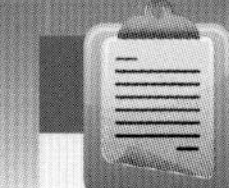

CLINICAL HISTORY

A 50-year-old male with metastatic melanoma hospitalized with shortness of breath.

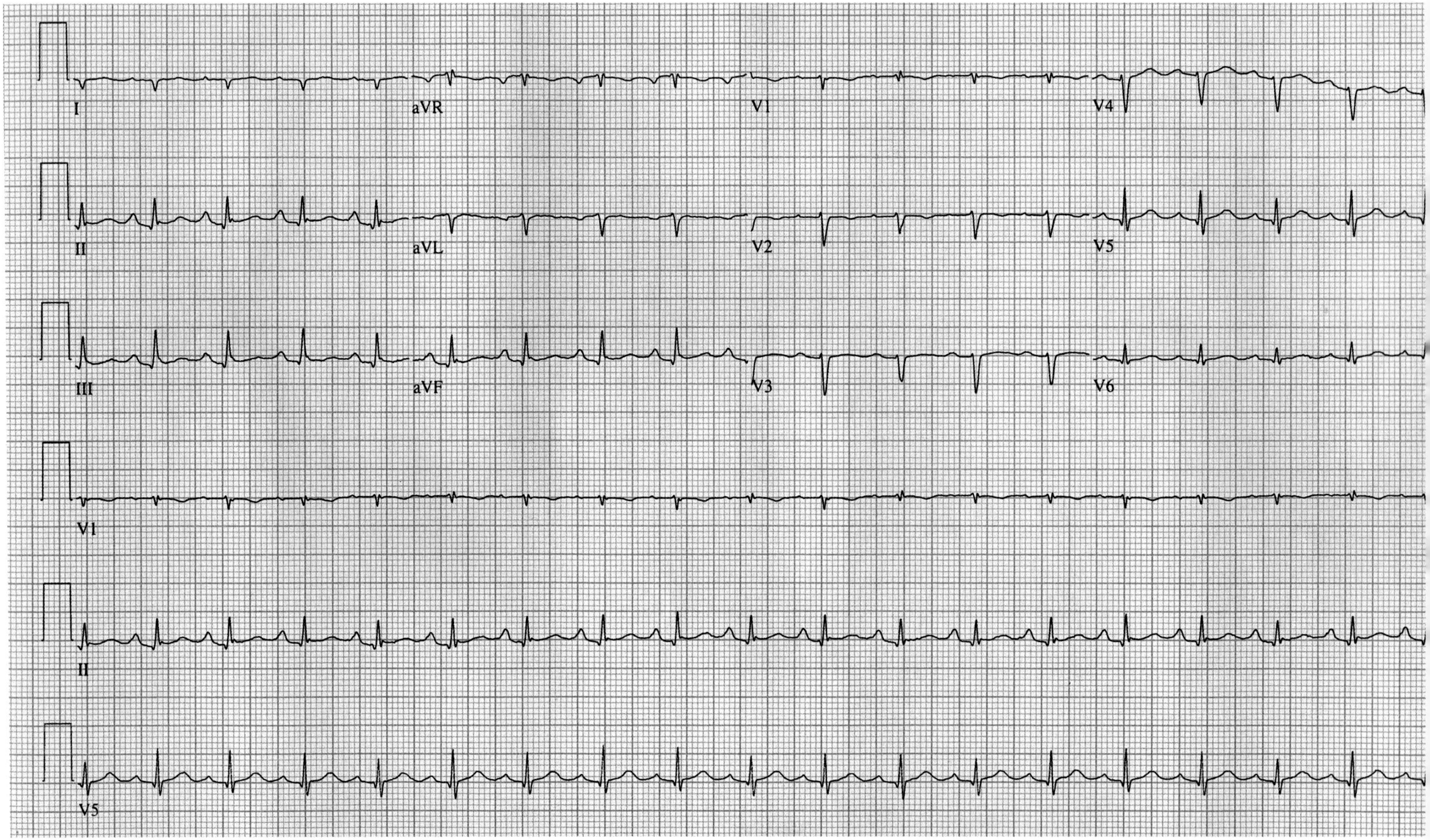

I aVR V1 V4

II aVL V2 V5

III aVF V3 V6

V1

II

V5

Interpretation Notes:

Electrocardiogram Case Study #27

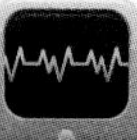

ELECTROCARDIOGRAM INTERPRETATION

This electrocardiogram demonstrates sinus tachycardia at an atrial rate of approximately 110 per minute. The QRS complex axis is deviated rightward to approximately +110 degrees. The chest leads demonstrate low-voltage QRS complexes, <1 mV in maximal amplitude. The limb leads possess low-voltage QRS complexes however, with an R wave >0.5 mV in amplitude, it does not officially meet the diagnostic criteria. A Q wave is seen in lead I and a small R wave is seen in lead aVL. This does not satisfy the criteria for a high lateral myocardial infarction. Most important, the QRS complex amplitude differs in an alternating QRS complex pattern. This is perhaps best seen in the lead V1 rhythm strip. It is also clearly evident in lead V3. This is consistent with electrical alternans and together with the low-voltage QRS complexes, supports the presence of a large pericardial effusion, confirmed in this patient by transthoracic echocardiography.

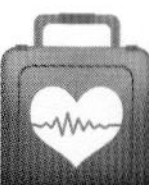

KEY DIAGNOSES

- Sinus tachycardia
- Low-voltage QRS complexes chest leads
- Electrical alternans
- QRS complex right-axis deviation
- Pericarditis
- Pericardial effusion

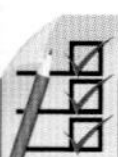

KEY TEACHING POINTS

- Electrical alternans as depicted on the electrocardiogram may be the first clinical indicator of a hemodynamically significant pericardial effusion
- The first clue is the low-voltage QRS complex morphology.
- J point and ST-segment elevation is seen particularly in leads II, III, and aVF. It is also seen in leads V5 and V6. Myocardial infarction was excluded by serial cardiac enzyme analysis. Instead, the ST-segment elevation reflects pericardial inflammation in the form of pericarditis.

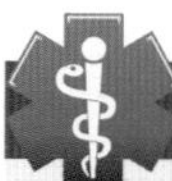

BOARD EXAMINATION ESSENTIALS

Electrical alternans reflecting a large pericardial effusion is likely to appear on the board exam. Ensure that you code for the heart rhythm, in this case sinus tachycardia. ST-segment elevation reflecting pericardial inflammation will often be found. If so, code for acute pericarditis. Also make sure to code for a pericardial effusion if electrical alternans is present. Low voltage is also commonly seen, in this case limited to the precordial leads. Lastly, QRS complex axis deviation can be present and if so, make sure you select the appropriate code. This is due to a change in cardiac position secondary to the large pericardial effusion.

Electrocardiogram Case Study #28

CLINICAL HISTORY

A 56-year-old male with known coronary artery disease admitted to the hospital with unstable angina. The patient underwent left heart catheterization, angioplasty, and stenting to the proximal right coronary artery. This electrocardiogram was obtained 4 hours after the percutaneous coronary revascularization procedure was completed.

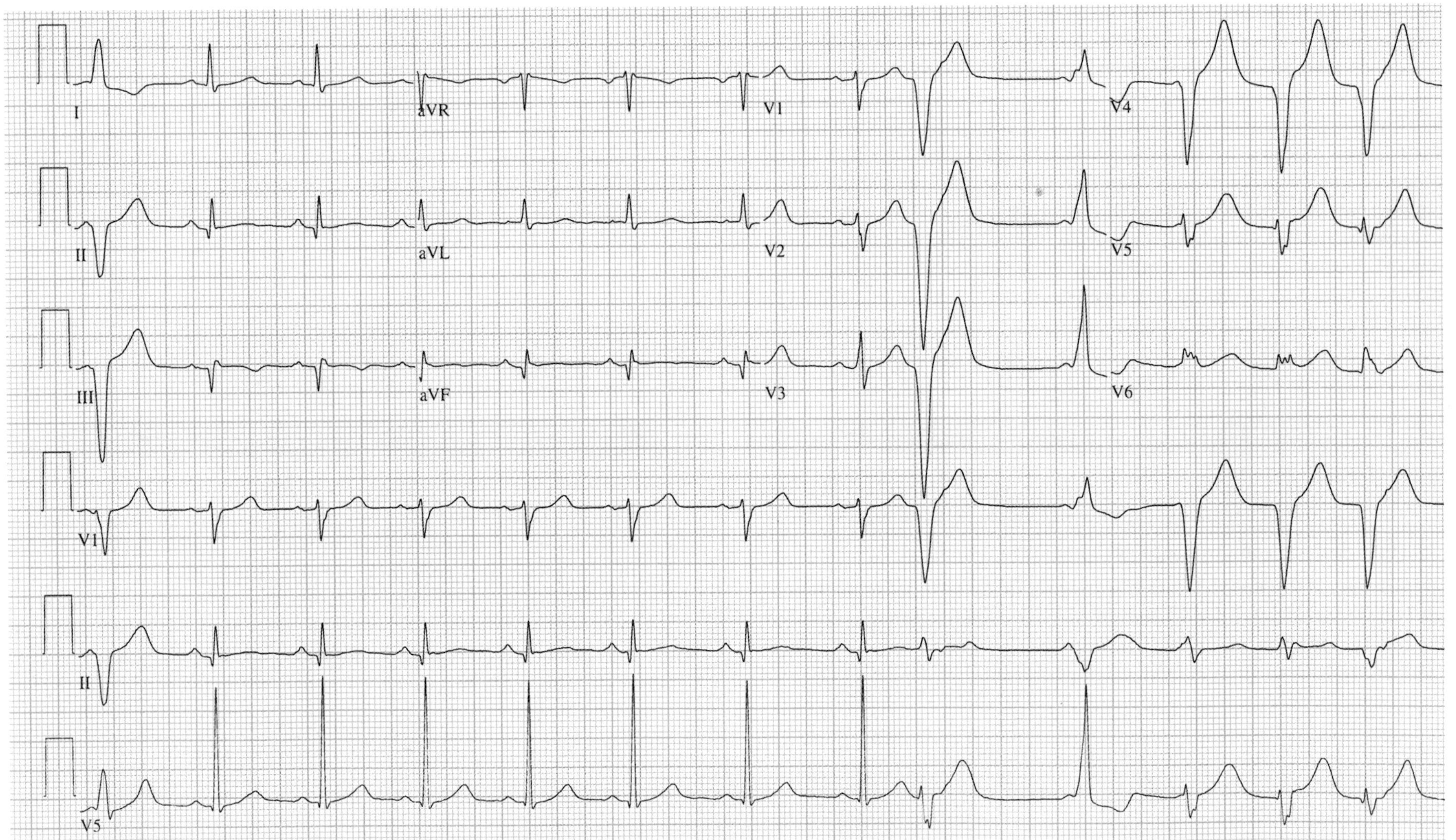

Interpretation Notes:

Electrocardiogram Case Study #28

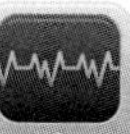

ELECTROCARDIOGRAM INTERPRETATION

This electrocardiogram demonstrates normal sinus rhythm at an atrial rate slightly >75 minutes. Q waves are seen in leads II, III, and aVF consistent with an age-indeterminate inferior myocardial infarction. The first QRS complex represents a premature ventricular complex as does the ninth QRS complex. The tenth QRS complex is widened and reflects a hybrid or a fusion complex between the ensuing accelerated idioventricular rhythm and the native QRS complex. The last three QRS complexes represent an accelerated idioventricular rhythm with a complete left bundle branch block QRS complex morphology consistent with a right ventricular origin.

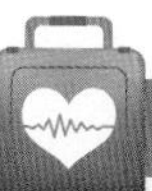

KEY DIAGNOSES

- Normal sinus rhythm
- Inferior myocardial infarction, age indeterminate
- Fusion complex
- Premature ventricular complex
- Accelerated idioventricular rhythm

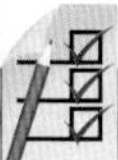

KEY TEACHING POINTS

- Accelerated idioventricular rhythm is a common arrhythmia in the presence of myocardial reperfusion. In this circumstance, this rhythm was observed shortly after percutaneous coronary intervention of a high-grade proximal right coronary artery stenosis.
- It is important not to confuse an accelerated idioventricular rhythm with ventricular tachycardia. Accelerated idioventricular rhythms are typically slower than ventricular tachycardia, and clinically, hemodynamic compromise is seldom observed.
- The tenth QRS complex, which represents a fusion complex, is due to simultaneous ventricular depolarization from a ventricular focus and via antegrade normal conduction via the atrioventricular node and His-Purkinje system.

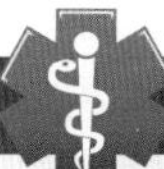

BOARD EXAMINATION ESSENTIALS

Appropriate board exam codes for this electrocardiogram include normal sinus rhythm; inferior myocardial infarction, acute; a ventricular premature complex; and accelerated idioventricular rhythm. The fusion complex suggests ventricular pre-excitation. This is not the case but instead secondary to the fusion complex. Should an accelerated idioventricular rhythm appear on the board exam, the most common association is ischemic heart disease. Since it is commonly clinically noted as a reperfusion arrhythmia, assess the electrocardiogram carefully for evidence of acute myocardial injury and infarction. On this electrocardiogram, ST-segment elevation is subtle but definitely present in leads II, III, and aVF. Remember to also code for ST- and/or T-wave abnormalities suggesting myocardial injury in the presence of a myocardial infarction acute.

Electrocardiogram Case Study #29

CLINICAL HISTORY

An 85-year-old male with acute chest pain and cardiogenic shock.

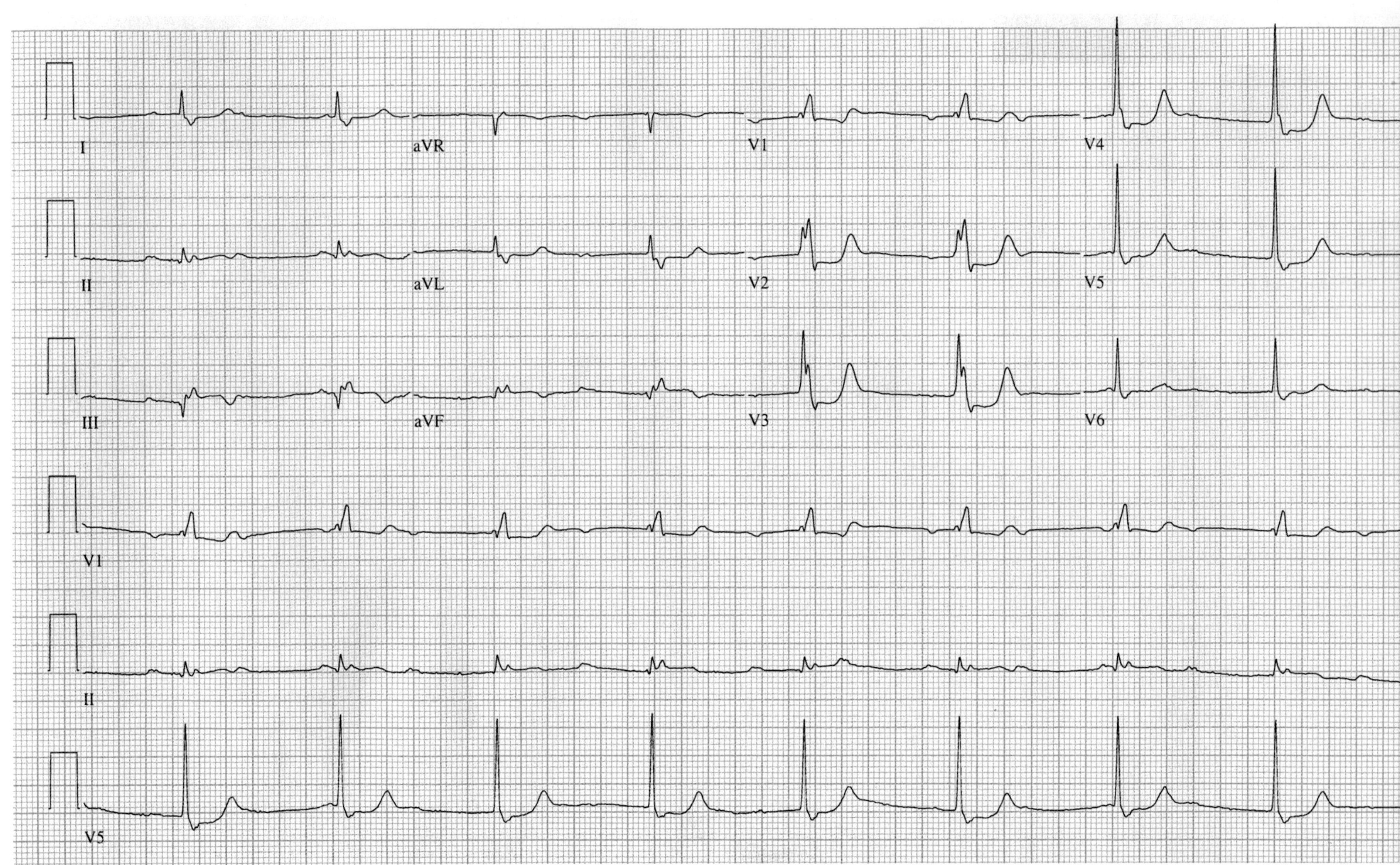

Interpretation Notes:

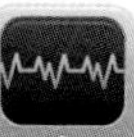

ELECTROCARDIOGRAM INTERPRETATION

This electrocardiogram demonstrates normal sinus rhythm at an atrial rate of approximately 85 per minute. The P waves demonstrate no temporal relationship to the QRS complexes. The QRS complexes demonstrate a constant R to R interval at a bradycardic rate slightly >50 per minute. This reflects a junctional rhythm and complete heart block. The QRS complex demonstrates prolongation >120 milliseconds in duration with a rSR' QRS complex morphology consistent with complete right bundle branch block. J point and ST-segment elevation is seen in leads II, III, and aVF with associated terminal T-wave inversion. Diminutive Q waves are also seen in these leads consistent with an acute inferior myocardial infarction. ST-segment depression is seen in leads V1, V2, V3, and V4. These findings, particularly in leads V1, V2, and V3 in the presence of an acute inferior myocardial infarction, suggest posterior myocardial injury and reciprocal ST-segment depression. Lending further credence to this suspicion is the presence of upright T waves in leads V1 and V2 that are not normally seen in the presence of complete right bundle branch block. This QRS complex T-wave concordance is best termed a primary T-wave change.

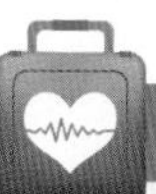

KEY DIAGNOSES

- Normal sinus rhythm
- Junctional rhythm
- Complete heart block
- Complete right bundle branch block
- Inferior myocardial infarction acute
- Posterior myocardial infarction acute

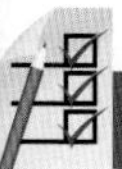

KEY TEACHING POINTS

- Serial electrocardiograms in this patient would be important to observe for R-wave amplitude growth in leads V1 and V2. If seen, this would further support the presence of a posterior myocardial infarction.
- The presence of a primary T-wave change, particularly if new during a period of acute chest discomfort, can be a helpful clue, especially when pre-existing conduction abnormalities are present. This is both true in the presence of complete right bundle branch block and also complete left bundle branch block.
- In the presence of an acute inferior myocardial infarction, it is of vital importance to assess contiguous myocardial territories for infarction involvement. For this patient, lateral ST-segment changes are seen but no discrete ST elevation or Q waves are noted precluding the diagnosis of a lateral myocardial infarction. In lead V1, there is no evidence of ST-segment elevation to support the presence of acute right ventricular myocardial injury. Instead, the findings as described above support posterior myocardial involvement.

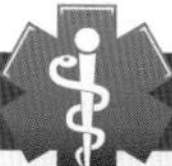

BOARD EXAMINATION ESSENTIALS

This electrocardiogram possesses the coding complexity similar to those found on the board exam. First, normal sinus rhythm is present as is complete heart block and an AV junctional rhythm. All of these diagnoses merit separate codes. The QRS complex morphology demonstrates complete right bundle branch block. In leads III and aVF, both Q waves and ST-segment elevation are noted consistent with inferior myocardial infarction, acute and ST- and/or T-wave abnormalities suggesting myocardial injury. The T waves are upright in leads V1, V2, and V3. This finding together with ST-segment depression in these leads and a prominent R wave in lead V2 supports the likelihood of a posterior myocardial infarction, acute.

Electrocardiogram Case Study **#30**

CLINICAL HISTORY

A 77-year-old male immediately postoperative mitral valve repair and coronary artery bypass grafting. The patient remains intubated in the surgical intensive care unit.

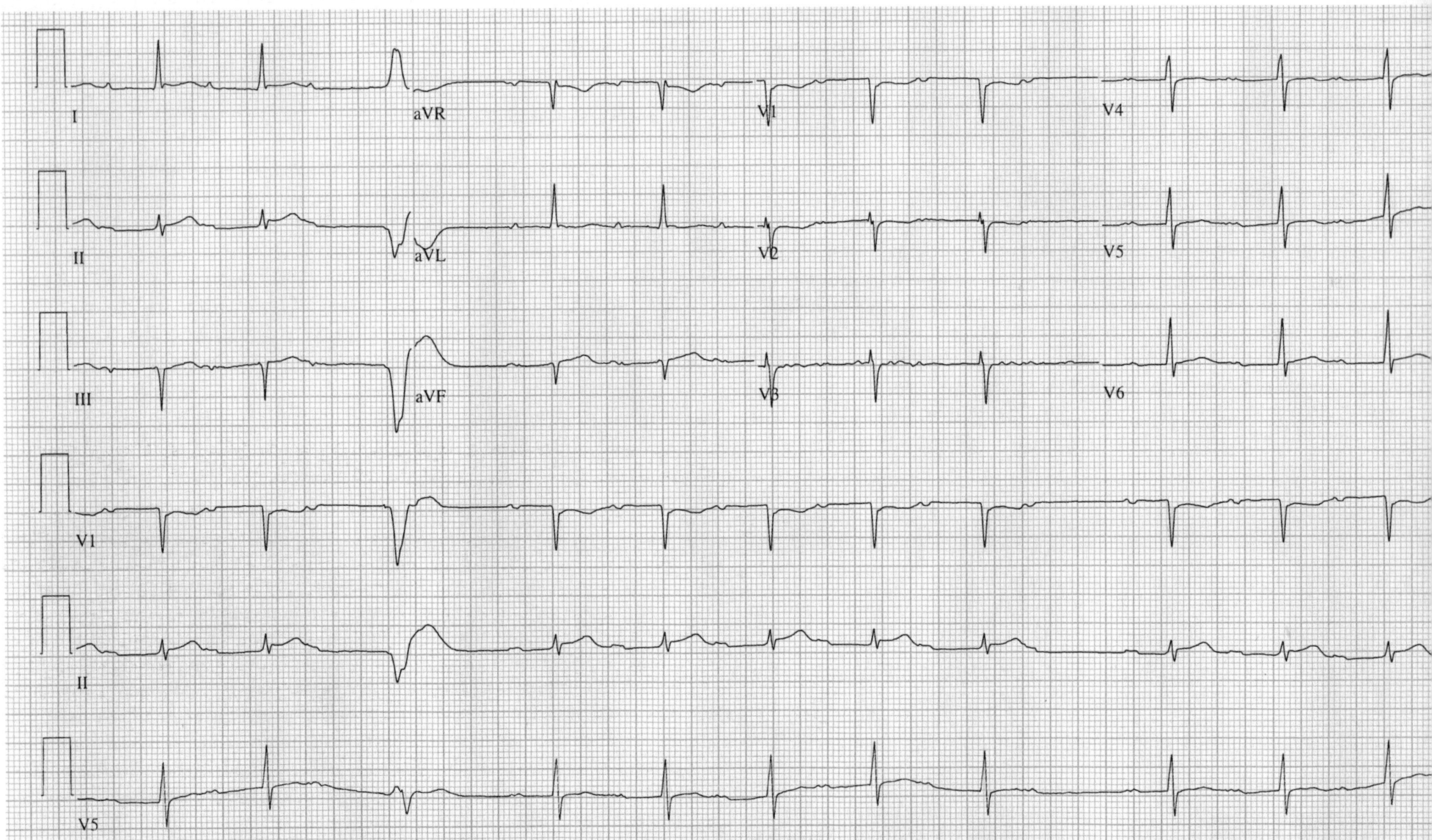

Interpretation Notes:

Electrocardiogram Case Study #30

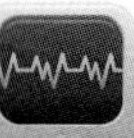

ELECTROCARDIOGRAM INTERPRETATION

This electrocardiogram demonstrates normal sinus rhythm at an atrial rate of 75 per minute. P waves are seen preceding each QRS complex with a progressively prolonging PR interval consistent with Mobitz type I Wenckebach atrioventricular block. ST-segment elevation is seen most notably in leads II, III, and aVF. ST-segment elevation is also present in leads I, V4, V5, and V6. PR-segment elevation is seen in lead aVR. Given the clinical history, these findings are most consistent with postoperative pericarditis and not myocardial injury. The third QRS complex is widened and it appears after a pause. In the lead V1 rhythm strip, a discrete deflection immediately prior to the QRS complex is seen most consistent with a ventricular paced complex. The terminal aspect of the ventricular paced complex demonstrates a deflection in its proximal ST segment consistent with a superimposed P wave. Diffuse nonspecific ST-T changes are also seen.

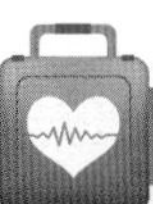

KEY DIAGNOSES

- Normal sinus rhythm
- Mobitz I Wenckebach atrioventricular block
- Pericarditis
- Ventricular pacemaker
- Nonspecific ST-T changes

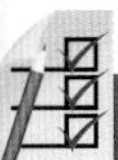

KEY TEACHING POINTS

- Atrioventricular conduction abnormalities are common after open-heart surgery. This is often a transient phenomenon that abates over time. Mobitz type I Wenckebach atrioventricular block does not warrant specific treatment other than avoiding AV nodal suppressing medications.
- The ventricular paced complex by clinical history represents a temporary epicardial pacemaker. It is not functioning in a completely normal fashion as a longer R to R interval exists toward the right hand portion of the electrocardiogram but no pacemaker discharge is seen. Epicardial pacemakers, in contrast to permanent pacemakers, are more frequently prone to malfunction.

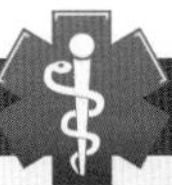

BOARD EXAMINATION ESSENTIALS

This electrocardiogram highlights several important principles for coding on the board exam. First, make sure that you code normal sinus rhythm. Next, code AV block, second degree—Mobitz type I (Wenckebach). Do not code AV block, first degree as the AV block, second degree, assumes precedence. While pericarditis is demonstrated, it is not a classic example and instead anticipate more pronounced J-point and ST-segment elevation on the board exam. Additionally, make certain to code pacemaker malfunction, not constantly sensing (atrium or ventricle). The first pacemaker deflection appropriately senses the pause at the end of the Wenckebach cycle, subsequently discharging and capturing the ventricle. After the second Wenckebach cycle concludes, there is no evidence of pacemaker discharge. This suggests abnormal sensing. Lastly, coding for nonspecific ST and/or T-wave abnormalities is correct, best seen in leads V2, V3, and V4. Q waves suggesting a myocardial infarction are not identified.

Electrocardiogram Case Study **#31**

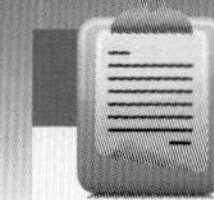

CLINICAL HISTORY

A 41-year-old male with an acute myocardial infarction and cardiogenic shock.

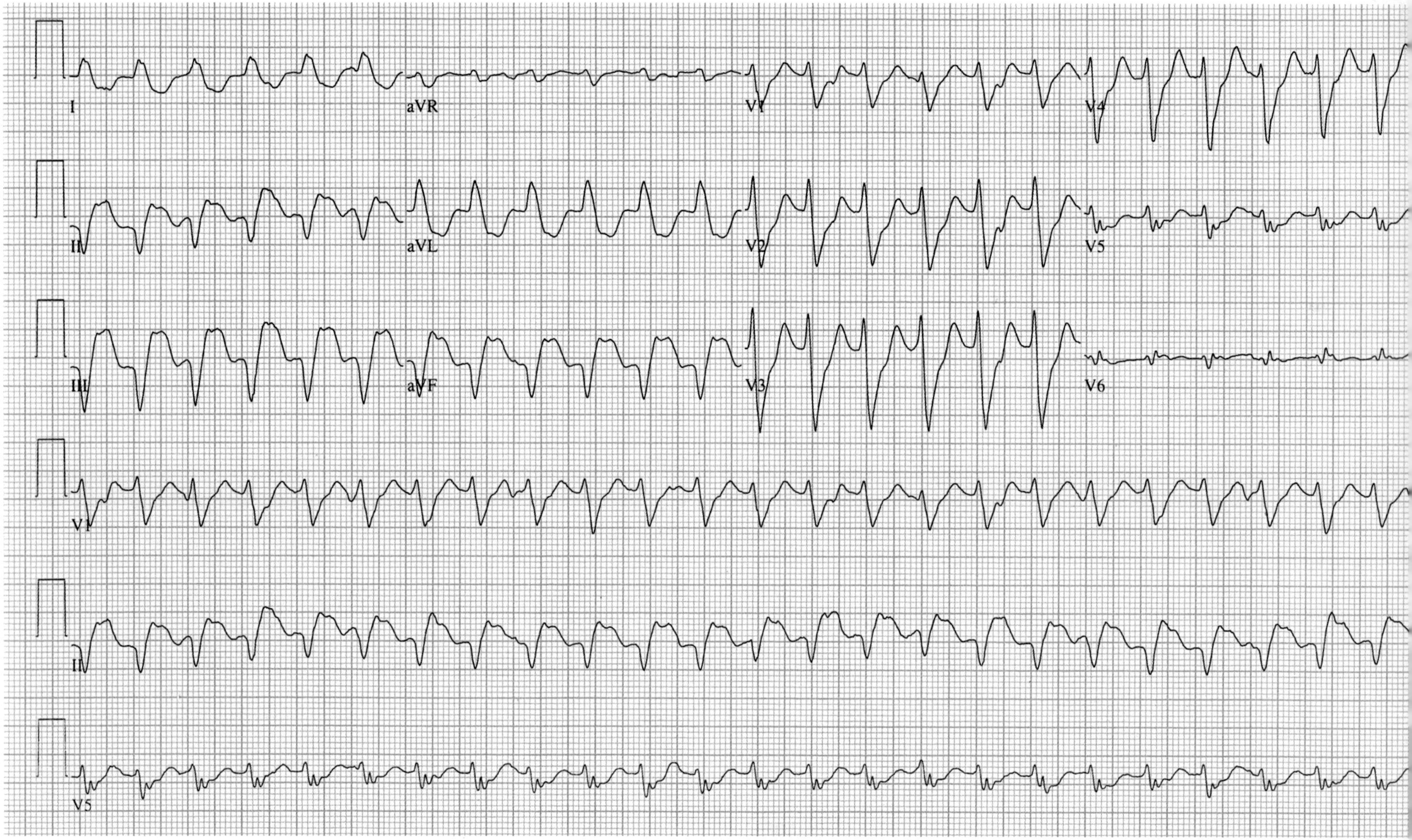

I aVR V1 V4

II aVL V2 V5

III aVF V3 V6

V1

II

V5

Interpretation Notes:

Electrocardiogram Case Study #31

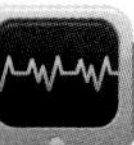

ELECTROCARDIOGRAM INTERPRETATION

This electrocardiogram demonstrates a widened QRS complex at a rate slightly <150 per minute. This is best termed a wide complex tachycardia. QRS complex left-axis deviation is present as the QRS complex vector is positive in lead I and negative in leads II, III, and aVF. P waves are intermittently seen, particularly in the lead V1 rhythm strip. There is intermittent deformation of the ST segment and, for instance, immediately preceding the twelfth QRS complex, a P wave is readily seen. This reflects an atrial rhythm, most likely sinus tachycardia with atrioventricular dissociation. This, in the presence of an acute myocardial injury and a wide complex tachycardia, renders the diagnosis of ventricular tachycardia with high probability. ST-segment elevation is seen in leads II, III, and aVF with ST-segment depression in leads I, aVL, V1, V2, and V3. This is consistent with acute inferior myocardial injury, high lateral reciprocal ST-segment depression, and possibly posterior myocardial injury. Repeating the electrocardiogram once the ventricular tachycardia resolves would be important to confirm the presence of inferior acute myocardial injury and also, the suspicion for posterior myocardial involvement.

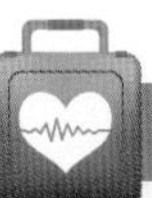

KEY DIAGNOSES

- Sinus tachycardia
- Ventricular tachycardia
- Atrioventricular dissociation
- Acute myocardial injury

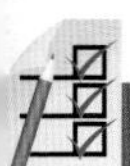

KEY TEACHING POINTS

- Ventricular tachycardia can be a difficult diagnosis to confirm on the 12-lead electrocardiogram. In this particular case, the presence of atrioventricular dissociation and a sinus mechanism confirms the diagnosis. The QRS complex morphology can also be helpful.
- Even in the presence of a wide complex rhythm, ST-segment deviation can sometimes be interpreted with confidence. In this particular patient, he presented with acute myocardial injury based on clinical symptoms and positive serum cardiac enzymes. The inferior ST-segment elevation was confirmed once the ventricular tachycardia resolved and a narrow QRS complex ensued. Additionally, posterior ST-segment depression was also seen, as suggested on this electrocardiogram.

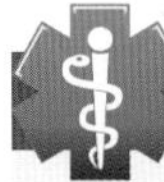

BOARD EXAMINATION ESSENTIALS

When coding for ventricular tachycardia, assess the electrocardiogram for evidence of atrial activity. If P waves are identified, next ascertain the shortest coupling interval. That will determine your atrial rate and should the P waves demonstrate a normal electrical axis (positive P-wave vector in lead II), code for a sinus mechanism—sinus tachycardia as is depicted here. This confirms the presence of atrioventricular dissociation. Even in the presence of a wide complex tachycardia, ST-segment deviation can be identified. This reflects acute myocardial injury, best observed in leads II, III, and aVF permitting the coding of ST- and/or T-wave abnormalities suggesting myocardial injury.

Electrocardiogram Case Study #32

CLINICAL HISTORY

A 56-year-old male who presented to the hospital emergency room with severe anterior chest pressure of 1-hour duration. This electrocardiogram was obtained in the emergency room.

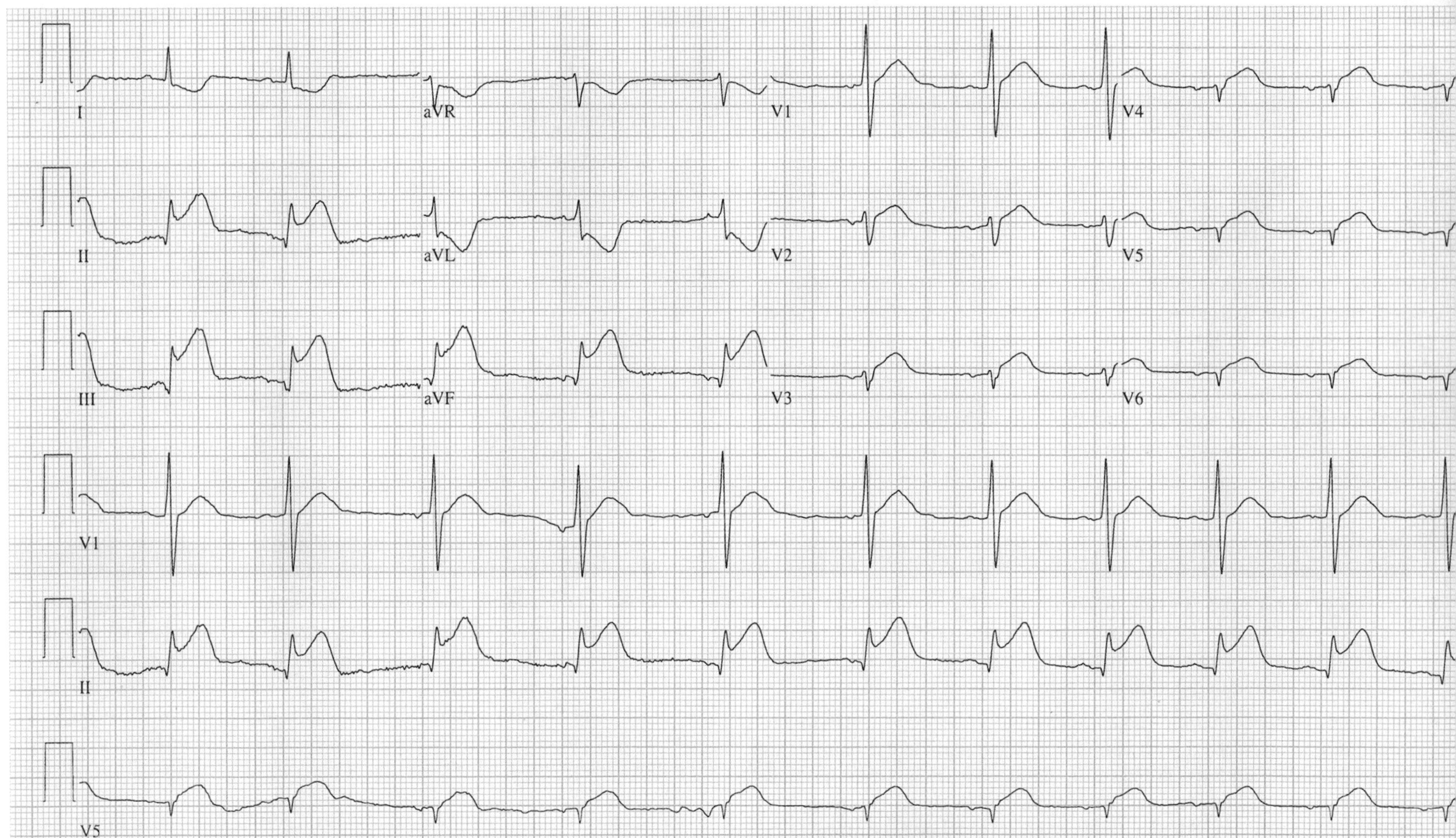

Interpretation Notes:

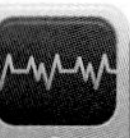

ELECTROCARDIOGRAM INTERPRETATION

This electrocardiogram demonstrates at least two different P-wave morphologies as depicted in the lead V1 rhythm strip. This is consistent with an ectopic atrial rhythm with two atrial foci. Q waves and marked J point and ST-segment elevation are seen in leads II, III, and aVF consistent with an acute inferior myocardial infarction. The precordial or chest leads are right-sided leads. A prominent R wave is present in lead V1 suggestive of a posterior myocardial infarction. J point and ST-segment elevation is seen in leads V2R through V6R confirming the presence of acute right ventricular myocardial injury. ST-segment depression is present in leads I and aVL. This reflects a reciprocal finding.

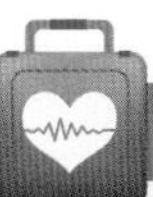

KEY DIAGNOSES

- Ectopic atrial rhythm
- Inferior myocardial infarction acute
- Posterior myocardial infarction acute
- Right ventricular myocardial injury
- Right-sided chest leads

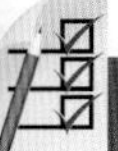

KEY TEACHING POINTS

- This patient demonstrated an acute proximal right coronary artery occlusion before the right ventricular marginal branch origin and takeoff. This resulted in an inferoposterior myocardial infarction and also acute right ventricular myocardial injury.
- On the patient's 12-lead electrocardiogram with a conventional hookup, lead V1 demonstrated ST-segment elevation. Since lead V1 directly overlies the right ventricle, it is the best lead positioned on the conventional 12-lead electrocardiogram to assess for the presence of acute right ventricular myocardial injury. When suspected, it is always best to perform an additional electrocardiogram as in this case with right-sided chest leads. Additionally, a transthoracic echocardiogram can also be helpful to assess for right ventricular hypokinesis and dilation.

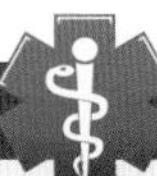

BOARD EXAMINATION ESSENTIALS

As mentioned above, an ectopic atrial rhythm is present. Since this is not an available code on the board exam, code normal sinus rhythm. Anticipate the possibility of an inferior myocardial infarction acute with right-sided chest leads. Q waves are present in leads II, III, and aVF with marked ST-segment elevation supporting coding inferior myocardial infarction, acute and ST- and/or T-wave abnormalities suggesting myocardial injury. While somewhat controversial, a prominent R wave is present in lead V1. This raises the likelihood of a posterior myocardial infarction, acute. This would need to be confirmed with a conventional 12-lead electrocardiogram.

Electrocardiogram Case Study #33

CLINICAL HISTORY

A 76-year-old female with severe mitral regurgitation immediately postoperative mitral valve repair.

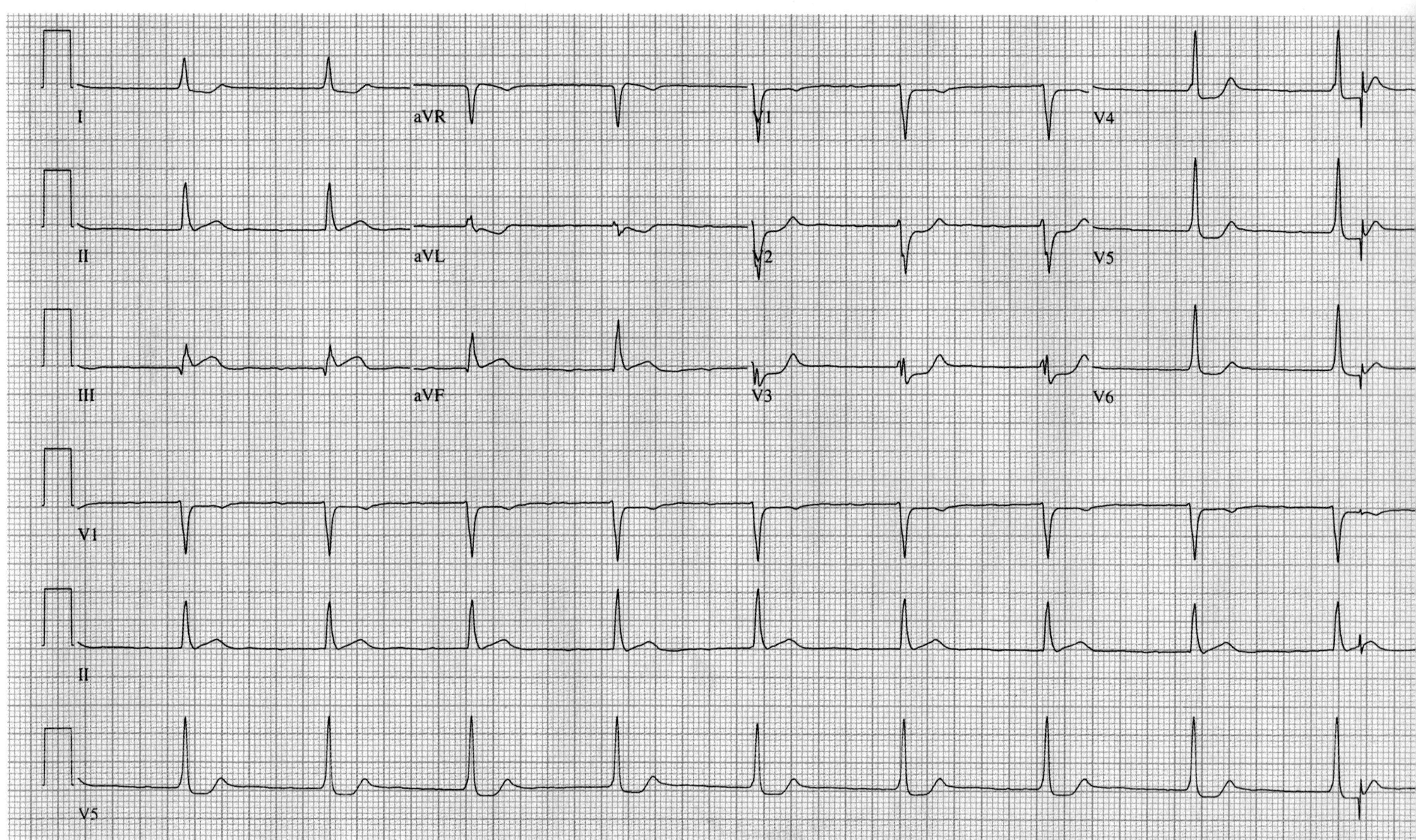

Interpretation Notes:____

Electrocardiogram Case Study #33

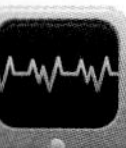

ELECTROCARDIOGRAM INTERPRETATION

This electrocardiogram demonstrates QRS complexes occurring at a regular interval at a rate of approximately 55 per minute. Atrial activity is not identified. The cardiac rhythm is most consistent with a junctional rhythm. The QRS complex duration is slightly >100 milliseconds consistent with a nonspecific intraventricular conduction delay. After the last QRS complex, a discrete deflection representing a pacemaker discharge is noted. This reflects an epicardial pacemaker that discharged inappropriately. J-point elevation, ST-segment straightening and elevation is seen in leads II, III, and aVF. Reciprocal ST-segment depression is seen in leads I and aVL. ST-segment depression is also seen in the precordial leads. This is consistent with an acute inferior myocardial injury pattern.

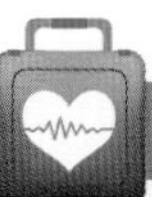

KEY DIAGNOSES

- Junctional rhythm
- Acute myocardial injury
- Ventricular pacemaker
- Nonspecific intraventricular conduction delay

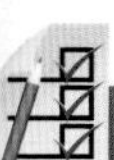

KEY TEACHING POINTS

- Junctional rhythms are a common finding after open-heart surgery, particularly in the immediate postoperative period.
- In the presence of J-point and ST-segment elevation, it is important to distinguish acute myocardial injury from pericarditis. This can be a particular challenge in the immediate post open-heart surgery timeframe. In this circumstance, regional ST-segment elevation and straightening of the ST segments are seen in the inferior leads with reciprocal high lateral ST-segment depression, best seen in leads I and aVL. In most circumstances when pericarditis is present, ST-segment elevation is a more diffuse process spanning multiple coronary artery territories.

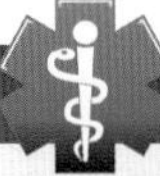

BOARD EXAMINATION ESSENTIALS

This electrocardiogram reflects an early form of myocardial injury with ST-segment straightening in leads II, III, and aVF and slight J-point elevation best seen in leads III and aVF. Diagnostic codes for the board exam include AV junctional rhythm and acute and ST- and/or T-wave abnormalities suggesting myocardial injury. No definite P waves are identified. There is a slight slurring to the QRS complex upstroke in leads V4, V5, and V6 and this may represent a superimposed P wave. The PR interval is too short to conduct to the ventricle and thus the heart rhythm is best coded as AV junctional rhythm. The ventricular pacemaker spike is ill timed and is best coded as pacemaker malfunction, not constantly sensing (atrium or ventricle).

Electrocardiogram Case Study #34

CLINICAL HISTORY

A 62-year-old female admitted to the hospital with suspected unstable angina. She has no known coronary artery disease.

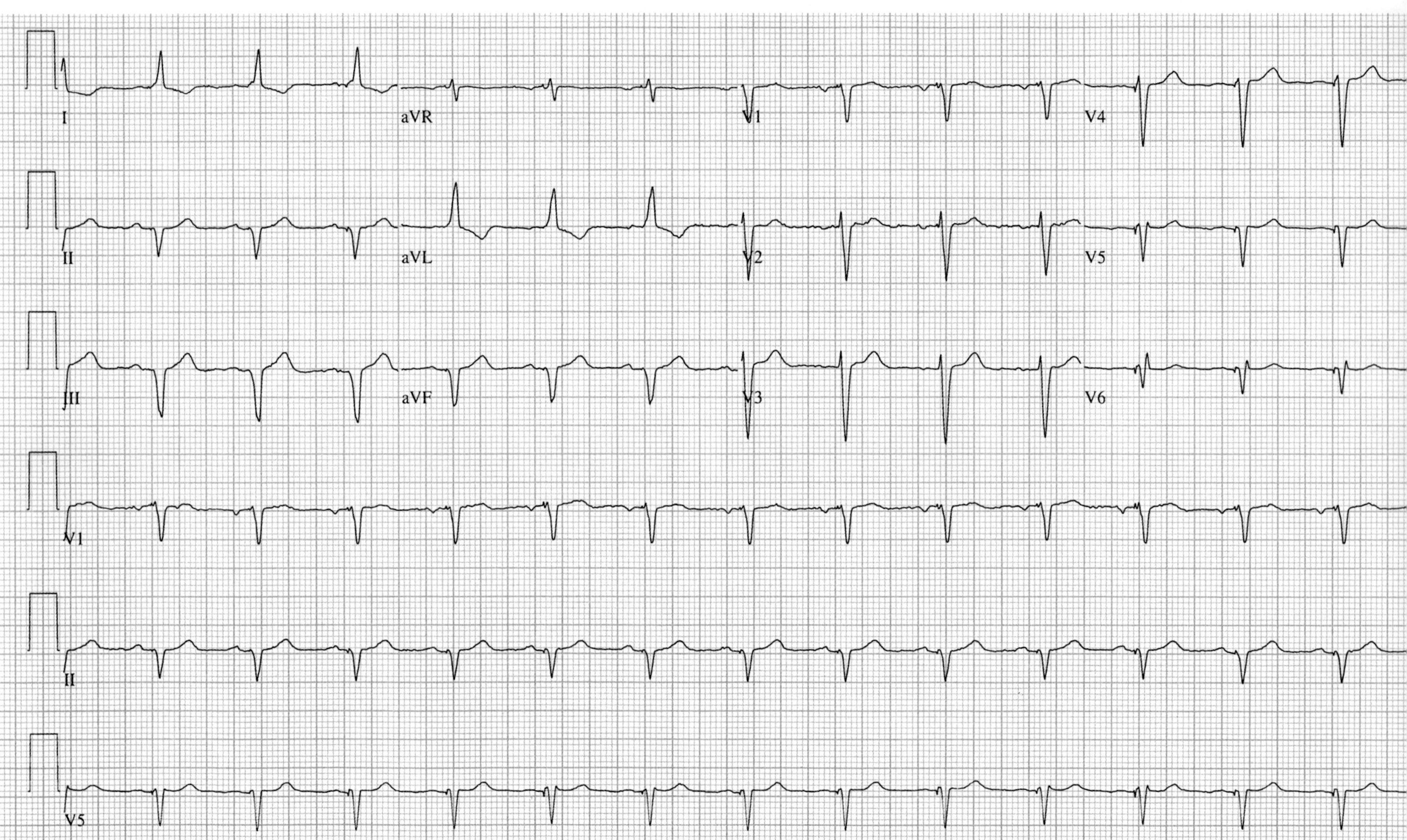

Interpretation Notes:

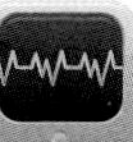

ELECTROCARDIOGRAM INTERPRETATION

This electrocardiogram demonstrates a normal P-wave axis with a P wave preceding each QRS complex at a rate slightly >80 per minute consistent with normal sinus rhythm. Discrete pacemaker deflections are seen before each QRS complex. This is most evident in leads V4, V5, and V6 and careful inspection of other leads including leads V1 and aVF reflects similar findings. This is consistent with an atrial tracking ventricular pacemaker. Q waves are seen in leads II, III, aVF, V5, and V6. The presence of a ventricular pacemaker precludes the diagnosis of an age-indeterminate myocardial infarction.

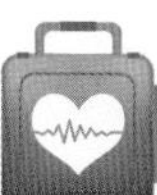

KEY DIAGNOSES

- Normal sinus rhythm
- Ventricular pacemaker

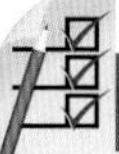

KEY TEACHING POINTS

- Pacemaker deflections can be diminutive and are often overlooked on the 12-lead electrocardiogram. It's important to note that pacemaker deflections may be seen in some leads better than others and that is why careful analysis of each QRS complex is important. Note the narrow QRS complex.
- Since the ventricular pacemaker lead is most typically placed in the right ventricular apex, right ventricular depolarization precedes left ventricular depolarization. Therefore, depolarization of the left ventricle is altered and the 12-lead electrocardiogram depiction of left ventricular depolarization is fraught with inaccuracy when considering age-indeterminate myocardial infarction patterns.
- When available, obtaining a past electrocardiogram without pacing can be exceedingly helpful to assess the native QRS complex morphology. Additionally, when safe, temporarily turning off the pacemaker to assess the native QRS complex can also be of clinical benefit.

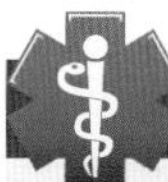

BOARD EXAMINATION ESSENTIALS

Pacemaker deflections can be subtle in appearance. When a ventricular pacemaker is identified, do not code an age-indeterminate myocardial infarction. Instead, focus on the atrial rhythm and code for it if it is identifiable, code for the ventricular pacemaker and assess its sensing and capturing capabilities. Doing so, the best codes for this electrocardiogram include normal sinus rhythm and ventricular demand pacemaker (VVI), normally functioning. This ventricular pacemaker lead was properly placed high up on the interventricular septum. Another possibility is coronary artery sinus pacing, not present in this circumstance.

Electrocardiogram Case Study #35

CLINICAL HISTORY

A 48-year-old female seen in the preoperative clinic prior to anticipated right knee surgery. The patient has no known cardiac history and with the exception of her knee abnormality maintains an excellent level of health.

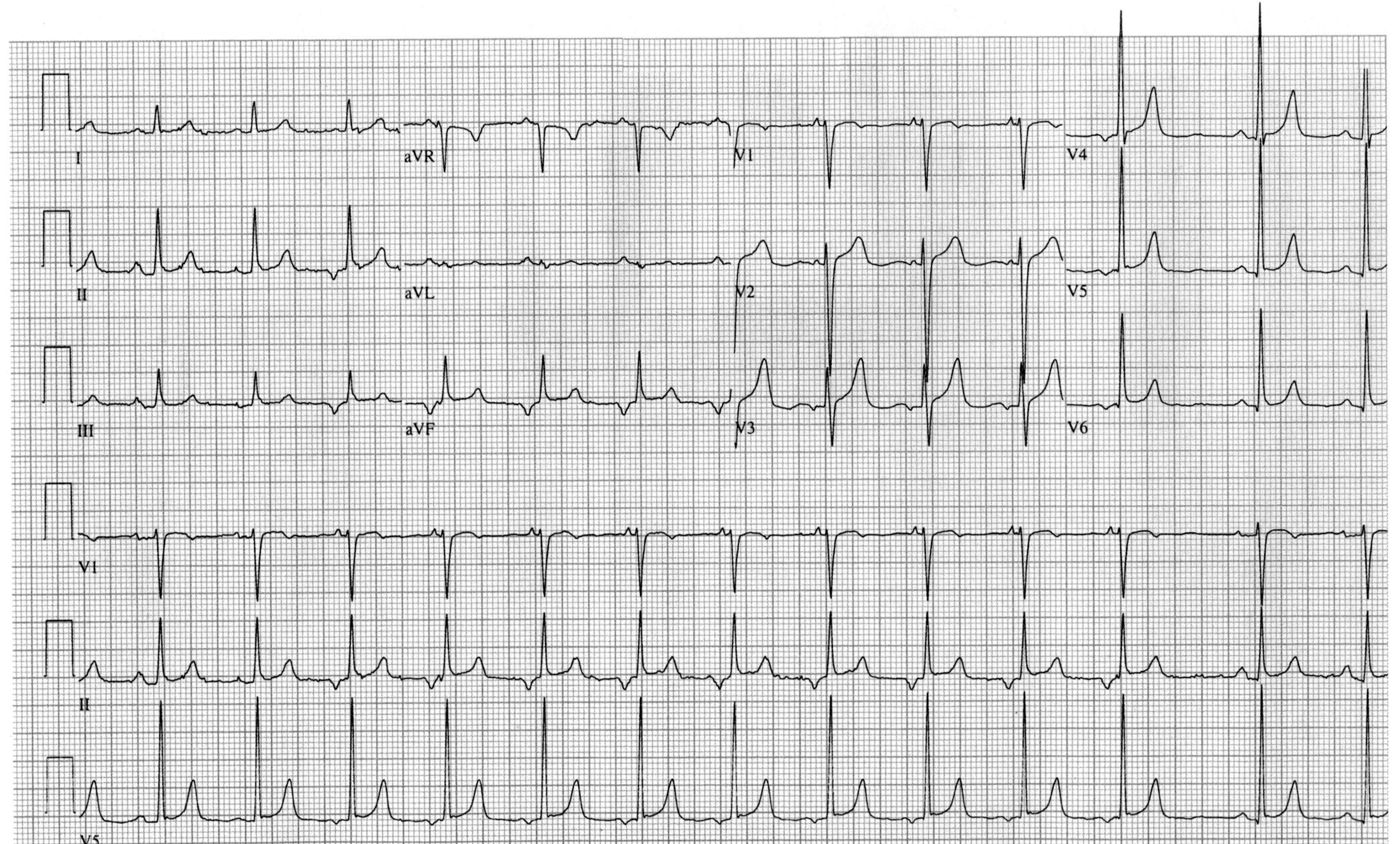

Interpretation Notes:

Electrocardiogram Case Study #35

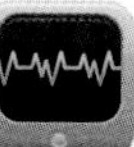

ELECTROCARDIOGRAM INTERPRETATION

This electrocardiogram demonstrates on the far right-hand portion preceding the last two QRS complexes a normal P-wave axis and normal sinus rhythm with an atrial rate of 75 per minute. The first P wave also appears to be of normal sinus origin. The second P wave is of different morphology and the 3rd through 11th P waves demonstrate a negative vector in lead aVF and a shortened PR interval consistent with a low atrial or ectopic atrial origin. The second P wave most likely represents an atrial fusion complex reflecting simultaneous atrial depolarization by both the sinus node and the ectopic atrial focus. The remainder of the electrocardiogram is normal.

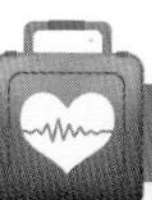

KEY DIAGNOSES

- Normal sinus rhythm
- Ectopic atrial rhythm
- Atrial fusion complex

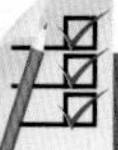

KEY TEACHING POINTS

- Ectopic atrial rhythms can be normal, particularly in physically well-conditioned patients with heightened vagal tone. In the absence of symptoms of systemic hypoperfusion, an ectopic atrial rhythm does not warrant further clinical evaluation.
- Atrial fusion complexes are rarely identified on the 12-lead electrocardiogram. This is a very nice example and reflects simultaneous "hybrid" depolarization of the atrium from two competing sources, creating a P wave of "merged" appearance.

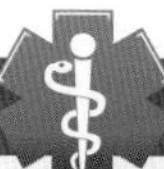

BOARD EXAMINATION ESSENTIALS

This is an excellent electrocardiogram example where close attention to the P-wave axis is important. Since no code exists for ectopic atrial rhythm on the board exam, it is unlikely an electrocardiogram with this combination of findings will be included. It still raises important concepts. This is not an AV junctional rhythm as the P wave clearly precedes the QRS complex, even when the P-wave axis is abnormal.

Electrocardiogram Case Study #36

CLINICAL HISTORY

A 78-year-old female with longstanding poorly controlled hypertension and nonischemic left ventricular systolic dysfunction.

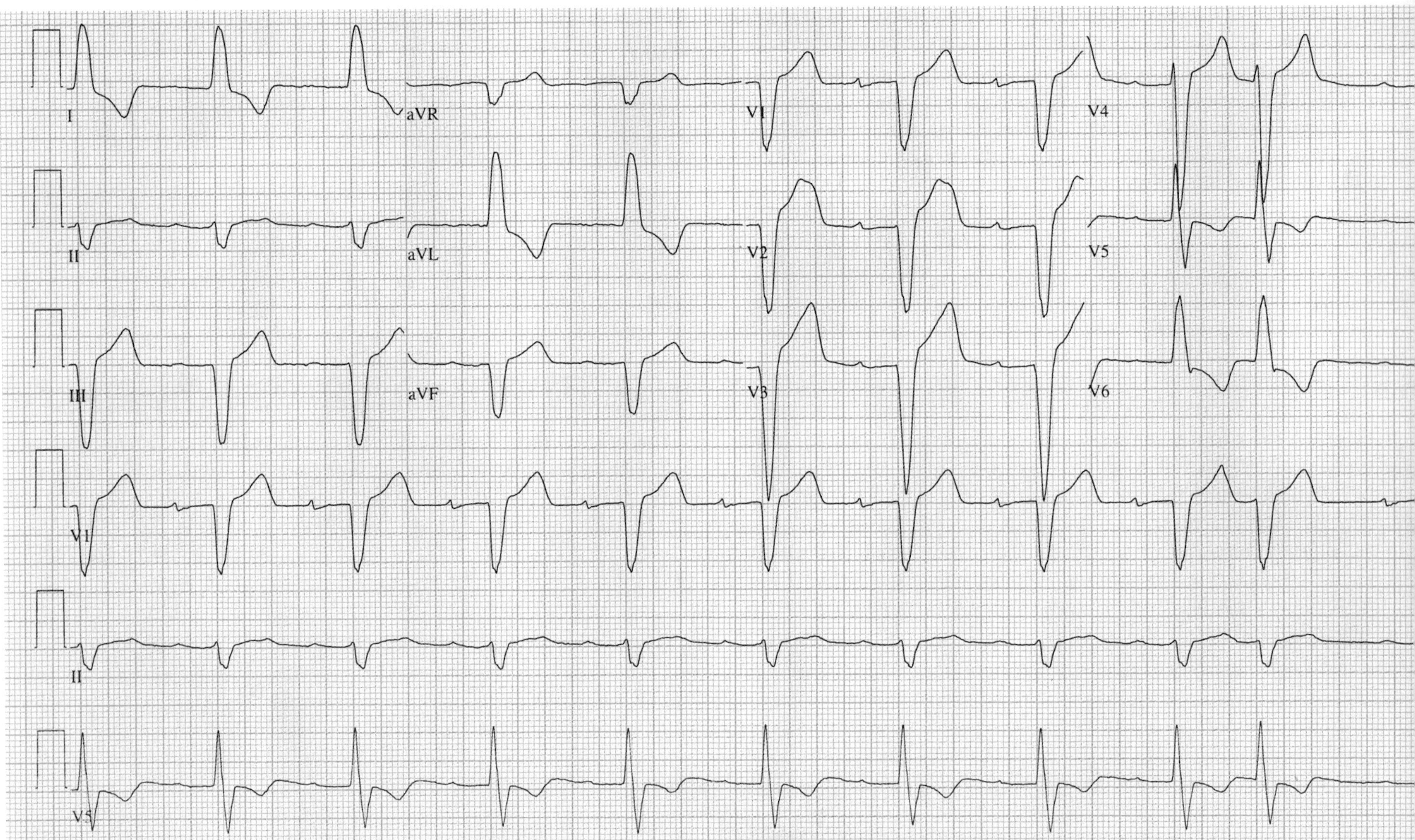

Interpretation Notes:

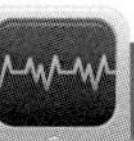

ELECTROCARDIOGRAM INTERPRETATION

This electrocardiogram demonstrates P waves with a normal axis at an atrial rate slightly >60 per minute consistent with normal sinus rhythm. There is marked prolongation of the PR interval approaching 300 milliseconds consistent with first-degree atrioventricular block. The QRS complex vector demonstrates left-axis deviation given the positive vector in lead I and negative vectors in leads II, III, and aVF. The QRS complex is widened at approximately 160 milliseconds. Q waves are not seen in leads I, aVL, V5, or V6 supporting a lack of left-to-right interventricular septal depolarization. These findings are consistent with complete left bundle branch block. On the far right-hand portion of the electrocardiogram, a QRS complex occurs prematurely. The immediately preceding T wave is peaked secondary to superimposition of the P wave on the preceding T wave. This is consistent with a premature atrial complex. In lead II, the P wave is prolonged at approximately 110 milliseconds. This supports slowed left atrial depolarization and conduction, meeting the criteria for left atrial abnormality.

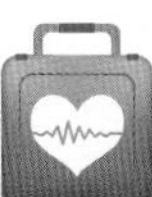

KEY DIAGNOSES

- Normal sinus rhythm
- QRS complex left-axis deviation
- First-degree atrioventricular block
- Complete left bundle branch block
- Premature atrial complex
- Left atrial abnormality

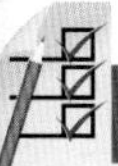

KEY TEACHING POINTS

- The presence of left atrial abnormality, first-degree atrioventricular block, and complete left bundle branch block with a significantly widened QRS complex all support organic heart disease, cardiac enlargement, and left ventricular systolic dysfunction.
- When considering the diagnosis of complete left bundle branch block, it is important to carefully assess for the presence of septal Q waves. An initial negative deflection in leads I, aVL, V5, or V6 supports left-to-right interventricular septal depolarization. When present in the setting of a QRS complex duration >120 milliseconds, it is best to ascribe the diagnosis of a nonspecific intraventricular conduction delay instead of complete left bundle branch block.

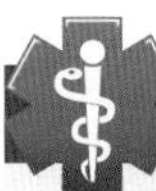

BOARD EXAMINATION ESSENTIALS

Several concepts presented on this electrocardiogram pertain to the board exam. Carefully assess the atrial rate. It is slightly >60 per minute and thus normal sinus rhythm should be coded. AV block, first degree, should also be coded. The last QRS complex is premature and proceeded by a P-wave consistent with a premature atrial complex. Complete left bundle branch block is present as is QRS complex left-axis deviation (> negative 30 degrees). Make sure not to code left anterior fascicular block. Lastly, left atrial abnormality/enlargement should be coded. This is based primarily on the P wave in lead II that demonstrates a prolonged duration >110 milliseconds. Lastly, do not code an infarction in the presence of complete left bundle branch block. First, a small R wave is present in leads II, III, and aVF plus even in the presence of Q waves, it is incorrect to code for an age-indeterminate myocardial infarction pattern in the presence of complete left bundle branch block.

Electrocardiogram Case Study #37

CLINICAL HISTORY

A 67-year-old male admitted via the emergency room with acute chest pain. The patient was taken immediately to the cardiac catheterization laboratory where an acute proximal left anterior descending coronary artery obstruction was identified. Balloon angioplasty and coronary artery stent placement was successfully undertaken.

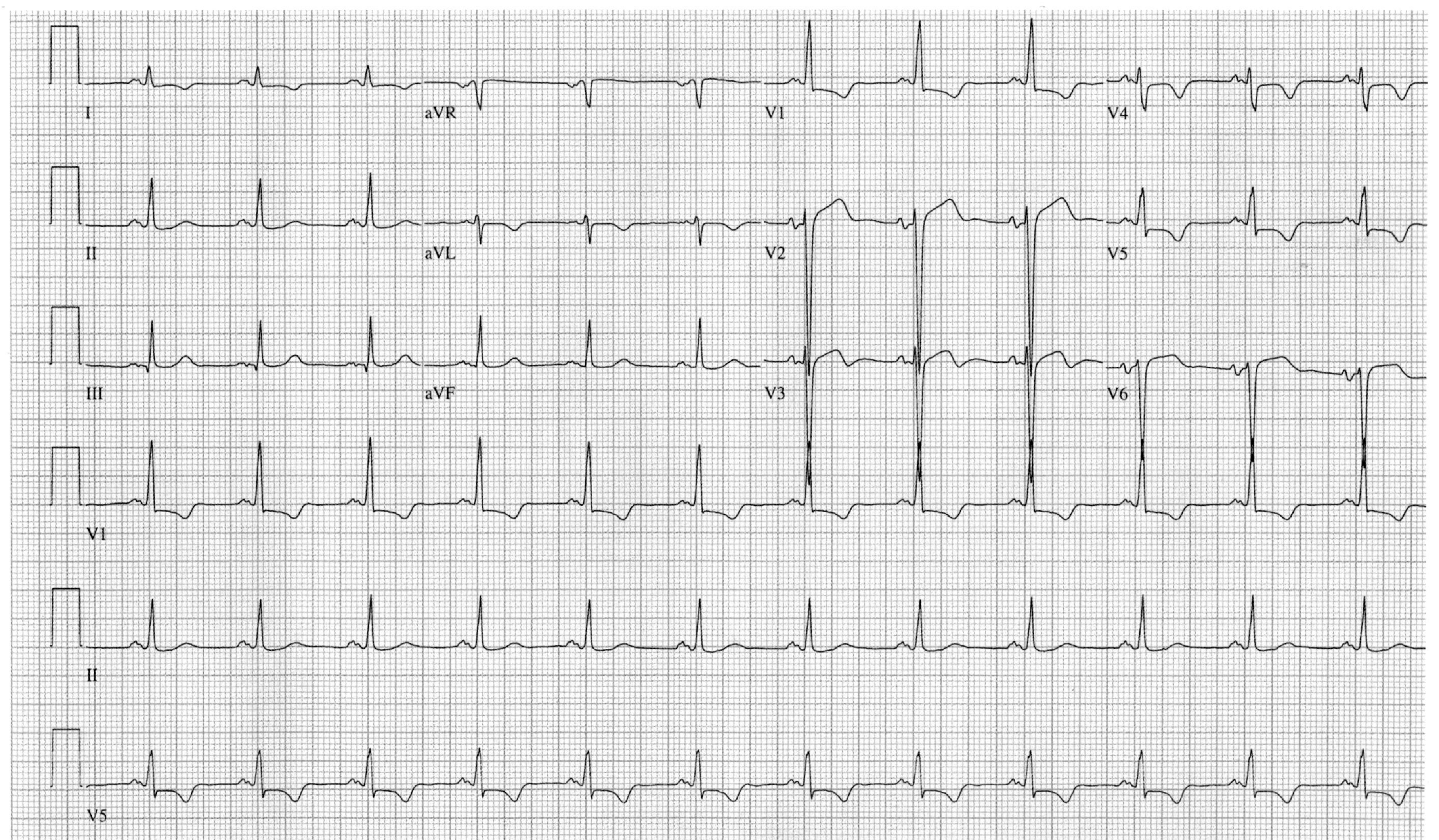

Interpretation Notes:____

Electrocardiogram Case Study #37

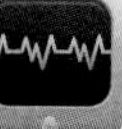

ELECTROCARDIOGRAM INTERPRETATION

This electrocardiogram demonstrates a normal P-wave axis at an atrial rate of 75 per minute reflecting normal sinus rhythm. A bifid P wave is present in lead II suggesting left atrial abnormality. The precordial leads demonstrate abnormal R-wave transition. A prominent R wave is present in lead V1 with regression of the R wave in leads V2, V3, and V4, reconstitution of the R wave in lead V5, and R-wave regression in lead V6. This represents switched or misplaced chest leads. Leads V1 and V6 are switched. Once this is identified, left atrial abnormality is seen as the P wave demonstrates terminal negativity of at least 1 mm^2 in area. J-point and ST-segment elevation is identified in leads V1, V2, and V3 with T-wave inversion in leads V4, V5, V6, I, and aVL. These findings are consistent with a proximal left anterior descending coronary artery occlusion and acute myocardial injury, confirmed at the time of his urgent heart catheterization.

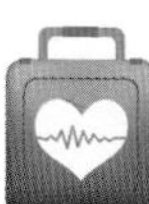

KEY DIAGNOSES

- Normal sinus rhythm
- Left atrial abnormality
- Acute myocardial injury
- Misplaced leads
- Left ventricular hypertrophy

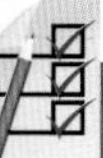

KEY TEACHING POINTS

- When interpreting an electrocardiogram, the first step should be to ensure the technical adequacy of the tracing. The most common error is to switch the left and the right arm leads resulting in a negative P-wave vector in leads I and aVL. The second most common mistake, switching chest leads, is identified on this electrocardiogram. If not identified, one might incorrectly consider the diagnosis of an age-indeterminate posterior myocardial infarction or right ventricular hypertrophy given the prominent R wave in lead V1.
- Once the misplaced chest leads are identified, J-point and ST-segment elevation is seen beginning in lead V1, represented as lead V6 on this electrocardiogram. This reflects a proximal left anterior descending coronary artery occlusion prior to the first septal perforator branch. A proximal left anterior descending coronary artery occlusion often carries adverse prognostic significance. It is thus important to identify.
- This patient was known to suffer from hypertension. The prominent voltage as seen in lead V2 summed with the QRS complex voltage as reflected in lead V1, which actually represents lead V6 (S wave + R wave > 35 mm), is consistent with left ventricular hypertrophy.

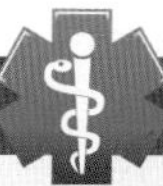

BOARD EXAMINATION ESSENTIALS

This electrocardiogram highlights several board exam relevant concepts. Incorrect electrode placement can occur in the limb leads or the precordial leads. If the R-wave transition from lead V1 to lead V6 does not make sense, consider incorrect electrode placement. J-point and ST-segment elevation coupled with ST-segment straightening/upward coving is demonstrated in leads V6 (actually this is misplaced lead V1), V2, and V3. This supports acute myocardial injury in the left anterior descending coronary artery distribution. Do not code for an infarction pattern in the absence of Q waves. Diagnostic codes for the board exam therefore include normal sinus rhythm, incorrect electrode placement, left atrial abnormality/enlargement, ST- and/or T-wave abnormalities suggesting myocardial injury and left ventricular hypertrophy.

Electrocardiogram Case Study #38

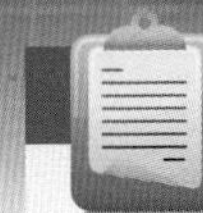

CLINICAL HISTORY

A 78-year-old female with intermittent lightheadedness and near fainting who presented to the emergency room with profound fatigue.

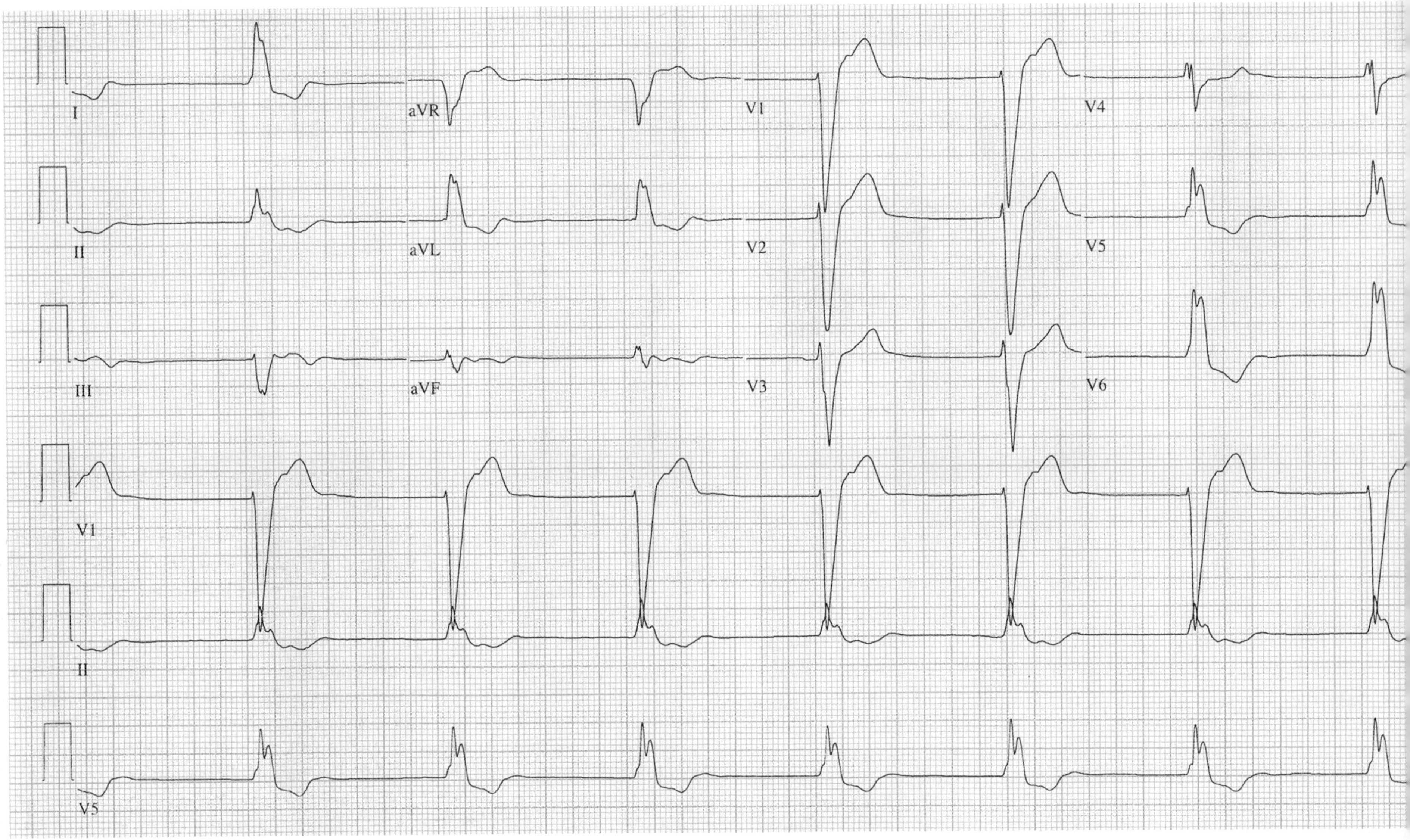

I aVR V1 V4
II aVL V2 V5
III aVF V3 V6
V1
II
V5

Interpretation Notes:

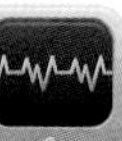

ELECTROCARDIOGRAM INTERPRETATION

This electrocardiogram demonstrates a wide QRS complex rhythm with a ventricular rate slightly >40 per minute reflecting junctional bradycardia. P waves are not identified preceding each QRS complex. Instead, consistent deformation of the ST segment before the peak or the apex of the T wave is seen reflecting retrograde atrial conduction and depolarization. The QRS complex is widened, significantly >120 milliseconds with a QRS complex morphology consistent with complete left bundle branch block. The complete left bundle branch block QRS complex supports initial right followed by left ventricular depolarization.

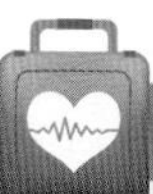

KEY DIAGNOSES

- Junctional bradycardia
- Retrograde P waves
- Complete left bundle branch block

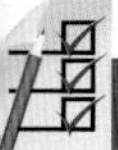

KEY TEACHING POINTS

- This is a significantly abnormal electrocardiogram and was responsible for the patient's intermittent lightheadedness, near fainting, and profound fatigue. Shortly after this electrocardiogram was obtained, the patient underwent permanent pacemaker placement with resolution of her symptoms.
- While it is reasonable to conclude that this electrocardiogram reflects a junctional rhythm, it is also possible that this dysrhythmia is an escape rhythm originating within the right ventricular Purkinje or fascicular system. It is difficult to make this distinction on this surface electrocardiogram and would require intracardiac catheter evaluation in the form of an electrophysiology study. Making this differentiation was not of clinical relevance as the patient had both a clear clinical and an electrocardiogram indication for permanent pacemaker implantation.

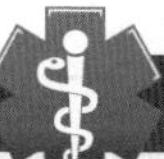

BOARD EXAMINATION ESSENTIALS

Appropriate codes for the board exam include AV junctional bradycardia and complete left bundle branch block. It is also important to assess the QRS complex axis—in this case it is normal. The retrograde P waves, while notable, do not possess a corresponding diagnostic code on the board exam scoring sheet.

Electrocardiogram Case Study #39

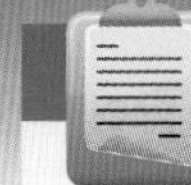

CLINICAL HISTORY

An 84-year-old male admitted to the hospital with acute decompensated systolic congestive heart failure. He has a known history of ischemic heart disease, past myocardial infarction, and left ventricular systolic dysfunction.

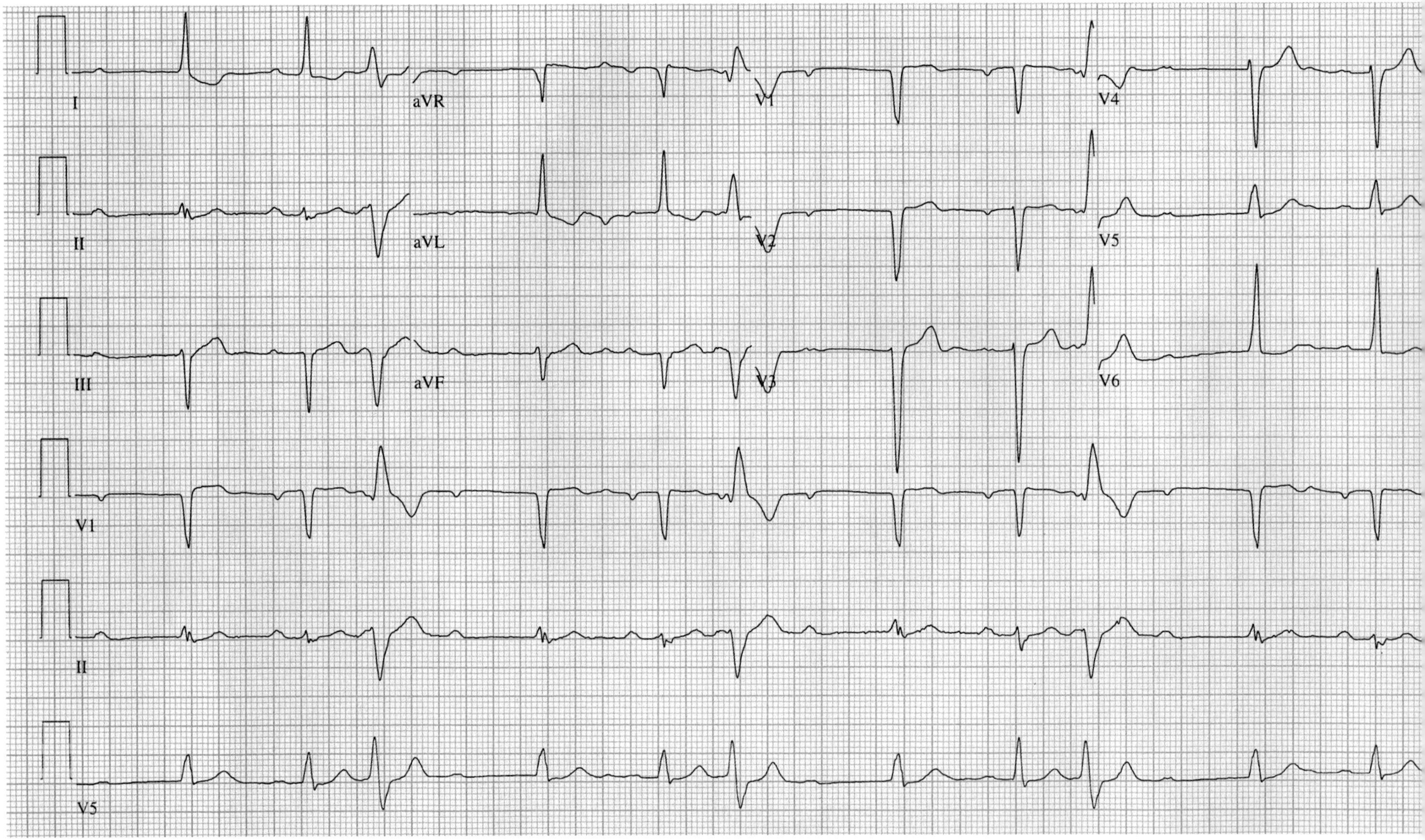

I aVR V1 V4

II aVL V2 V5

III aVF V3 V6

V1

II

V5

Interpretation Notes:

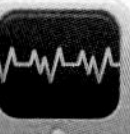

ELECTROCARDIOGRAM INTERPRETATION

This electrocardiogram demonstrates a normal P-wave axis at an atrial rate of approximately 90 per minute consistent with normal sinus rhythm. The PR interval is >200 milliseconds reflecting first-degree atrioventricular block. Left atrial abnormality is suspected given the P-wave terminal negativity in lead V1 and prolonged duration in leads II and aVF. Premature ventricular complexes are identified in a trigeminal pattern with a qR pattern in lead V1 reflecting right ventricular conduction delay and therefore a left ventricular origin. Post PVC, a P wave is identified that either conducts with a markedly prolonged PR interval or is blocked with the subsequent QRS complex representing a junctional escape complex. It is not possible to distinguish between these two possibilities on the surface electrocardiogram, requiring an intracardiac recording in the form of an electrophysiology study. This is a consistent finding on this electrocardiogram. In lead aVF, the initial QRS complex demonstrates an R wave that is in fact a superimposed P wave with the second QRS complex demonstrating a Q wave. The premature ventricular complex as reflected in lead aVF also reflects a Q wave. Since the premature ventricular complex is of left ventricular origin, initial ventricular forces solely reflect left ventricular events raising the likelihood of an age-indeterminate inferior myocardial infarction, consistent with the patient's known history of ischemic heart disease. Lateral and high lateral nonspecific ST-T changes are also identified.

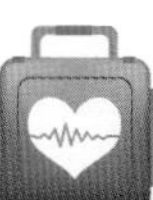

KEY DIAGNOSES

- Normal sinus rhythm
- First-degree atrioventricular block
- Left atrial abnormality
- Inferior myocardial infarction, age indeterminate
- Premature ventricular complexes
- Nonspecific ST-T changes
- Junctional escape complexes

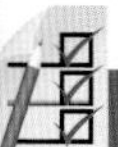

KEY TEACHING POINTS

- Premature ventricular complexes can unmask underlying conduction system disease, in this circumstance with retrograde ventriculoatrial conduction penetrating the atrioventricular node impeding antegrade atrioventricular conduction. In this circumstance, this results in probable junctional escape complexes.
- Conduction system disease is suggested based on the presence of first-degree atrioventricular block.
- This is another example where a premature ventricular complex of left ventricular origin helps contribute to the diagnosis of an age-indeterminate myocardial infarction, most likely reflecting in this circumstance the right coronary artery distribution.

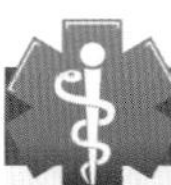

BOARD EXAMINATION ESSENTIALS

Appropriate codes for the board exam include normal sinus rhythm, AV block, first degree, left atrial abnormality/enlargement, premature ventricular complexes (unlikely to reflect ventricular parasystole given the fixed coupling interval to the QRS complex just prior), and AV junctional escape complexes. An intraventricular conduction disturbance, nonspecific type is suggested but since the QRS complex duration is <100 milliseconds, it is not coded. Nonspecific ST- and/or T-wave abnormalities are also present.

Electrocardiogram Case Study #40

CLINICAL HISTORY

A 66-year-old female with lung cancer undergoing chemotherapy who is acutely hospitalized with nausea, vomiting, and severe dehydration.

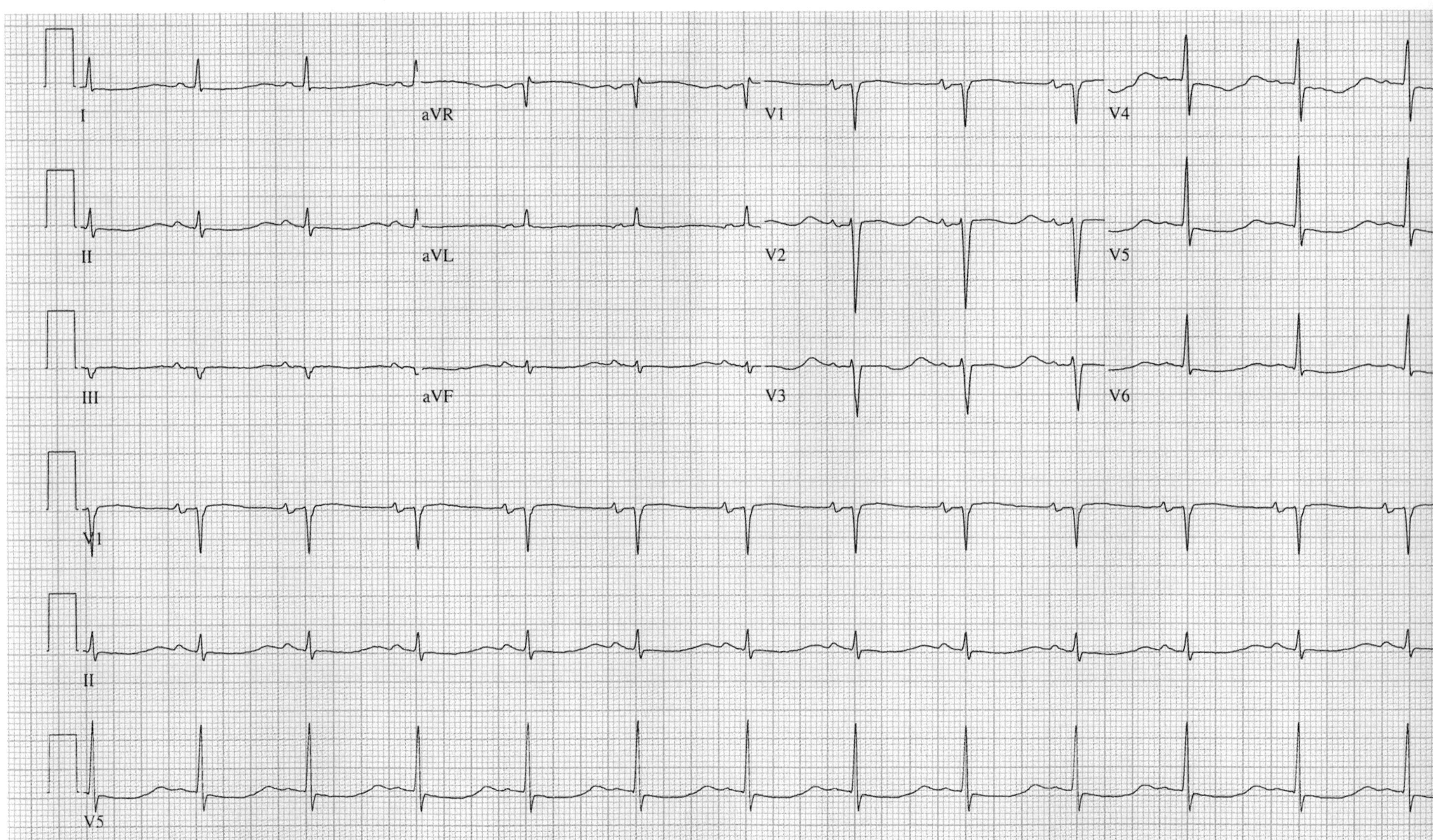

Interpretation Notes:

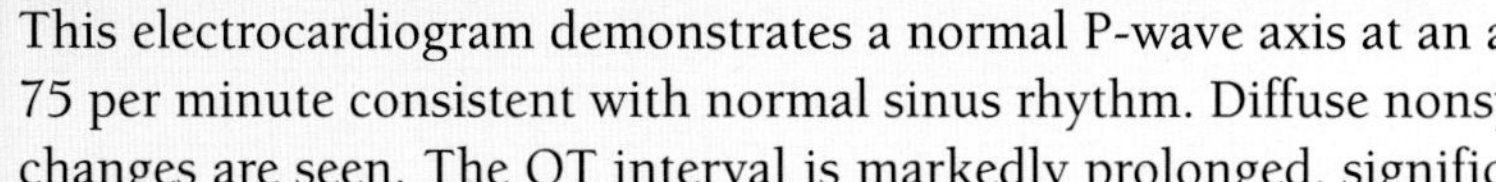

Electrocardiogram Case Study #40

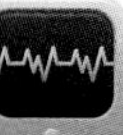

ELECTROCARDIOGRAM INTERPRETATION

This electrocardiogram demonstrates a normal P-wave axis at an atrial rate of 75 per minute consistent with normal sinus rhythm. Diffuse nonspecific ST-T changes are seen. The QT interval is markedly prolonged, significantly >50% of the R to R interval. In leads V2, V3, V4, V5, and V6 at the terminal aspect of the QT interval, a prominent positive deflection is identified. This is a positive U wave. A markedly prolonged QT interval with terminal U-wave positivity is consistent with profound hypokalemia. At the time of this electrocardiogram, this patient's serum potassium level was 2.6 mEq per L.

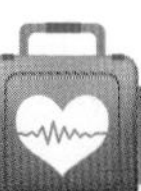

KEY DIAGNOSES

- Normal sinus rhythm
- Nonspecific ST-T changes
- Prolonged QT-U interval
- Positive U waves
- Hypokalemia

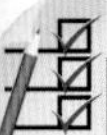

KEY TEACHING POINTS

- The initial manifestation of an electrolyte abnormality is often identified on the 12-lead electrocardiogram.
- Both potassium and calcium disorders can be distinguished on the 12-lead electrocardiogram. Potassium disorders typically impact the T wave and the U wave sparing the ST segment. In contrast, calcium disorders spare the T and the U waves, impacting the ST segment and thus QT interval duration.

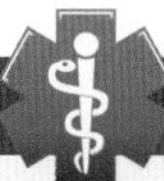

BOARD EXAMINATION ESSENTIALS

For the board exam, anticipate 12-lead electrocardiogram manifestations of potassium and calcium disorders. This electrocardiogram demonstrates the following board exam codes including normal sinus rhythm, prolonged QT interval, ST- and/or T-wave abnormalities suggesting electrolyte disturbances and under clinical disorders, hypokalemia. Prominent U waves should also be coded.

Electrocardiogram Case Study #41

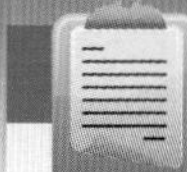

CLINICAL HISTORY

A 51-year-old female with mitral valve prolapse and severe mitral regurgitation. The patient presents with exertional intolerance, new-onset palpitations, and signs and symptoms consistent with decompensated congestive heart failure.

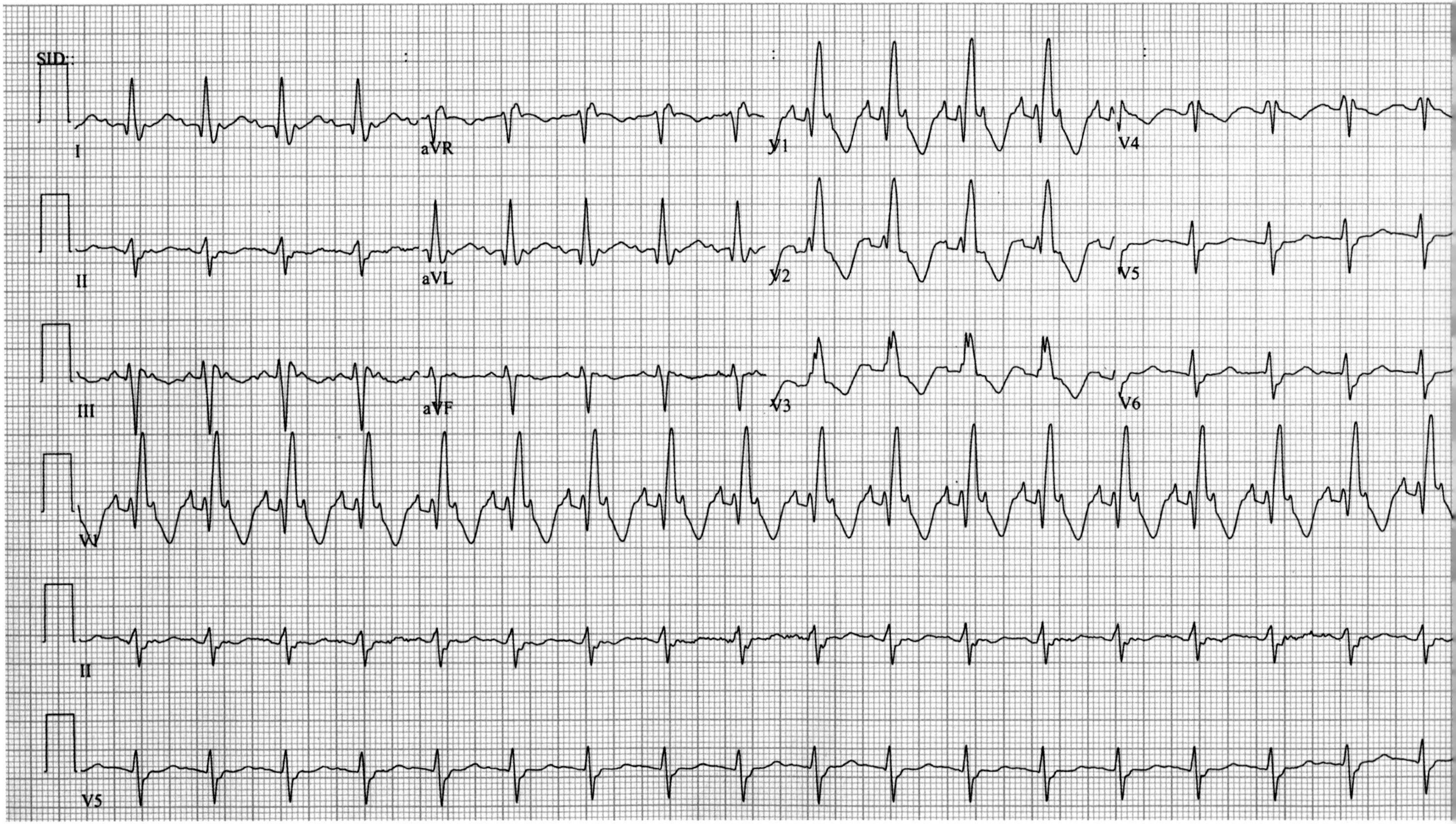

SID: I aVR V1 V4 II aVL V2 V5 III aVF V3 V6 V1 II V5

Interpretation Notes:

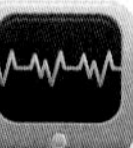

ELECTROCARDIOGRAM INTERPRETATION

This electrocardiogram demonstrates a tachycardic heart rhythm with two discrete atrial depolarizations for each QRS complex. The atrial rate is approximately 220 per minute with an atrial depolarization identified both before and immediately after the QRS complex best seen in the lead V1 rhythm strip consistent with atrial tachycardia and 2:1 atrioventricular conduction. A rsR' pattern is seen in lead V1 with a QRS complex duration approaching 140 milliseconds consistent with complete right bundle branch block. The QRS complex demonstrates a positive QRS complex vector in lead I and negative QRS complex vectors in leads II, III, and aVF consistent with left anterior hemiblock. Q waves are seen in leads I and aVL. In this instance, the q waves do not likely represent an age-indeterminate high lateral myocardial infarction but instead are due to the QRS complex axis deviation as seen with left anterior fascicular block. Inferior nonspecific ST-T changes are also identified.

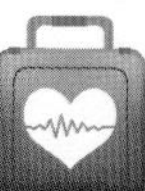

KEY DIAGNOSES

- Ectopic Atrial tachycardia
- 2:1 atrioventricular conduction
- Left anterior fascicular block
- Complete right bundle branch block
- Nonspecific ST-T changes

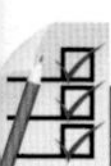

KEY TEACHING POINTS

- Atrial dysrhythmias are commonly identified in the presence of mitral valve disease. In this patient, when in normal sinus rhythm, she was relatively asymptomatic despite the presence of severe mitral regurgitation. In the presence of an atrial tachycardic heart rhythm with associated impaired left ventricular diastolic filling, the patient experienced a profound decline in functional capacity.
- This electrocardiogram was exceedingly helpful in this circumstance. After documenting the atrial tachycardic rhythm, it was decided to proceed with mitral valve reparative surgery. This was successfully undertaken with a significant improvement in symptomatology.
- This electrocardiogram highlights the importance of utilizing calipers when assessing intracardiac intervals. An atrial depolarization is readily identified before each QRS complex. Sinus tachycardia is a reasonable consideration. The second P wave is partially superimposed on the terminal aspect of the QRS complex and without the use of calipers, could easily be ascribed to terminal QRS complex conduction delay. Calipers demonstrate the constant atrial depolarization to atrial depolarization interval, securing the diagnosis of atrial tachycardia and therefore explaining the patient's precipitous symptomatic decline.

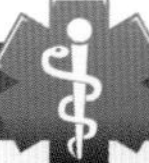

BOARD EXAMINATION ESSENTIALS

Relevant diagnostic codes for the board exam include atrial tachycardia, AV block, 2:1, left anterior fascicular block, complete right bundle branch block, and nonspecific ST-and/or T-wave abnormalities. In the presence of atrial tachycardia, it is important to recognize the P wave as an ectopic focus and resist coding for atrial abnormality/enlargement patterns.

Electrocardiogram Case Study #42

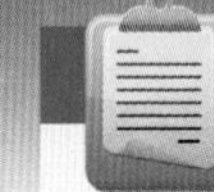

CLINICAL HISTORY

A 54-year-old male with dialysis requiring end-stage renal disease admitted to the medical intensive care unit after presenting to the hospital with acute delirium.

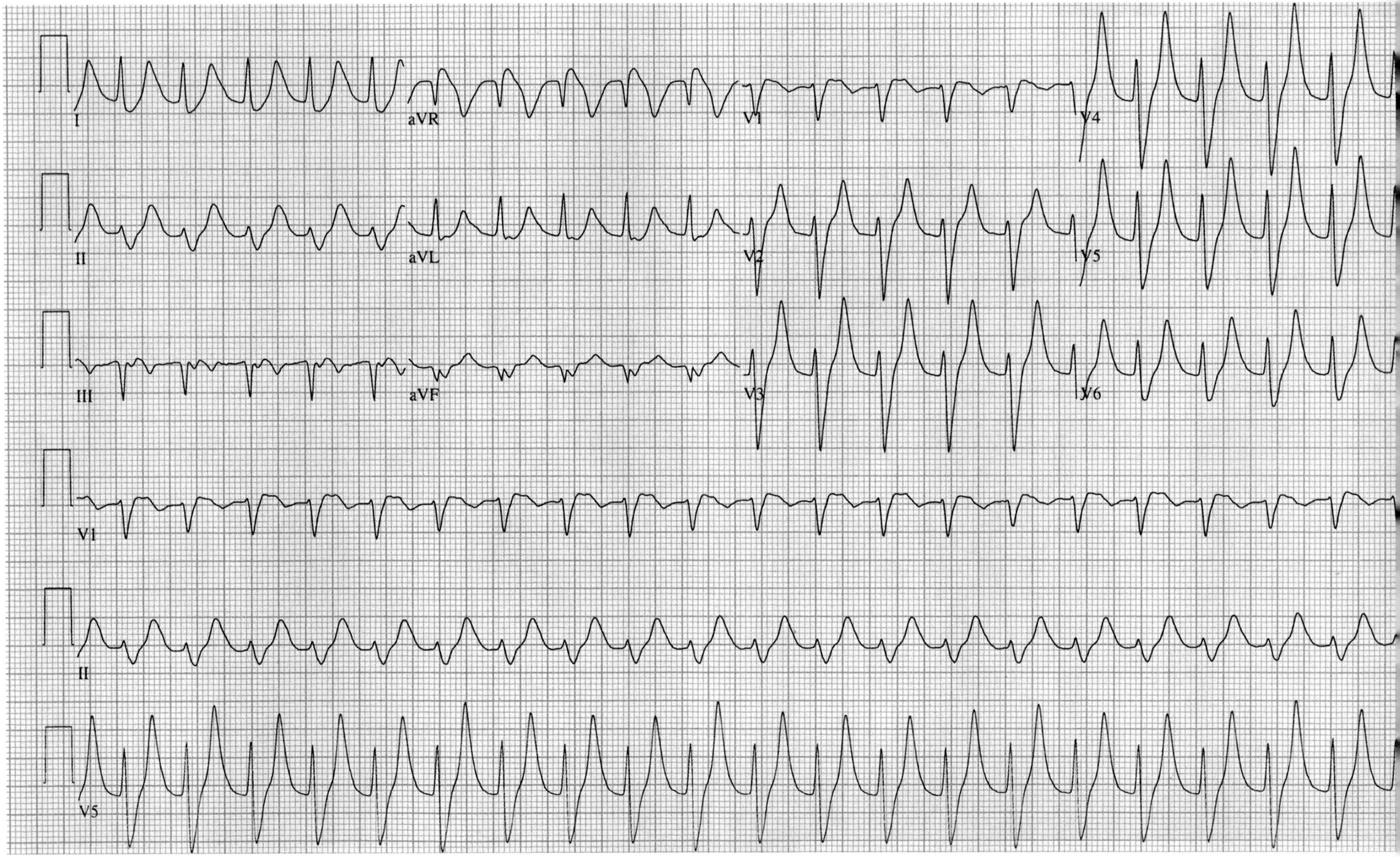

I aVR V1 V4
II aVL V2 V5
III aVF V3 V6
V1
II
V5

Interpretation Notes:

Electrocardiogram Case Study #42

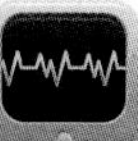

ELECTROCARDIOGRAM INTERPRETATION

This electrocardiogram demonstrates widened QRS complexes at a ventricular rate of approximately 125 per minute. P waves are not identified with certainty. A P wave may in fact be superimposed on the T wave best seen in lead V1. If so, this would reflect sinus tachycardia with first-degree atrioventricular block. It is best not to make this definitive conclusion. Instead, this electrocardiogram is most consistent with junctional tachycardia. The QRS complex is widened approaching 150 milliseconds consistent with a nonspecific intraventricular conduction delay. The QRS complex morphology does not support the presence of complete right or left bundle branch block. There appears to be an equal conduction delay within the early, middle, and terminal portions of the QRS complex. The QT interval is also prolonged and the T waves are symmetric and peaked. Q waves in leads III and aVF are present suggestive but not diagnostic of an age-indeterminate inferior myocardial infarction given the presence of the markedly prolonged QRS complex. Considering the collective presence of QRS complex interval prolongation, QT interval prolongation with peaked and symmetric T waves, this electrocardiogram is consistent with profound hyperkalemia. This patient's serum potassium level was 7.1 mEq per L.

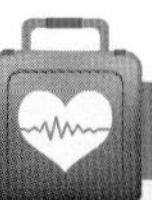

KEY DIAGNOSES

- Junctional tachycardia
- Nonspecific intraventricular conduction delay
- Prolonged QT interval
- Hyperkalemia

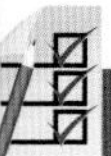

KEY TEACHING POINTS

- Potassium disorders typically spare the ST segment. In this case, the QT interval prolongation is due to the QRS complex interval being markedly prolonged, not the ST segment.
- In the presence of hyperkalemia, T-wave symmetry can be as important as T-wave amplitude in securing this diagnosis. Increased T-wave amplitude is not always present in the setting of hyperkalemia. Careful examination of the T-wave morphology for a symmetric appearance can be extremely helpful.
- The fact that the QRS complex duration is prolonged as if the entire electrocardiogram was spread apart or recorded at a faster paper speed suggests profound hyperkalemia. When this type of electrocardiogram pattern is seen, ensure that the paper speed has been correctly set. This electrocardiogram was properly performed at 25 mm per second.

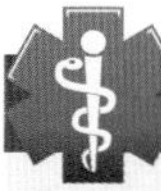

BOARD EXAMINATION ESSENTIALS

P waves are not identified. QRS complexes occur at regular intervals at a rate >100 per minute satisfying the board exam diagnostic code for AV junctional rhythm/tachycardia. Additional diagnostic codes include intraventricular conduction disturbance, nonspecific type, ST- and/or T-wave abnormalities suggesting electrolyte disturbances and under clinical diagnoses, hyperkalemia. Given the abnormal QRS complex and the profound hyperkalemia, resist coding a myocardial infarction pattern in this circumstance.

Electrocardiogram Case Study #43

CLINICAL HISTORY

A 79-year-old male with recurrent syncope, status post recent permanent pacemaker implantation.

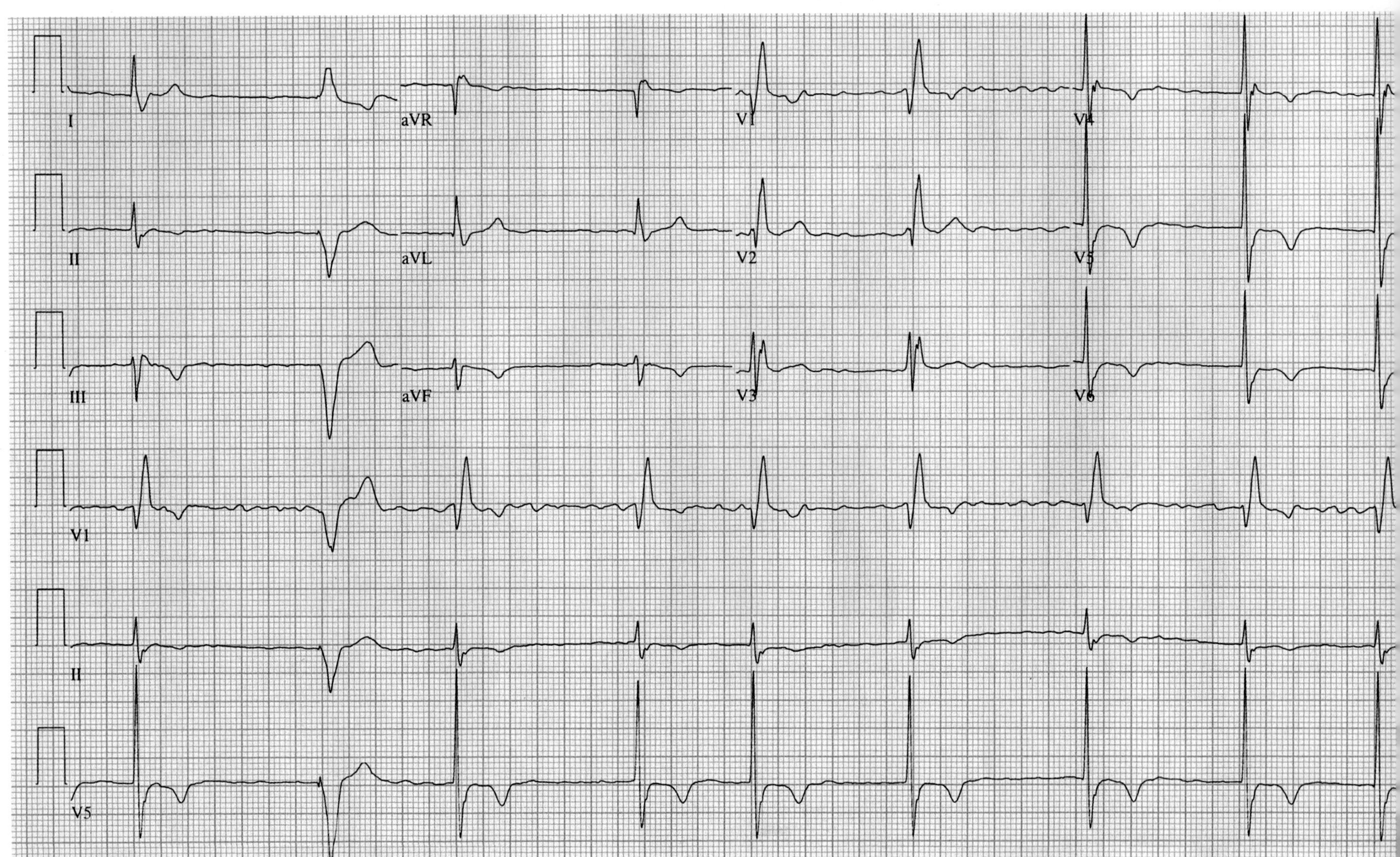

Interpretation Notes:

Electrocardiogram Case Study #43

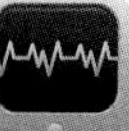

ELECTROCARDIOGRAM INTERPRETATION

This electrocardiogram demonstrates atrial fibrillation as no identifiable discrete atrial activity is present. The ventricular response averages approximately 50 per minute consistent with a slow ventricular response. The QRS complex is widened with a rsR' pattern in leads V1 and V2 with terminal conduction delay evidenced by a prolonged S wave in leads I and aVL supporting complete right bundle branch block. T-wave inversion is seen in leads II, III, aVF, V4, V5, and V6. The second QRS complex is seen after a longer R to R interval and demonstrates an initial discrete deflection consistent with a ventricular paced complex. The ventricular paced complex exhibits complete left bundle branch block morphology consistent with the pacemaker lead tip located within the right ventricular apex.

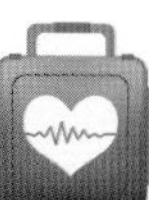

KEY DIAGNOSES

- Atrial fibrillation
- Complete right bundle branch block
- Nonspecific ST-T changes
- Ventricular paced complex

KEY TEACHING POINTS

- This patient demonstrates significant conduction system disease given the presence of atrial fibrillation with a slow ventricular response and complete right bundle branch block.
- The ventricular paced complex is appropriately timed after a lengthy interval, following the initial QRS complex devoid of subsequent native ventricular depolarization.
- The patient is intermittently utilizing the pacemaker with predominant ventricular depolarization via preserved atrioventricular conduction.

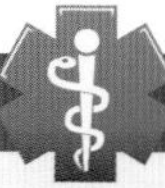

BOARD EXAMINATION ESSENTIALS

Appropriate diagnostic codes for the board exam include atrial fibrillation, complete right bundle branch block, nonspecific ST- and/or T-wave changes, and ventricular demand pacemaker (VVI), normally functioning. It is important to identify the pacemaker deflection and not mistakenly code for a ventricular escape complex. In the absence of the pacemaker spike, this finding would reflect a ventricular escape complex.

Electrocardiogram Case Study #44

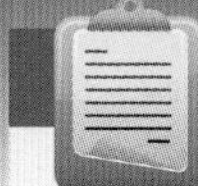

CLINICAL HISTORY

A 16-year-old male admitted to the hospital with a cerebral hemorrhage due to an arteriovenous malformation. He subsequently expired.

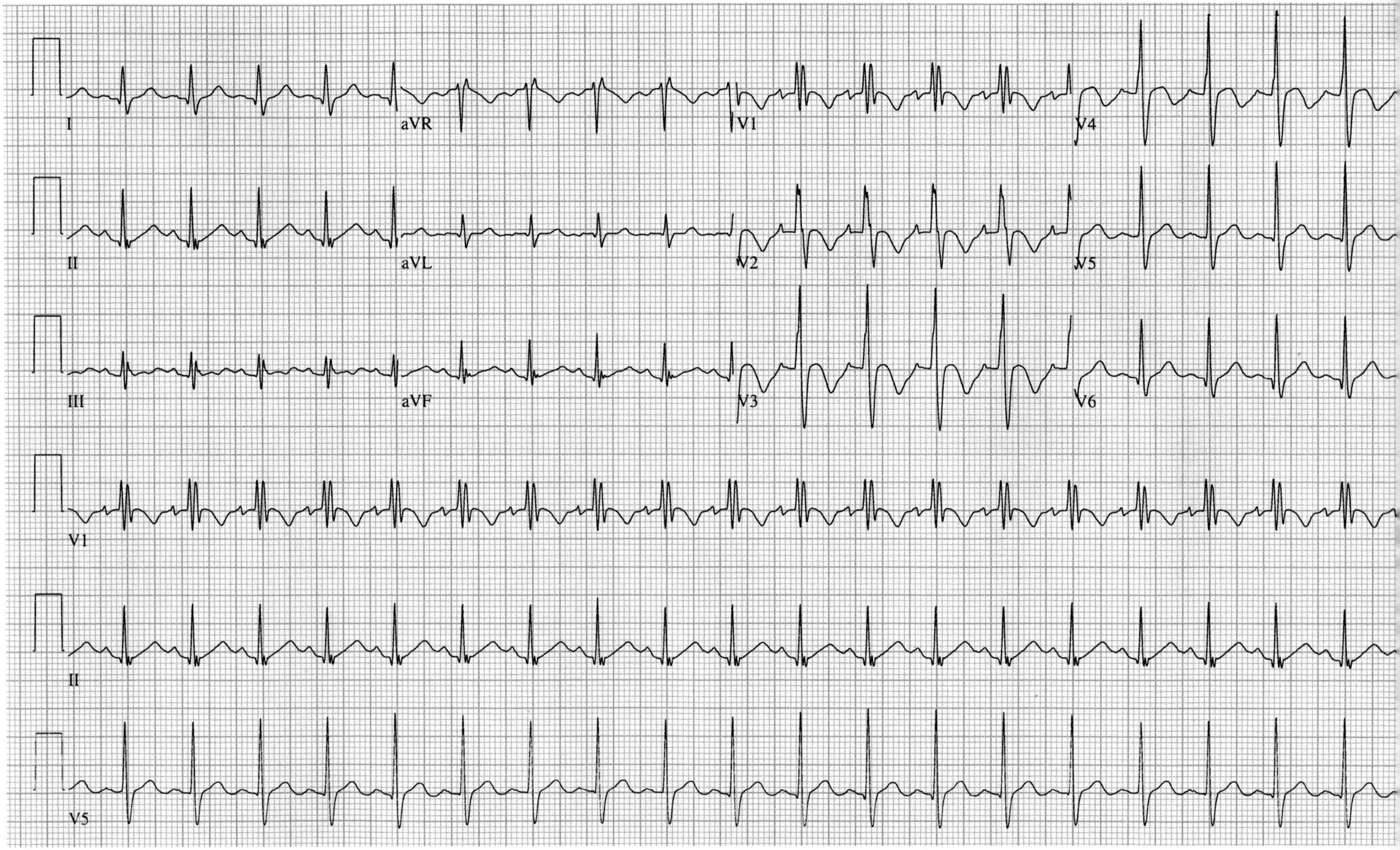

I aVR V1 V4
II aVL V2 V5
III aVF V3 V6
V1
II
V5

Interpretation Notes:

Electrocardiogram Case Study #44

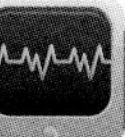

ELECTROCARDIOGRAM INTERPRETATION

This electrocardiogram demonstrates P waves preceding each QRS complex with a normal P-wave axis at an atrial rate close to 120 per minute consistent with sinus tachycardia. The QRS complex duration is slightly >100 milliseconds. Right ventricular conduction delay is evidenced by an RSR' QRS complex morphology as seen in lead V1 and delayed terminally negative S waves as seen in leads I, V4, V5, and V6. This is consistent with incomplete right bundle branch block. T-wave inversion is noted in leads V2, V3, and V4, which is a nonspecific finding and is likely secondary to the patient's known increased intracranial pressure. The QT interval is prolonged, best seen in lead II and also in leads V2, V3, and V4 being >50% of the R to R interval.

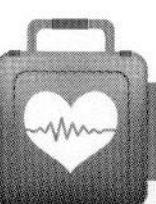

KEY DIAGNOSES

- Sinus tachycardia
- Incomplete right bundle branch block
- Nonspecific ST-T changes
- Prolonged QT interval
- Central nervous system event

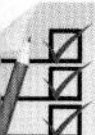

KEY TEACHING POINTS

- T-wave inversion and a prolonged QT interval are commonly seen in the presence of an acute rise of intracranial pressure.
- The pattern of right ventricular conduction delay as evidenced in lead V1 can be seen in the presence of an atrial septal defect. This patient did not undergo cardiac imaging and, therefore, it is not known if an atrial septal defect was present.

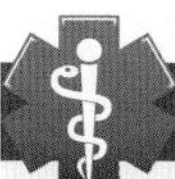

BOARD EXAMINATION ESSENTIALS

The cardiac rhythm should be coded as sinus tachycardia given the normal P-wave axis at an atrial rate >100 per minute. In the context of the clinical history, under the clinical disorders section, central nervous system disorder should be coded. Right bundle branch block, incomplete and a prolonged QT interval are also applicable. None of the ST- and/or T-wave abnormality options strictly apply as the T-wave inversion is specific to the central nervous system event. One could consider coding nonspecific ST-and/or T-wave abnormalities although, in fact, the findings are specific.

Electrocardiogram Case Study **#45**

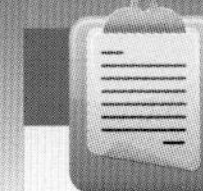

CLINICAL HISTORY

An 18-year-old male with an unrepaired ventricular septal defect, moderately severe pulmonary hypertension, and activity-related oxygen desaturation now being seen in follow-up outpatient evaluation.

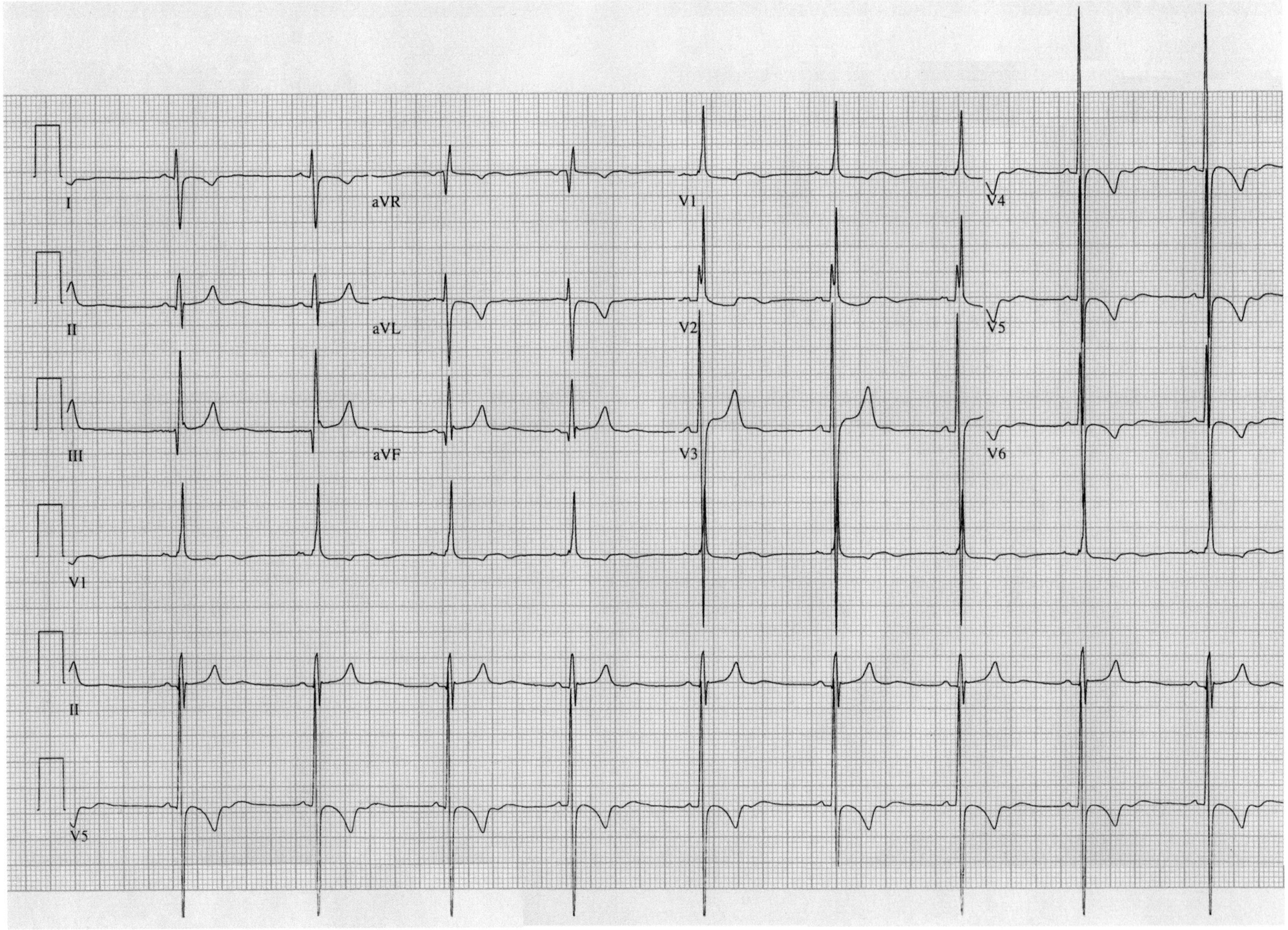

Interpretation Notes:____

____

Electrocardiogram Case Study #45

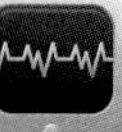

ELECTROCARDIOGRAM INTERPRETATION

This electrocardiogram demonstrates an abnormal P-wave axis at an atrial rate of approximately 55 per minute consistent with an ectopic atrial bradycardia. The QRS complex is of normal duration. QRS complex right-axis deviation is seen as a negative QRS complex vector is present in lead I and positive QRS complex vectors are seen in leads II, III, and aVF, most positive toward lead III. The approximate QRS complex axis is +130 degrees. A prominent R wave is seen in leads V1, V2, and V3. The R wave remains prominent in leads V4, V5, and V6 with asymmetric T-wave inversion in the lateral precordial leads. This is also seen in leads I and aVL. These findings are consistent with both left and right ventricular hypertrophy.

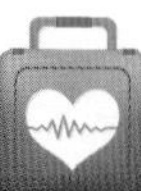

KEY DIAGNOSES

- Ectopic atrial bradycardia
- QRS complex right-axis deviation
- Right ventricular hypertrophy
- Left ventricular hypertrophy
- Biventricular hypertrophy
- Secondary ST-T changes

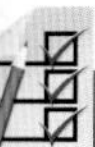

KEY TEACHING POINTS

- QRS complex right-axis deviation suggests right greater than left ventricular hypertrophy. That is suspected given the moderately severe pulmonary hypertension by history.
- Left ventricular hypertrophy is due to the volume overload of the left ventricle given the ventricular septal defect and resultant increased left ventricular mass with the reversal of blood flow in a right to left ventricular direction due to advanced pulmonary hypertension.
- Left or right atrial abnormality is not identified on this electrocardiogram due to the ectopic atrial bradycardia.

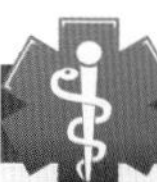

BOARD EXAMINATION ESSENTIALS

Board exam diagnostic codes for this electrocardiogram include sinus bradycardia (sinus rate < 60 per minute) as no ectopic bradycardia exists, right-axis deviation (>100 degrees), combined ventricular hypertrophy, and ST- and/or T-wave abnormalities secondary to hypertrophy. There is no electrocardiogram evidence for atrial abnormality/enlargement. For the board exam, this latter diagnosis should always be sought, particularly in the presence of hypertrophy patterns where elevated intracardiac pressures are suggested.

Electrocardiogram Case Study #46

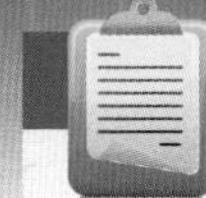

CLINICAL HISTORY

An 86-year-old male with fatigue, shortness of breath, and lightheadedness who was admitted to the coronary intensive care unit. Shortly after this electrocardiogram was obtained, a ventricular pacemaker was implanted.

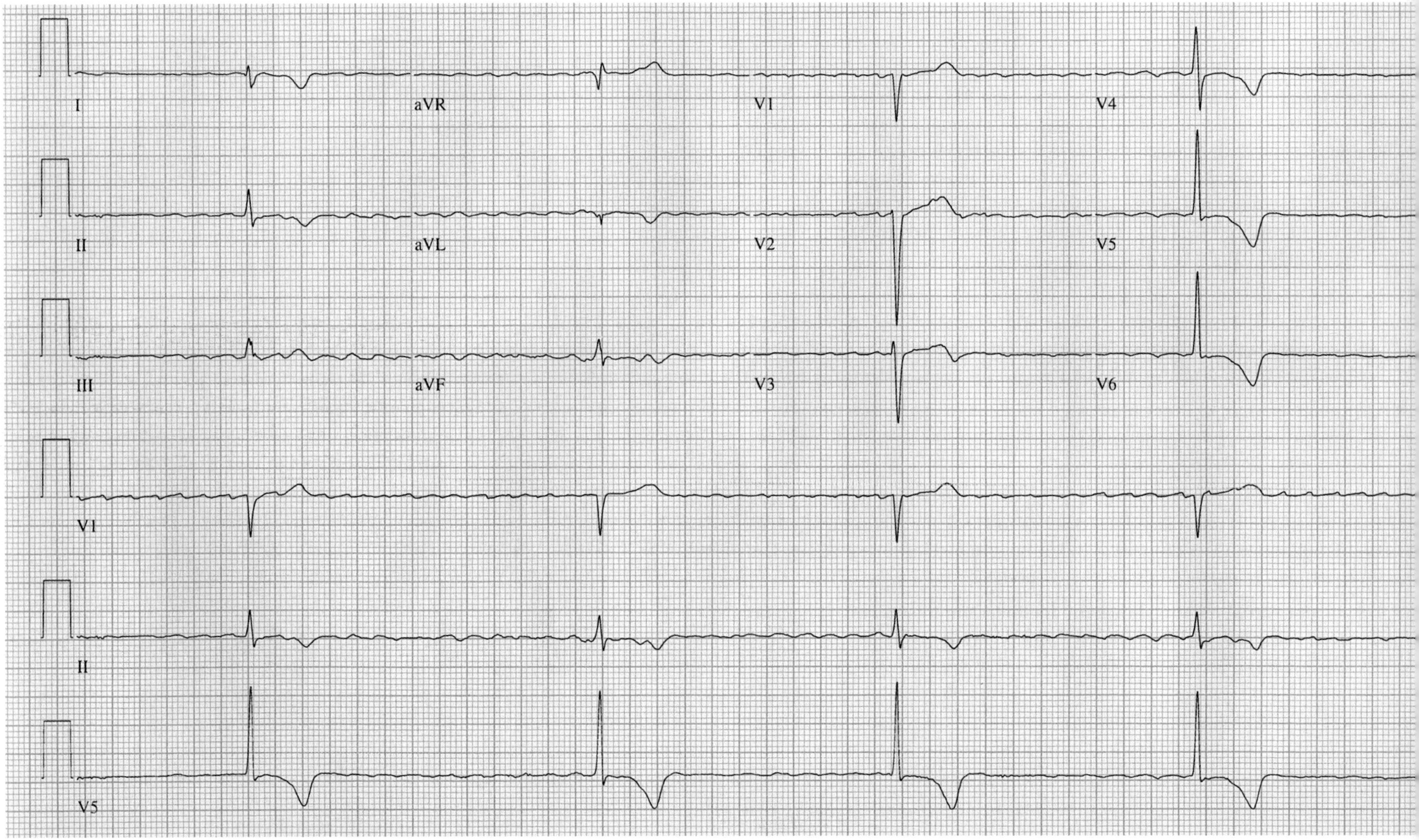

I aVR V1 V4

II aVL V2 V5

III aVF V3 V6

V1

II

V5

Interpretation Notes:

Electrocardiogram Case Study #46

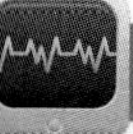

ELECTROCARDIOGRAM INTERPRETATION

This electrocardiogram demonstrates no discernible discrete atrial activity. Instead, atrial fibrillation is present. The ventricular response is markedly slowed with an inconstant R to R interval at a rate of approximately 25 per minute. QRS complex right-axis deviation is present as the QRS complex is negative in lead I and positive in leads II, III, and aVF. Nonspecific T-wave inversion is diffusely present. The R to R intervals between the second, third, and fourth QRS complexes are constant supporting a brief paroxysm of junctional escape complexes/junctional escape rhythm.

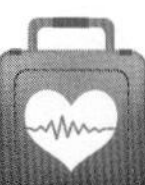

KEY DIAGNOSES

- Atrial fibrillation
- Slow ventricular response
- Junctional escape complexes/junctional escape rhythm
- QRS complex right-axis deviation
- T-wave abnormality

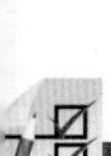

KEY TEACHING POINTS

- This electrocardiogram requires careful evaluation of the R to R interval. The R to R interval spanning the second, third, and fourth QRS complexes is constant suggesting a paroxysmal junctional escape rhythm. A longer rhythm strip would be helpful to confirm or refute this suspicion.
- The Q wave in lead aVL is not diagnostic of a high lateral myocardial infarction as this Q wave is present in isolation without evidence of an additional Q wave in a contiguous lead. Instead, this Q wave is secondary to the right-axis QRS complex deviation.

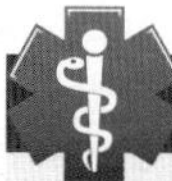

BOARD EXAMINATION ESSENTIALS

Board exam codes include atrial fibrillation, right-axis deviation (>100 degrees), nonspecific ST- and/or T-wave abnormalities, and AV junctional rhythm. This latter diagnostic code is the most challenging aspect of this electrocardiogram and requires precise measurement of the R to R intervals to demonstrate the short period where the R to R intervals are constant. While the asymmetric T-wave inversion has a pattern suggesting ventricular hypertrophy, QRS complex voltage criteria are not met (S-wave lead V2 + R-wave lead V6 < 35 mm) and therefore coding as a nonspecific ST-and/or T-wave abnormality is most accurate.

Electrocardiogram Case Study #47

CLINICAL HISTORY

A 52-year-old female who is postoperative day 2 status post mechanical aortic valve replacement secondary to congenital bicuspid aortic valve stenosis.

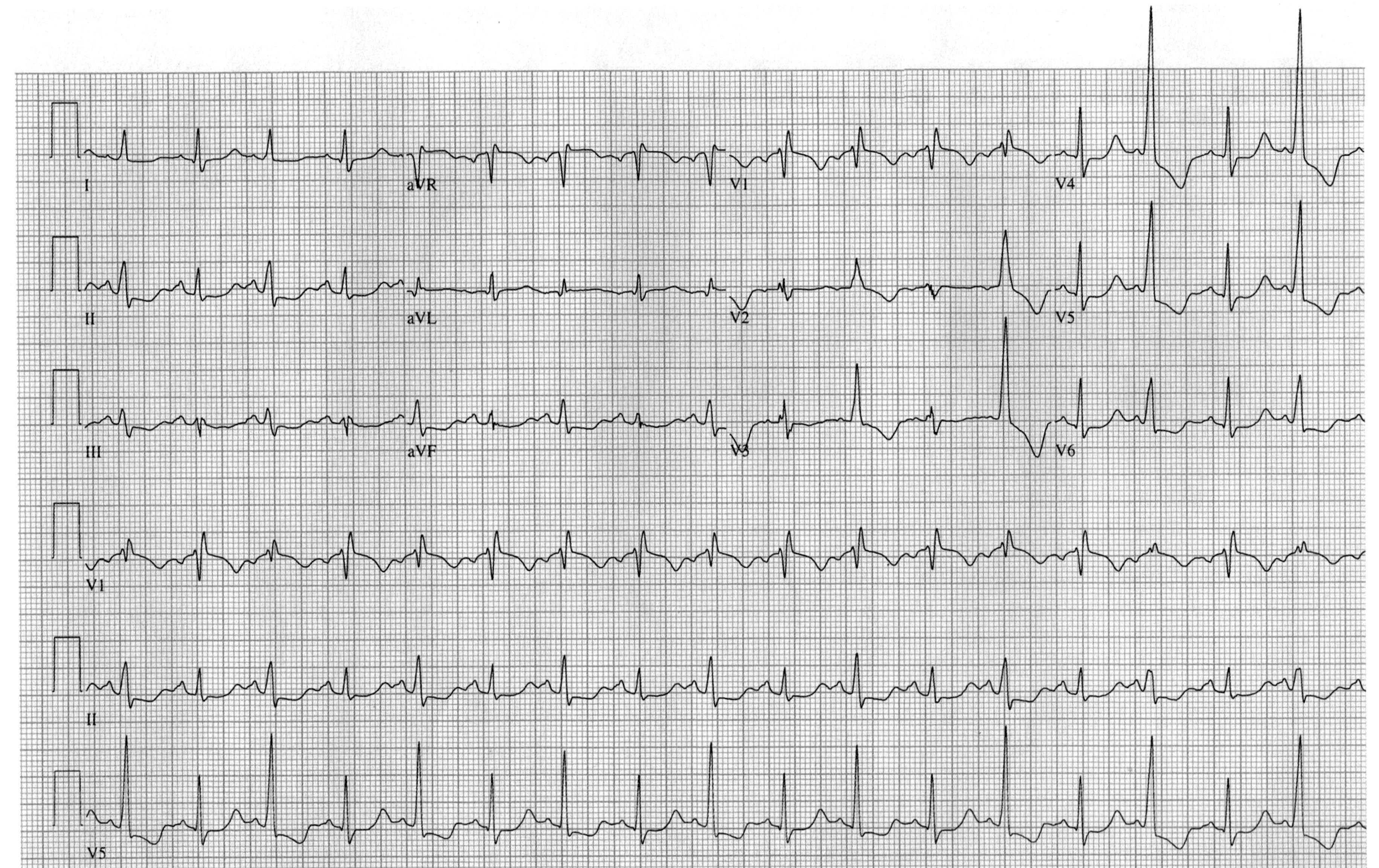

Interpretation Notes:

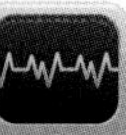

ELECTROCARDIOGRAM INTERPRETATION

This electrocardiogram demonstrates a normal P-wave axis at a constant atrial rate slightly >100 per minute reflecting sinus tachycardia. In lead II, a bifid P wave with left atrial prominence is noted as is a terminally negative P wave in lead V1 supporting left atrial abnormality. In lead V1, incomplete right bundle branch block is seen as the QRS complex duration is <120 milliseconds and the QRS complex morphology demonstrates an rsr' QRS complex pattern. Diffuse nonspecific ST-T changes are present as is QT interval prolongation, seen in most leads as greater than fifty percent of the R to R interval. In the lead V5 rhythm strip, QRS complexes of alternating amplitude are identified. This is consistent with electrical alternans in this recently postoperative cardiothoracic surgical patient who was found to have a large pericardial effusion with echocardiographic evidence of increased intrapericardial pressures. The patient underwent urgent pericardiocentesis with resolution of the electrical alternans finding.

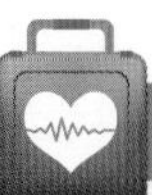

KEY DIAGNOSES

- Sinus tachycardia
- Left atrial abnormality
- Incomplete right bundle branch block
- Nonspecific ST-T changes
- Prolonged QT interval
- Electrical alternans

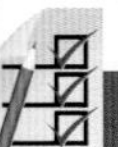

KEY TEACHING POINTS

- Electrocardiogram evidence of electrical alternans is secondary to the changing cardiac position within a large pericardial fluid collection. Reproducible beat-to-beat variability of cardiac position is demonstrated echocardiographically and reflected electrocardiographically as electrical alternans.
- Despite the longstanding presence of aortic stenosis, left ventricular hypertrophy is not seen on this electrocardiogram. Preoperative electrocardiography demonstrated increased QRS complex voltage consistent with left ventricular hypertrophy. Given the presence of a large pericardial effusion, the QRS complex amplitude was likely reduced secondary to the interposed fluid collection between the heart and the chest surface.

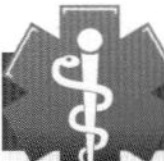

BOARD EXAMINATION ESSENTIALS

Applicable board exam diagnostic codes for this electrocardiogram include sinus tachycardia, left atrial abnormality/enlargement, prolonged QT interval, pericardial effusion, electrical alternans, right bundle branch block, incomplete, and nonspecific ST-and/or T-wave abnormalities. Pericarditis is not definitively demonstrated and therefore not coded. The abnormal QRS complexes are due to an electrical axis shift, are not premature, and should not be confused with functional (rate-related) aberrancy or premature ventricular complexes.

Electrocardiogram Case Study #48

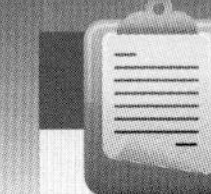

CLINICAL HISTORY

A 66-year-old male with known coronary artery disease who is acutely admitted to the hospital after presenting to the emergency room with a 10-hour history of incessant rapid heart beating, shortness of breath, and chest tightness.

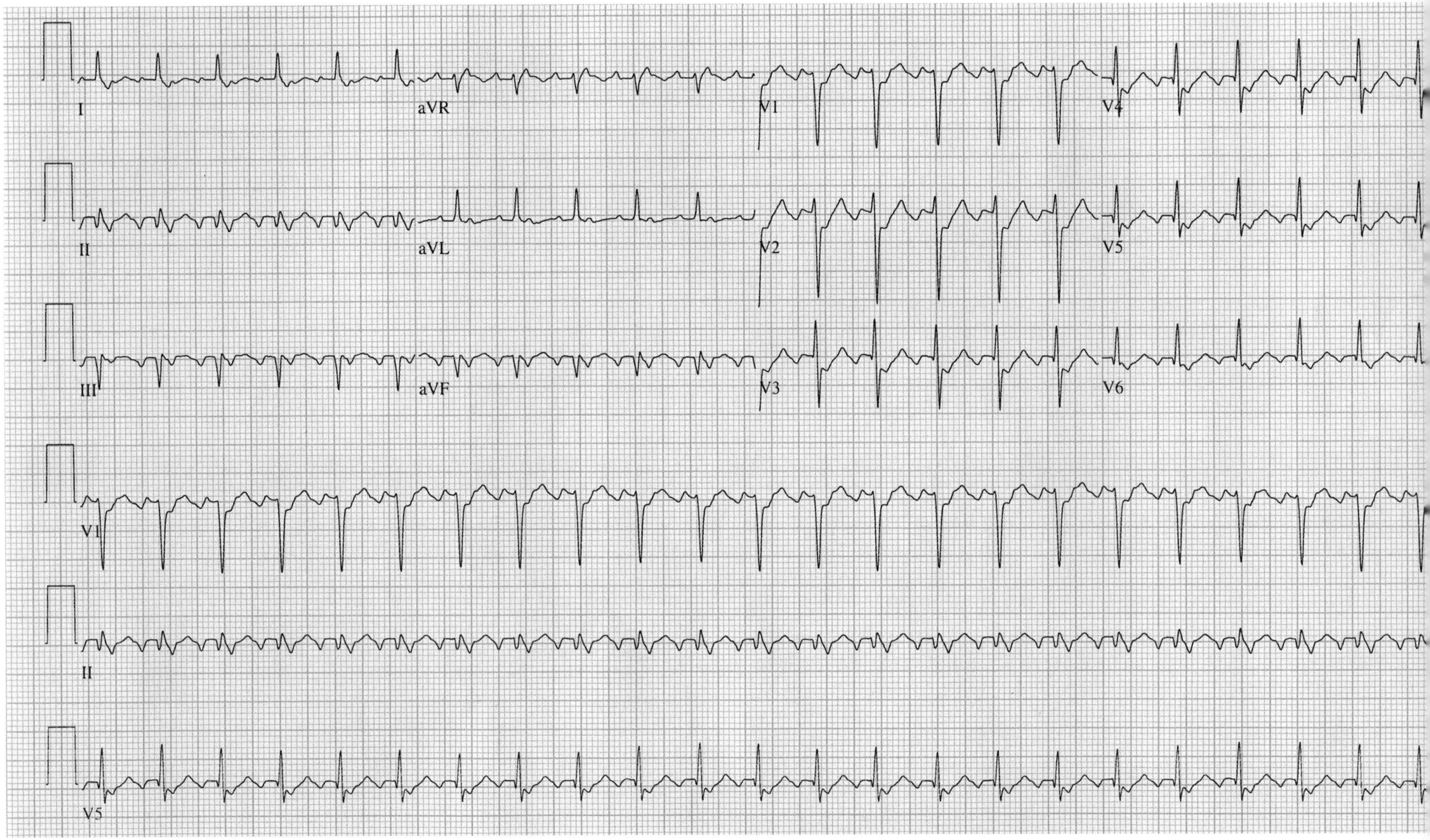

I aVR V1 V4
II aVL V2 V5
III aVF V3 V6
V1
II
V5

Interpretation Notes:

Electrocardiogram Case Study #48

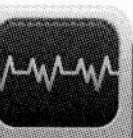

ELECTROCARDIOGRAM INTERPRETATION

This electrocardiogram demonstrates a regular narrow complex tachycardia with a ventricular rate of approximately 135 per minute. Discrete atrial depolarizations are seen in a repetitive manner with a negative vector in leads II, III, and aVF preceding and immediately following each QRS complex with a 2:1 atrioventricular conduction ratio. This is most consistent with atrial flutter and the typical sawtoothed pattern in the inferior leads. Q waves >40-millisecond duration are seen in leads II, III, and aVF consistent with an age-indeterminate inferior myocardial infarction.

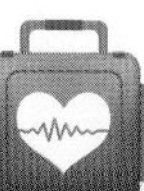

KEY DIAGNOSES

- Atrial flutter
- 2:1 atrioventricular conduction
- Inferior myocardial infarction, age indeterminate

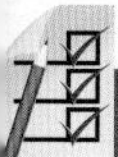

KEY TEACHING POINTS

- In the presence of atrial dysrhythmias, it is important to pursue an underlying cause. This electrocardiogram strongly supports ischemic heart disease as the underlying mechanism for atrial flutter given the finding of an age-indeterminate inferior myocardial infarction.
- Once a myocardial infarction is diagnosed, it is equally important to assess contiguous leads for infarction involvement. Lead V1 does not demonstrate a prominent R wave therefore not supporting an age-indeterminate posterior myocardial infarction. Leads V5 and V6 likewise do not demonstrate diagnostic Q waves therefore not supporting lateral myocardial involvement. On the basis of this electrocardiogram, the myocardial infarction is limited to the inferior territory or in this case, as confirmed by a cardiac catheterization, the right coronary artery distribution.

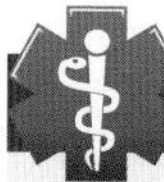

BOARD EXAMINATION ESSENTIALS

When assessing this electrocardiogram, it is important to identify two atrial depolarizations for each QRS complex. The saw-toothed atrial depolarization satisfies the board exam diagnostic code criteria for atrial flutter and AV block, 2:1. This latter diagnosis is best termed 2:1 AV conduction as it represents physiologic, not pathologic block but for the purposes of the board exam, AV block is the best choice. An inferior myocardial infarction, age indeterminate, should also be coded. The apparent ST-T changes are due to the impact of the atrial flutter waves on the electrocardiogram baseline and therefore should not be coded.

Electrocardiogram Case Study #49

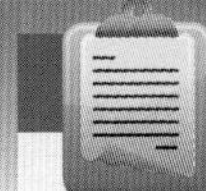

CLINICAL HISTORY

An 81-year-old female with severe coronary artery disease who is post-operative day 3 after multivessel coronary artery bypass grafting. Both preoperative left heart catheterization and echocardiogram confirmed normal left ventricular systolic function.

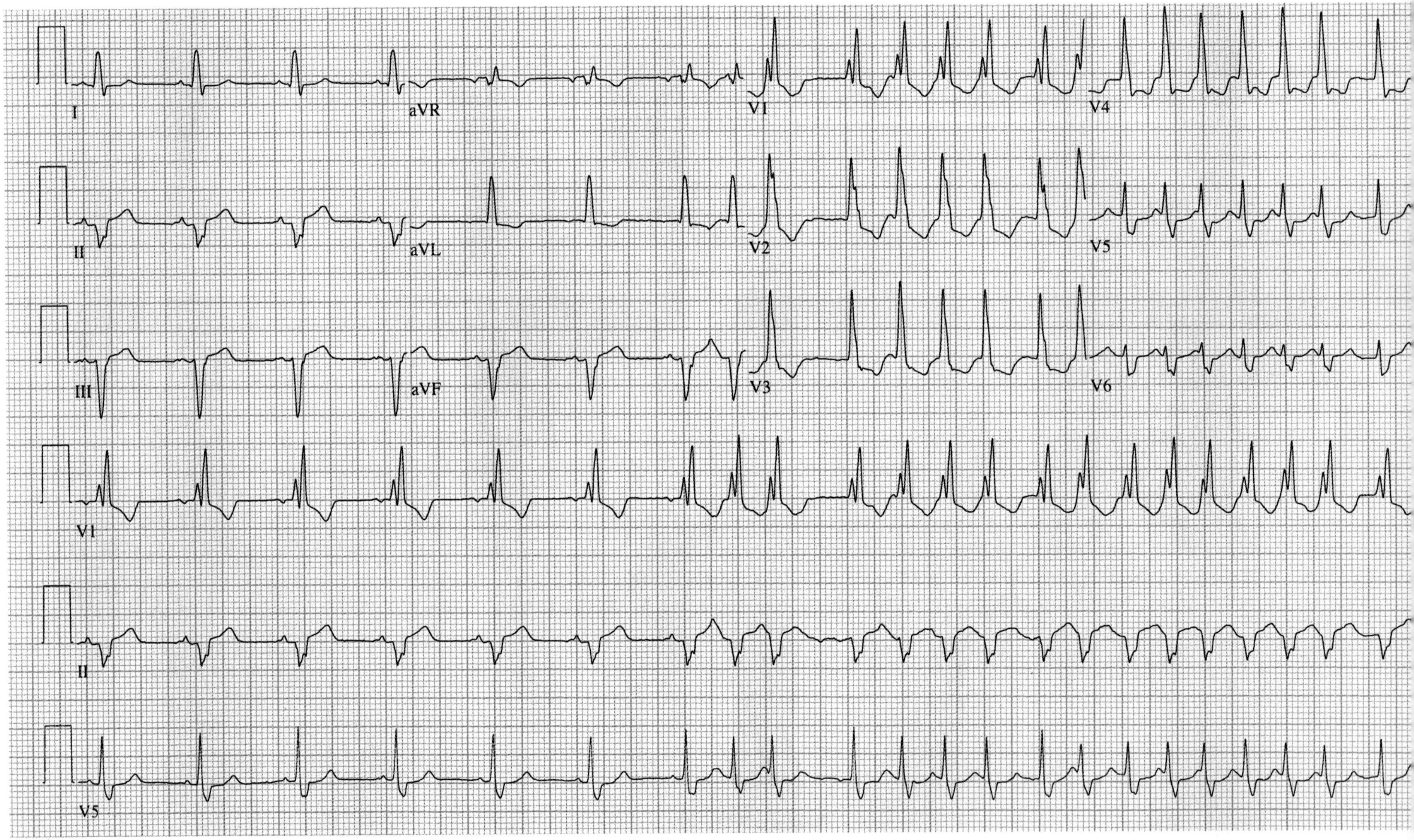

I aVR V1 V4
II aVL V2 V5
III aVF V3 V6
V1
II
V5

Interpretation Notes:

Electrocardiogram Case Study #49

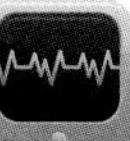

ELECTROCARDIOGRAM INTERPRETATION

This electrocardiogram demonstrates on the left-hand portion P waves of normal axis preceding each QRS complex at an atrial rate of approximately 85 per minute consistent with normal sinus rhythm. The QRS complex vector is deviated leftward as it is positive in lead I and negative in leads II, III, and aVF consistent with left anterior fascicular block. The QRS complex duration is >100 milliseconds and <120 milliseconds with an rsR' QRS complex morphology best seen in lead V1 consistent with incomplete right bundle branch block. In the middle of the electrocardiogram, the atrial rhythm abruptly changes; the ventricular response is tachycardic reflecting atrial fibrillation with a rapid ventricular response. This is initiated by a premature atrial complex as the last QRS complex in lead aVF is preceded by a premature P wave that is superimposed on the T wave. This is best seen in lead aVF and rhythm strip lead II. Nonspecific ST-T changes are demonstrated in lead aVL.

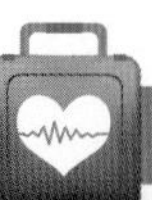

KEY DIAGNOSES

- Normal sinus rhythm
- Left anterior fascicular block
- Incomplete right bundle branch block
- Premature atrial complex
- Paroxysmal atrial fibrillation
- Rapid ventricular response
- Nonspecific ST-T changes

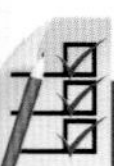

KEY TEACHING POINTS

- This is an excellent example of paroxysmal atrial fibrillation, initiated by a premature atrial complex. This is a common clinical occurrence and was serendipitously captured on this 12-lead electrocardiogram.
- Atrial dysrhythmias are commonly observed in the immediate postoperative period due to heightened circulating catecholamine levels coupled with pericardial inflammation and electrolyte abnormalities.

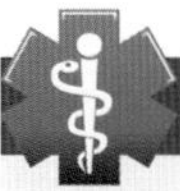

BOARD EXAMINATION ESSENTIALS

This electrocardiogram demonstrates several important board exam diagnostic codes including normal sinus rhythm, left anterior fascicular block, right bundle branch block, incomplete, as the QRS complex duration is <120 milliseconds, atrial fibrillation—in this case new onset—initiated by an atrial premature complex. Nonspecific ST- and/or T-wave abnormality is clearly demonstrated in lead aVL. Note the small r wave in lead aVF precluding the diagnosis of an inferior myocardial infarction, age indeterminate.

Electrocardiogram Case Study #50

CLINICAL HISTORY

A 61-year-old male with known coronary artery disease acutely admitted to the hospital after experiencing an episode of syncope. The patient underwent successful permanent pacemaker placement with symptomatic improvement.

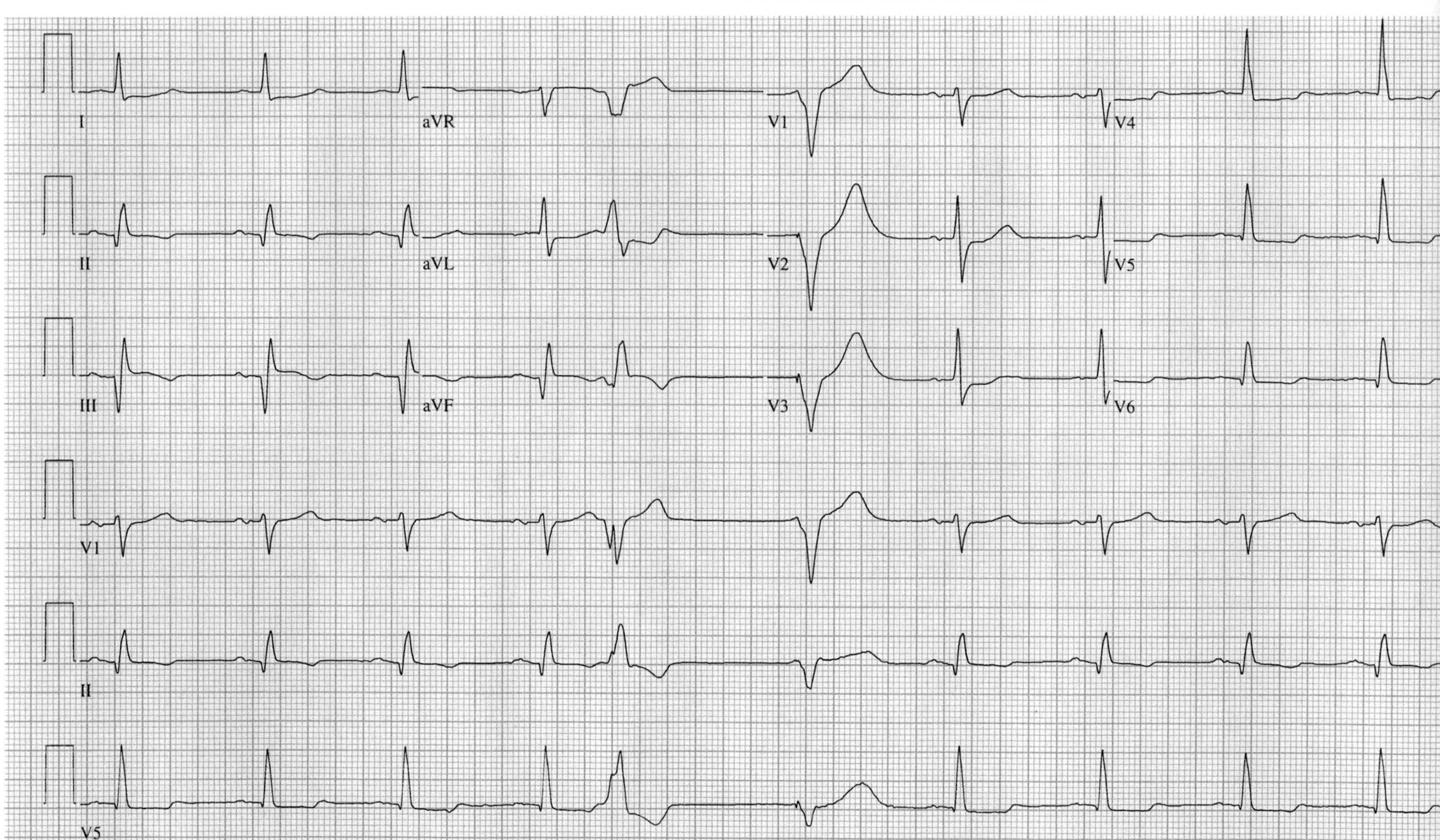

Interpretation Notes:

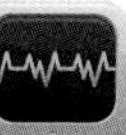

ELECTROCARDIOGRAM INTERPRETATION

This electrocardiogram demonstrates a normal P-wave axis at an atrial rate slightly <60 per minute consistent with sinus bradycardia. The QRS complex is prolonged with a duration of approximately 120 milliseconds. Deep and wide Q waves are identified in leads II, III, and aVF consistent with an inferior myocardial infarction of indeterminate age. Assessing contiguous leads, R-wave regression is noted from lead V4 to V5 to V6. As one transitions to leads V5 and V6, a Q wave emerges. This is consistent with a lateral myocardial infarction of indeterminate age. Most likely, this is one myocardial infarction, spanning the inferolateral distribution. The fifth QRS complex represents a premature ventricular complex of right ventricular origin provided its complete left bundle branch block morphology as assessed in the lead V5 rhythm strip. Following the premature ventricular complex, a sinus pause ensues with the pause terminated with a ventricular paced complex. The prolonged QRS complex duration is due to terminal conduction delay toward the infarct zone demonstrating a terminal positive vector in leads II, III, and aVF. This is consistent with peri-infarction block. This is similarly manifest in leads V5 and V6.

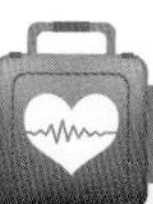

KEY DIAGNOSES

- Sinus bradycardia
- Premature ventricular complex
- Inferior myocardial infarction age indeterminate
- Lateral myocardial infarction age indeterminate
- Ventricular pacemaker
- Peri-infarction block
- Left ventricular aneurysm

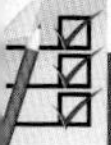

KEY TEACHING POINTS

- This is another example of an age-indeterminate myocardial infarction and the importance of assessing contiguous electrocardiogram leads. An age-indeterminate inferior myocardial infarction is present. R-wave regression is noted in the lateral chest leads with Q-wave formation as the precordial leads transition to lead V6. This R-wave regression coupled with Q-wave formation finalizes the diagnosis of a lateral myocardial infarction.
- This patient underwent a diagnostic left heart catheterization previously. Findings included a proximal right coronary artery occlusion. This was a dominant right coronary artery supplying both the inferior and the lateral aspects of the heart explaining the electrocardiogram myocardial infarction pattern.
- J-point and ST-segment elevation is suggested particularly in leads III and aVF. At the time of the left heart catheterization, an inferobasal left ventricular aneurysm was noted. This was a sequela of the prior inferior myocardial infarction and explains the persistent J-point and ST-segment elevation as demonstrated on this electrocardiogram.

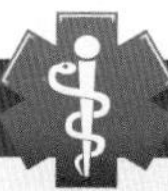

BOARD EXAMINATION ESSENTIALS

Board exam diagnostic codes for this electrocardiogram include sinus bradycardia (atrial rate just slightly <60 per minute); ventricular premature complex; ventricular demand pacemaker (VVI), normally functioning; inferior myocardial infarction, age indeterminate; lateral myocardial infarction, age indeterminate; intraventricular conduction disturbance, nonspecific type. One can also consider sinus pause or arrest as evidenced after the ventricular premature complex.

Electrocardiogram Case Study #51

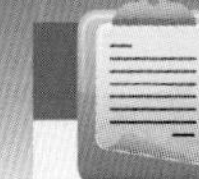

CLINICAL HISTORY

An 85-year-old male with intermittent chest pain and shortness of breath. He underwent permanent pacemaker placement 5 years prior to this electrocardiogram.

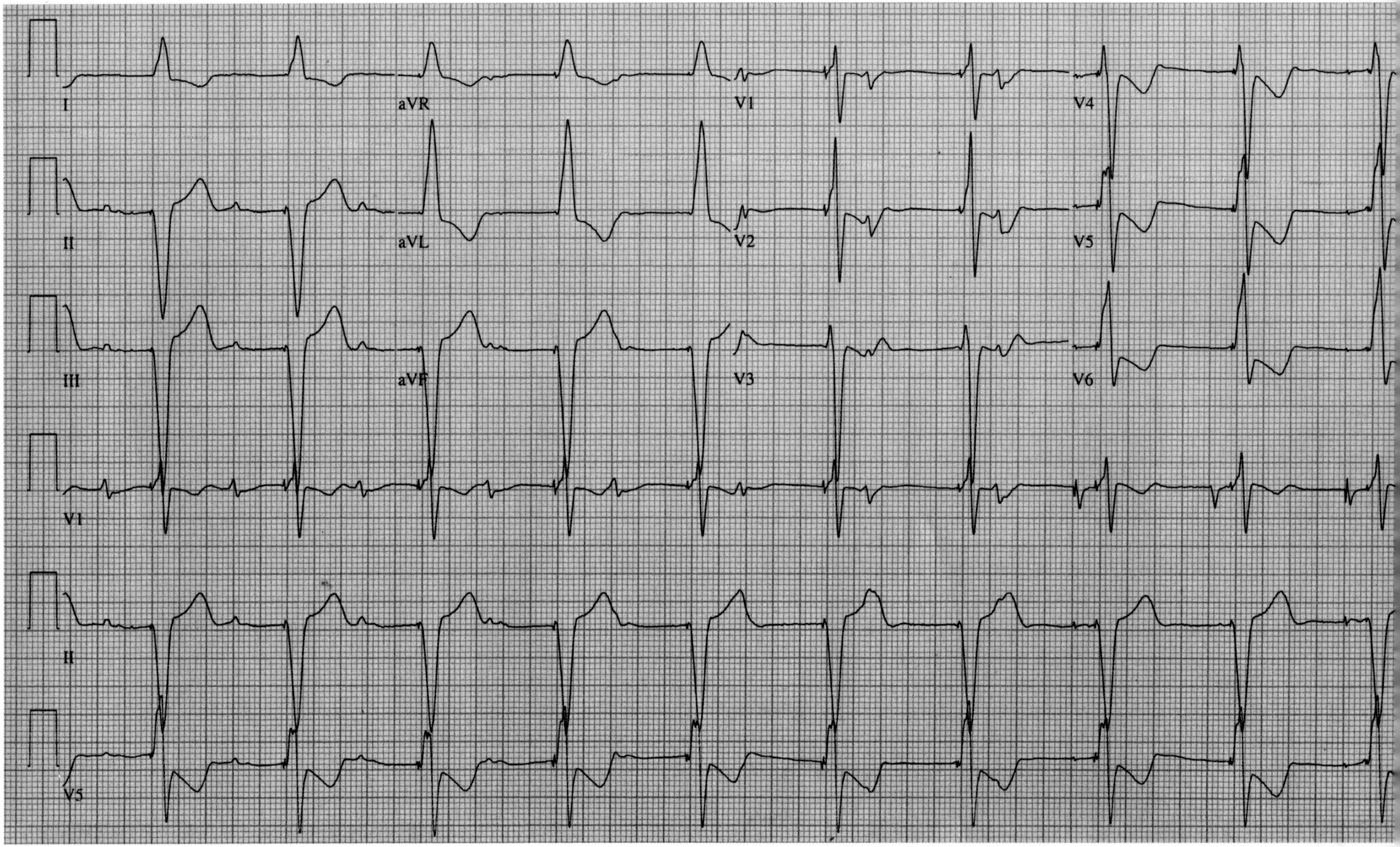

Interpretation Notes:

Electrocardiogram Case Study #51

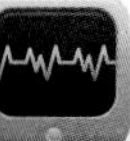

ELECTROCARDIOGRAM INTERPRETATION

This electrocardiogram demonstrates regularly occurring P waves at an atrial rate slightly >60 per minute. The P-wave axis is abnormal demonstrating a near isoelectric vector in leads 1 and aVL. This is best characterized as an ectopic atrial rhythm. The P waves do not appear to be associated with the QRS complexes as there is no constant PR interval. This is consistent with complete heart block. The QRS complexes occur at a regular interval at a rate of 60 per minute and are preceded by a discrete deflection consistent with ventricular pacing. Preceding the eighth QRS complex, a second pacemaker deflection is seen and this reflects atrial and ventricular pacing. Before the last QRS complex, atrioventricular pacing is also seen.

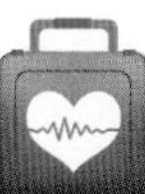

KEY DIAGNOSES

- Ectopic atrial rhythm
- Complete heart block
- Ventricular pacemaker
- Atrioventricular pacemaker

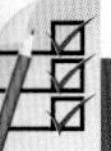

KEY TEACHING POINTS

- The instances of atrial pacing reflect normal pacemaker function and normal atrial pacemaker lead sensing. Given the perceived delay of native ectopic atrial focus discharge, the atrial component of the pacemaker discharges depolarizing the atrium. This is most notable when the P wave is at a significant distance from the subsequent QRS complex. With a tighter P wave to QRS complex coupling interval, atrial sensing inhibits atrial pacemaker discharge.
- Distinguishing complete heart block from atrioventricular dissociation can be difficult and often requires a longer rhythm strip. In this circumstance, numerous potential PR intervals exist and there is no evidence of atrioventricular conduction. Given this finding coupled with the known history of permanent pacemaker placement, this renders a higher likelihood and confidence to the diagnosis of complete heart block.

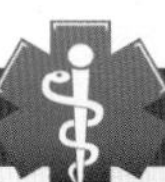

BOARD EXAMINATION ESSENTIALS

This electrocardiogram example once again highlights the importance of identifying P waves, calculating the P to P interval and assessing the P-wave axis. The P waves demonstrate no relationship to the QRS complexes supporting the board exam diagnostic code of complete heart block. Even though the electrical axis of the P wave is abnormal, the best code for the board exam would be normal sinus rhythm as ectopic atrial rhythm is not an available code. If normal sinus rhythm is coded, left atrial abnormality/enlargement would also be appropriate to code given the terminal negativity of the P wave in lead V1 and the bifid appearance of the P wave in lead II. Both ventricular demand pacemaker (VVI), normally functioning; and dual chamber pacemaker (DDD), normally functioning, should be coded.

Electrocardiogram Case Study #52

CLINICAL HISTORY

A 62-year-old female with sudden-onset severe chest discomfort and diaphoresis of 90-minute duration. She was directly admitted from the emergency room to the coronary intensive care unit.

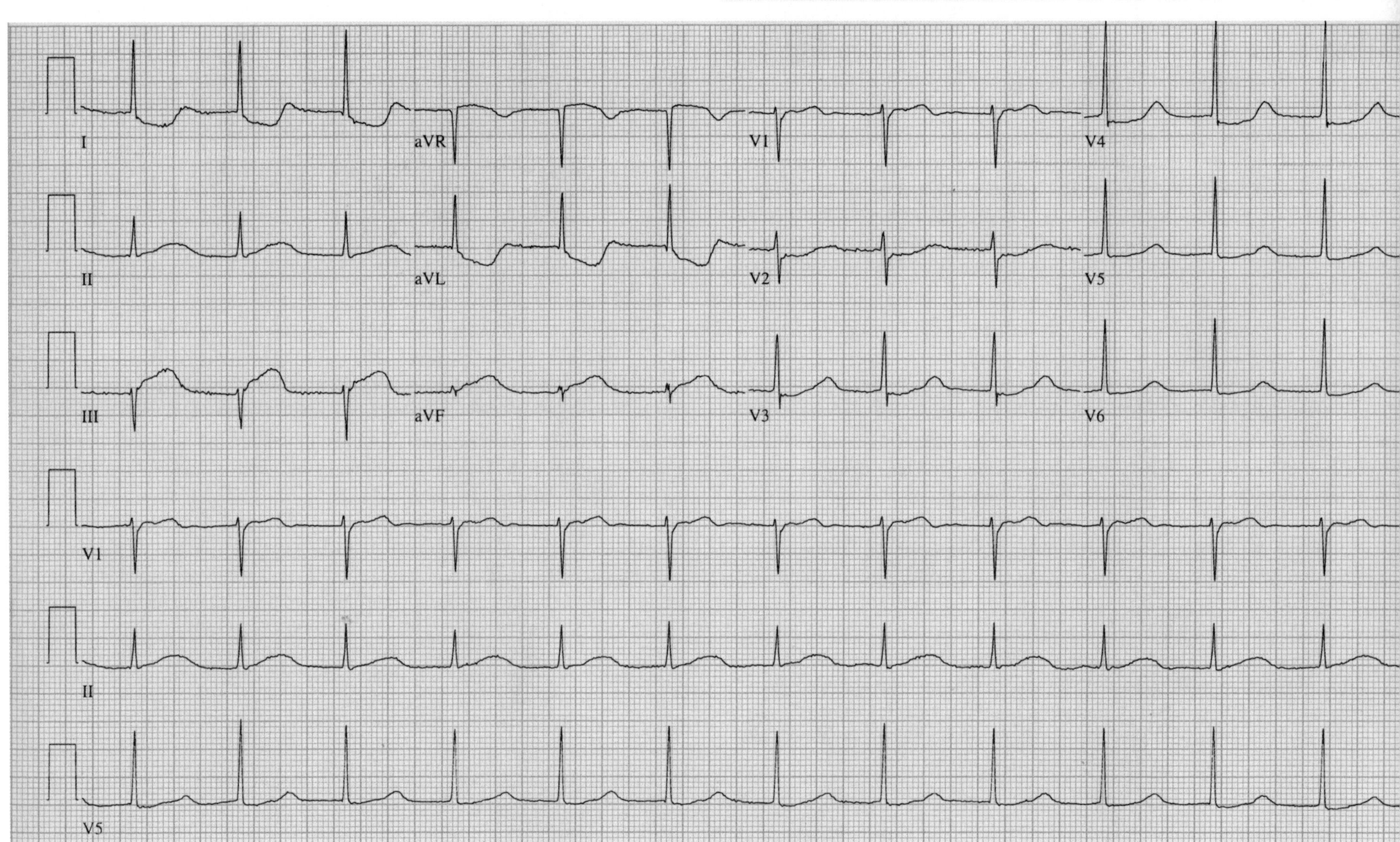

Interpretation Notes:

Electrocardiogram Case Study #52

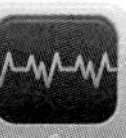

ELECTROCARDIOGRAM INTERPRETATION

This electrocardiogram demonstrates narrow QRS complexes at a constant R to R interval at a rate of 75 per minute, devoid of identifiable atrial activity. This is consistent with an accelerated junctional rhythm. Most prominent on this electrocardiogram is the downsloping ST-segment depression seen in leads I and aVL. This is actually a reciprocal finding as J- point and ST-segment elevation and ST-segment straightening is identified in leads II, III, and aVF consistent with acute inferior myocardial injury. Q waves are not identified. Subtle ST-segment elevation is present in lead V1 possibly indicating an acute right ventricular myocardial injury pattern. Serial electrocardiograms or right-sided precordial lead placement would be appropriate in this circumstance. Slight ST-segment depression is seen in leads V2, V3, V4, V5, and V6. A prolonged QT interval is identified, best discerned in lead II. This is not a prolonged QT-U interval as U waves are not clearly identifiable in the precordial leads.

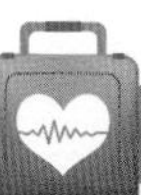

KEY DIAGNOSES

- Accelerated junctional rhythm
- Acute myocardial injury
- Prolonged QT interval
- Right ventricular myocardial injury

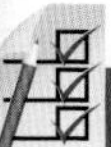

KEY TEACHING POINTS

- A follow-up electrocardiogram demonstrated more prominent ST-segment elevation in lead V1 consistent with acute right ventricular myocardial injury.
- A variety of abnormal supraventricular arrhythmias are observed in the setting of acute myocardial injury. This electrocardiogram provides an example of an accelerated junctional rhythm prior to the patient undergoing a left heart catheterization and successful urgent percutaneous coronary revascularization to a proximal right coronary artery 100% stenosis. Once his procedure was completed, the patient reverted to normal sinus rhythm.

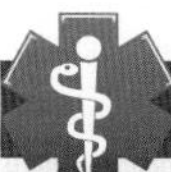

BOARD EXAMINATION ESSENTIALS

For the board exam, the cardiac rhythm supports coding AV junctional rhythm and acute myocardial injury. It is important to code ST- and/or T-wave abnormalities suggesting myocardial injury. The high lateral ST depression is abnormal and reflects a reciprocal change from the acute ST elevation observed in the inferior leads. Coding ST- and/or T-wave abnormalities supporting myocardial ischemia is not recommended as this is a secondary finding. Also, prolonged QT interval should be coded as the QT interval is >50% of the R to R interval. No definite Q waves are identified to code for a myocardial infarction. No U waves are identified.

Electrocardiogram Case Study #53

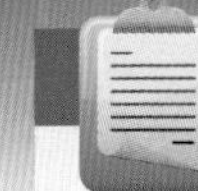

CLINICAL HISTORY

A 60-year-old female with nonischemic severe left ventricular systolic dysfunction who is status post a heart transplantation procedure 2 years before this electrocardiogram was obtained.

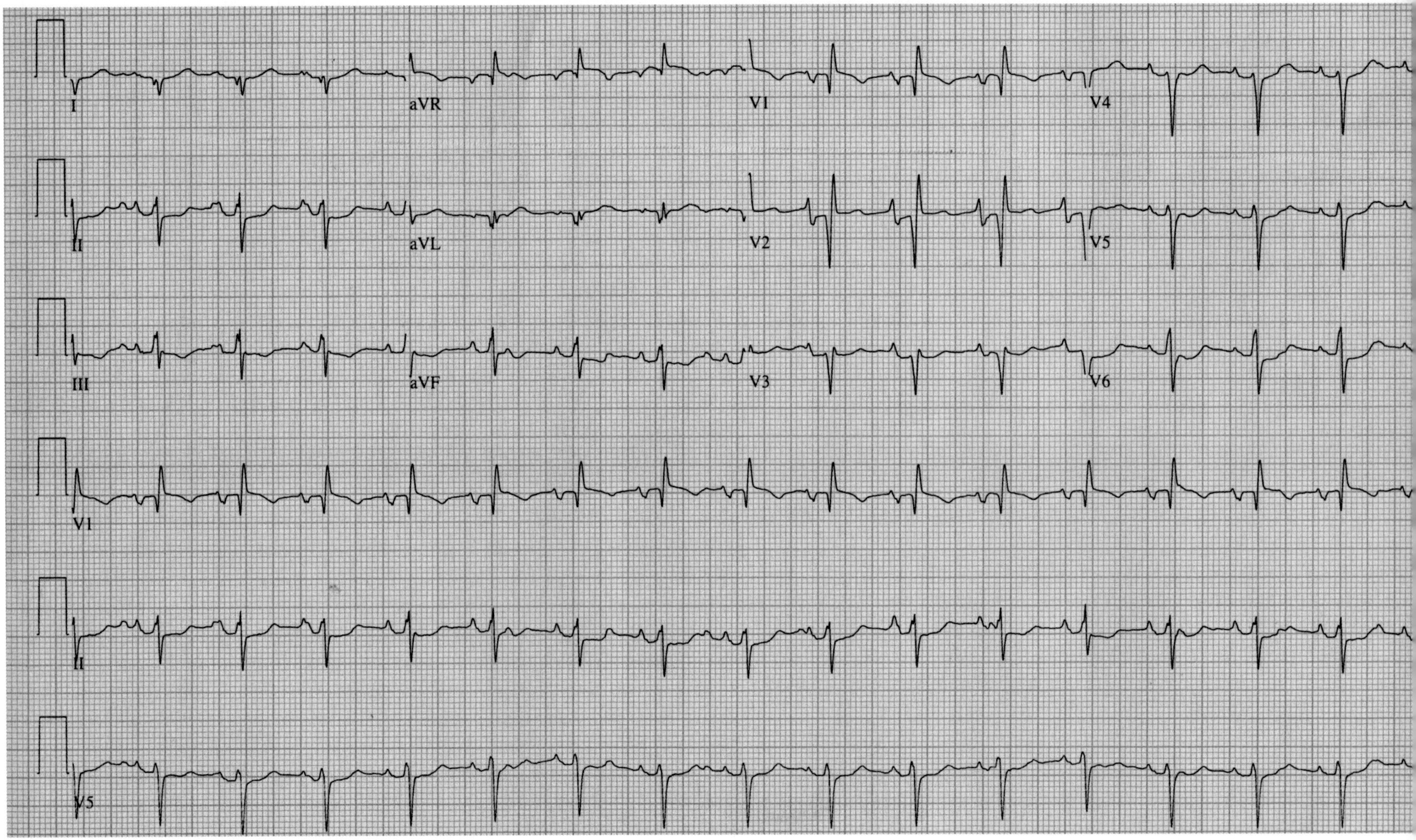

I aVR V1 V4

II aVL V2 V5

III aVF V3 V6

V1

II

V5

Interpretation Notes:

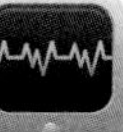

ELECTROCARDIOGRAM INTERPRETATION

This electrocardiogram demonstrates a normal P-wave axis at an atrial rate slightly <100 per minute consistent with normal sinus rhythm. The P waves as assessed in leads V1 and V2 demonstrate prominent terminal negativity consistent with left atrial abnormality. A second P wave is seen preceding the first QRS complex in leads II and III. This identifies this patient as a cardiac transplantation patient with both donor and native atrial electrical activity persisting. The QRS complex duration is <100 milliseconds. A qr pattern is seen in lead V1 with the R wave being approximately 40 milliseconds in duration fulfilling the criteria for incomplete right bundle branch block. Q waves are seen in leads I and aVL supporting a high lateral myocardial infarction of indeterminate age. Q waves are also seen in leads V2 and V3 consistent with an anteroseptal myocardial infarction of indeterminate age.

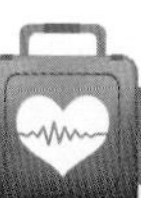

KEY DIAGNOSES

- Normal sinus rhythm
- Left atrial abnormality
- Cardiac transplant
- High lateral myocardial infarction, age indeterminate
- Anteroseptal myocardial infarction, age indeterminate
- Incomplete right bundle branch block

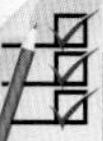

KEY TEACHING POINTS

- Atrial abnormality and incomplete right bundle branch block patterns are commonly seen in cardiac transplant patients.
- This patient was known to suffer from an accelerated form of transplant vasculopathy and diffuse coronary artery disease. Echocardiography confirmed wall motion abnormalities in the left anterior descending and the left circumflex coronary artery distributions. A left heart catheterization demonstrated severe diffuse coronary artery disease.

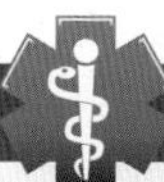

BOARD EXAMINATION ESSENTIALS

This electrocardiogram demonstrates an example of a cardiac transplant patient. A diagnostic code for cardiac transplant does not exist on the board exam. Diagnostic codes other than cardiac transplant include normal sinus rhythm; left atrial abnormality/enlargement; anteroseptal myocardial infarction, age indeterminate; and lateral myocardial infarction, age indeterminate. For this electrocardiogram, do not code left anterior fascicular block. The abnormal QRS complex axis is secondary to the myocardial infarction and supersedes coding abnormal QRS complex axis deviation. Right bundle branch block, incomplete, is also present.

Electrocardiogram Case Study #54

CLINICAL HISTORY

A 42-year-old male with a known ostium secundum atrial septal defect, status post repair 2 years prior to this electrocardiogram who returns for cardiovascular medicine outpatient follow-up evaluation.

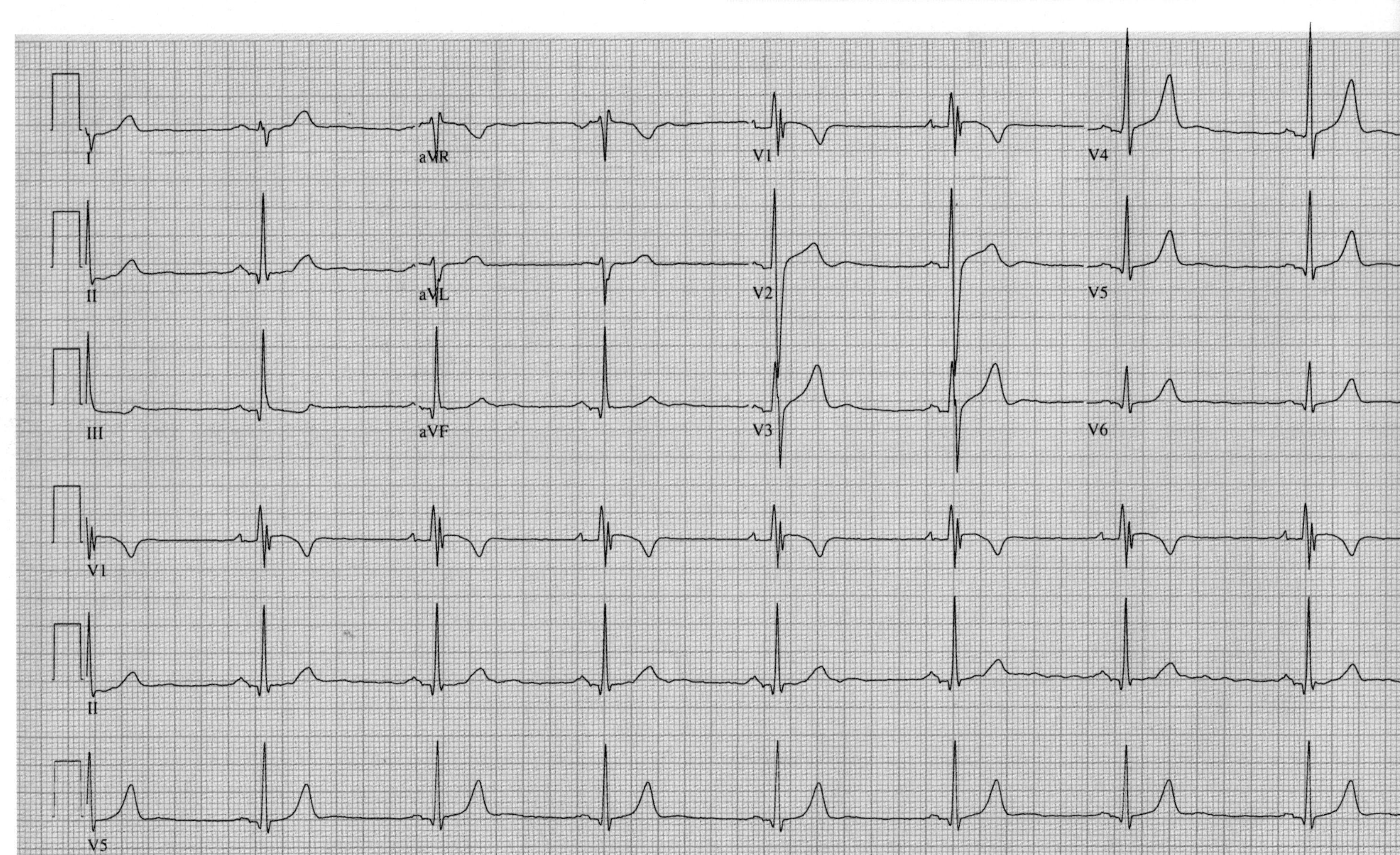

Interpretation Notes:

Electrocardiogram Case Study #54

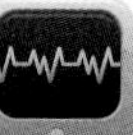

ELECTROCARDIOGRAM INTERPRETATION

This electrocardiogram demonstrates P waves of normal axis at a regular atrial rate slightly <50 per minute consistent with sinus bradycardia. The QRS complex axis demonstrates right axis deviation given the negative QRS complex vector in lead I and positive QRS complex vectors in leads II, III, and aVF. Q waves are identified in the inferior leads; however, these are not of diagnostic duration and do not reflect underlying ischemic heart disease. Right ventricular conduction delay is noted in lead V1 with a characteristic pattern often seen in patients with an atrial septal defect. The P-wave duration in lead II is >110 milliseconds supporting left atrial abnormality.

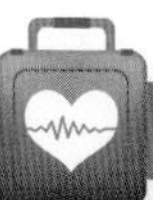

KEY DIAGNOSES

- Sinus bradycardia
- QRS complex right-axis deviation
- Ostium secundum atrial septal defect
- Left atrial abnormality

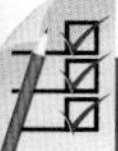

KEY TEACHING POINTS

- This electrocardiogram is consistent with an ostium secundum atrial septal defect given the right-axis QRS complex deviation coupled with the characteristic right ventricular conduction delay as demonstrated in lead V1. A notched upstroke to the S wave in lead aVL and terminal S-wave slowing in lead V6 is also indicative of right ventricular conduction delay.
- The right ventricular conduction delay in this circumstance is due to right ventricular dilatation and a longstanding left-to-right atrial shunt present prior to surgical repair of the ostium secundum atrial septal defect. In contrast, this should not be confused with conduction block within the right bundle branch.
- The QRS complex right-axis deviation is consistent with right ventricular enlargement and rightward displacement of the frontal plane QRS complex vector.

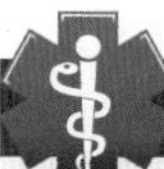

BOARD EXAMINATION ESSENTIALS

This is an important electrocardiogram to consider for the board exam. Anticipate an atrial septal defect example as part of the exam but less likely in the electrocardiogram section as no code for an atrial septal defect exists. Diagnostic codes for the board exam include sinus bradycardia, right-axis deviation (greater than +100 degrees), and characteristic QRS complex conduction delay is seen in lead V1 consistent with an atrial septal defect, best coded as an intraventricular conduction disturbance, nonspecific type. Since QRS complex right-axis deviation is present, considering atrial septal defect, secundum is most appropriate. Lastly, left atrial abnormality/enlargement should be coded.

Electrocardiogram Case Study #55

CLINICAL HISTORY

A 50-year-old male with known coronary artery disease and a prior myocardial infarction who is postoperative day 1 following coronary artery bypass grafting surgery.

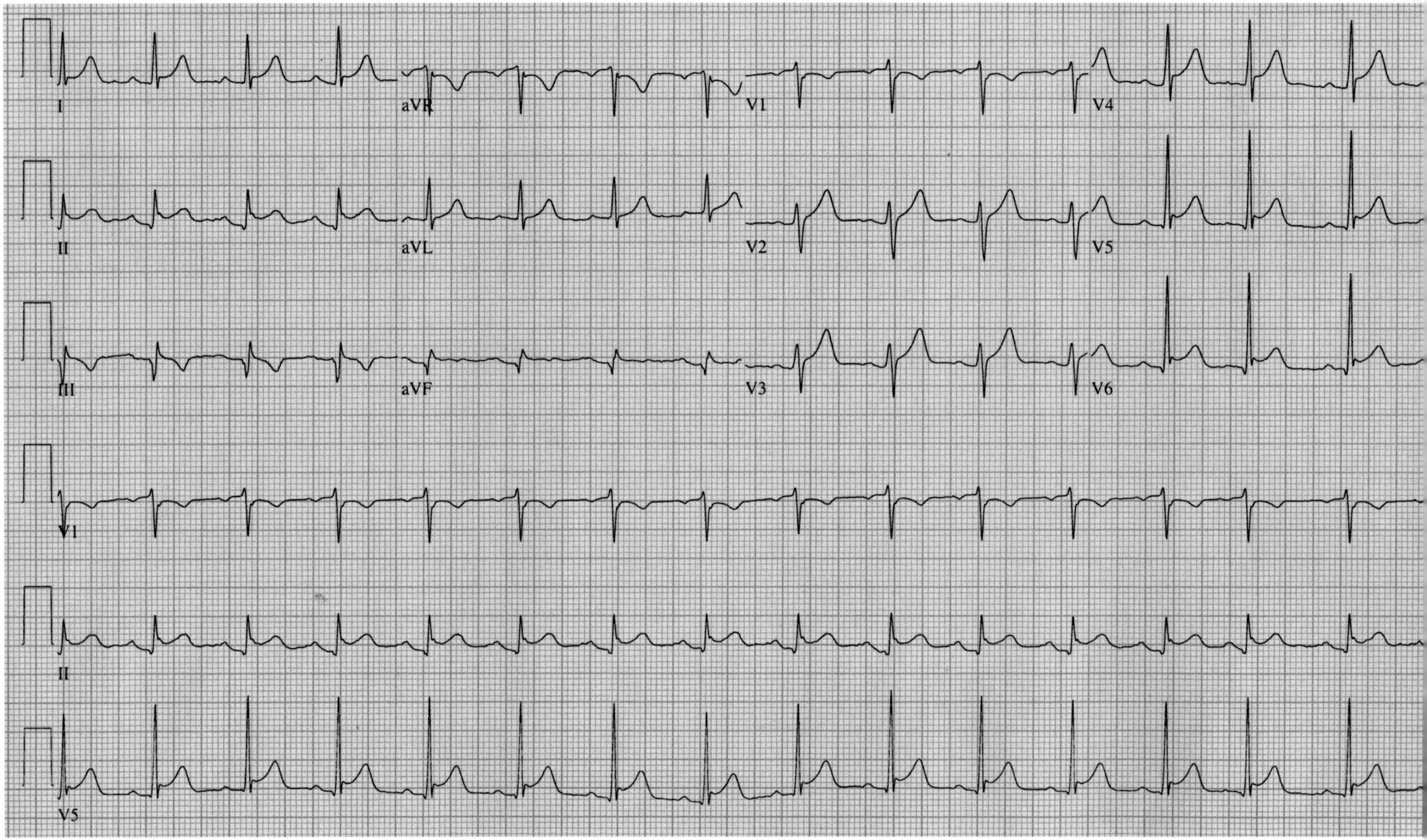

I aVR V1 V4

II aVL V2 V5

III aVF V3 V6

V1

II

V5

Interpretation Notes: __________

Electrocardiogram Case Study #55

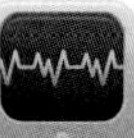

ELECTROCARDIOGRAM INTERPRETATION

This electrocardiogram demonstrates P waves of normal axis at an atrial rate of approximately 90 per minute supporting normal sinus rhythm. Diffuse J-point and ST-segment elevation is identified. Elevation of the PR segment in lead aVR is also seen. These findings collectively support pericarditis in this immediately postoperative open-heart surgical patient. Q waves are also identified in leads II, III, and aVF. The QRS complexes are diminutive as are the Q waves. The Q waves are of diagnostic duration being 40 milliseconds, supporting the presence of an age-indeterminate inferior myocardial infarction. The second to last QRS complex is premature reflecting a premature atrial complex with normal antegrade ventricular conduction.

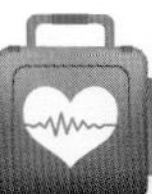

KEY DIAGNOSES

- Normal sinus rhythm
- Pericarditis
- Inferior myocardial infarction, age indeterminate
- Premature atrial complex

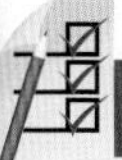

KEY TEACHING POINTS

- Lead aVR can be exceedingly helpful when assessing for the presence of pericarditis. Elevation of the PR segment is highly specific for pericarditis and can be an important differentiator when pericarditis and acute myocardial injury are under simultaneous consideration. Additionally, pericarditis does not typically demonstrate reciprocal ST-T changes as seen with acute myocardial injury.
- Q-wave duration is more important than depth in terms of diagnostic significance. This is well illustrated on this electrocardiogram as the Q-wave depth is quite shallow, yet the 40 millisecond Q-wave duration is diagnostic of an age-indeterminate myocardial infarction. This is consistent with the patient's known history of coronary artery disease and a previous myocardial infarction. Cardiac catheterization confirmed a chronically occluded right coronary artery in the setting of multivessel coronary artery disease. Acute myocardial injury was excluded by serial cardiac enzymes.

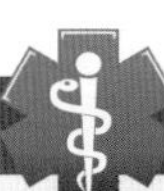

BOARD EXAMINATION ESSENTIALS

This electrocardiogram demonstrates normal sinus rhythm; inferior myocardial infarction, age indeterminate; and diffuse J-point and ST-segment elevation including the PR segment in lead aVR consistent with pericarditis. The ST-segment elevation in the inferior leads reflects superimposed pericarditis and does not support acute myocardial injury. The diffuseness of the J-point and the ST-segment elevation coupled with the clinical history supports this assertion. Diagnostic codes for the board exam would normal sinus rhythm; inferior myocardial infarction, age indeterminate; and pericarditis. There is no evidence of electrical alternans to support the presence of a hemodynamically significant pericardial effusion. The second to last QRS complex is slightly premature proceeded by a premature P wave of slightly differing morphology. This supports coding an atrial premature complex.

Electrocardiogram Case Study #56

CLINICAL HISTORY

A 64-year-old female with a history of hypertension and moderately severe aortic stenosis seen in cardiovascular medicine follow-up.

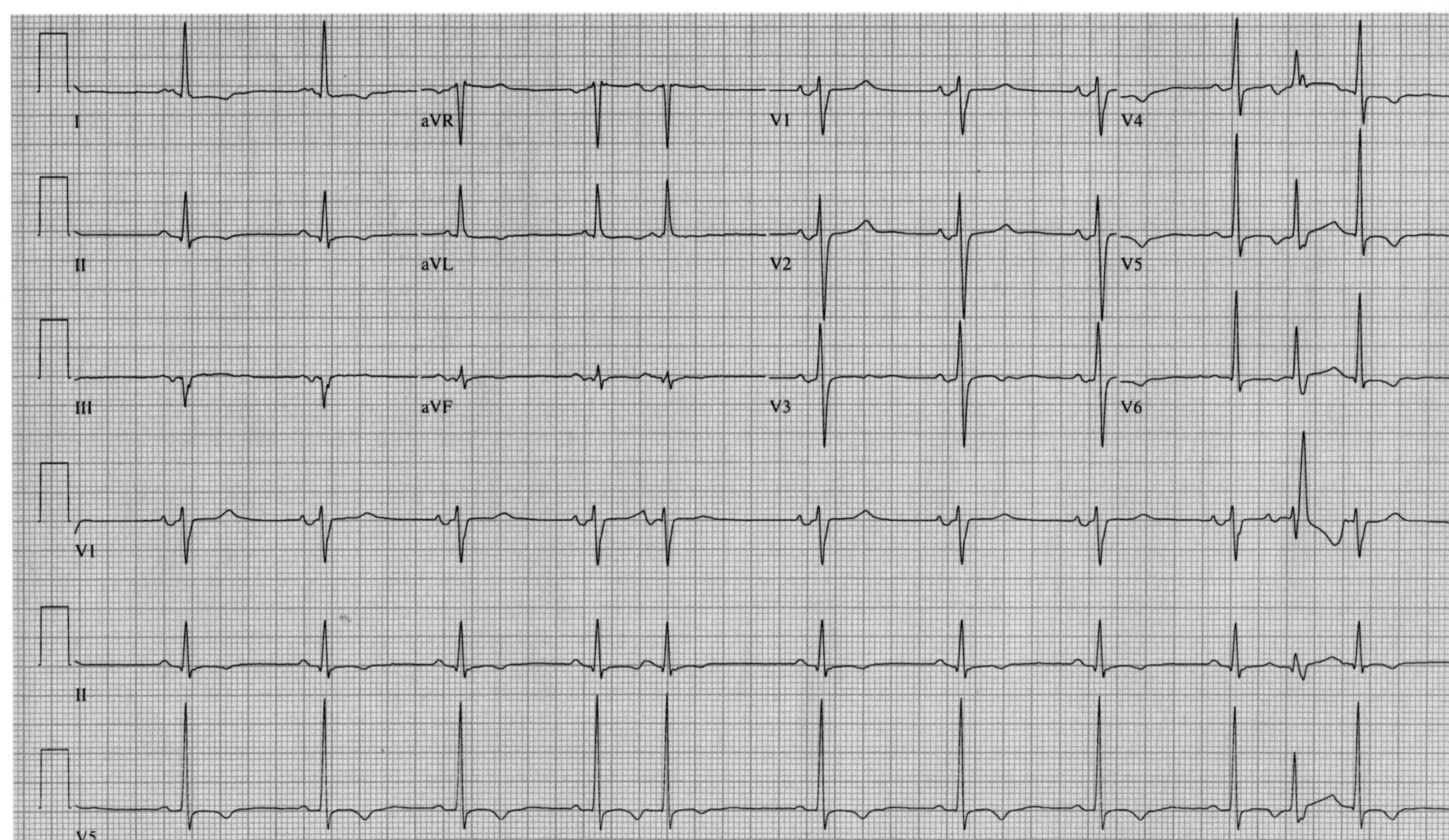

Interpretation Notes:

Electrocardiogram Case Study #56

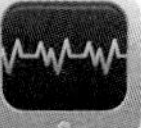

ELECTROCARDIOGRAM INTERPRETATION

This electrocardiogram demonstrates P waves of normal axis at an atrial rate of 70 per minute consistent with normal sinus rhythm. In the lead V1 rhythm strip, the fifth P wave is premature followed by prompt antegrade conduction to the ventricle. This reflects a premature atrial complex. The 10th P wave is also premature and also reflects a premature atrial complex. This P-wave conducts to the ventricle with complete right bundle branch block aberrancy. Unlike the first premature atrial complex, which is followed by a compensatory pause, the second premature atrial complex does not reset the sinus node cycle length. This latter premature atrial complex is best categorized as an interpolated premature atrial complex. The native P wave in lead V1 demonstrates terminal negativity suggesting left atrial abnormality. Diffuse nonspecific ST-T changes are also present. There is no clearly identified myocardial infarction pattern.

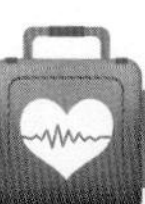

KEY DIAGNOSES

- Normal sinus rhythm
- Premature atrial complex
- Premature atrial complex interpolated
- Left atrial abnormality
- Nonspecific ST-T changes
- Complete right bundle branch block aberrancy

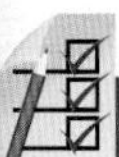

KEY TEACHING POINTS

- Interpolated premature atrial complexes are less common than noninterpolated premature atrial complexes. Clinically, the differences are not known to be significant.
- Left atrial abnormality is observed that may in fact represent the substrate for premature atrial activity.
- Premature atrial complexes with right bundle branch block aberration are more common than left bundle branch block aberration given the longer refractory period of the right bundle branch.

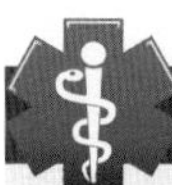

BOARD EXAMINATION ESSENTIALS

This electrocardiogram highlights an example of aberrant conduction. Anticipate at least one form of aberrant conduction on the board exam. Board exam diagnostic codes include normal sinus rhythm, atrial premature complexes, left atrial abnormality/enlargement, nonspecific ST- and/or T-wave abnormalities, and aberrant conduction. For the board exam electrocardiogram section, differentiating interpolated from noninterpolated premature atrial complexes is not necessary.

Electrocardiogram Case Study #57

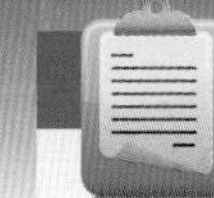

CLINICAL HISTORY

A 79-year-old female with intermittent palpitations who is seen preoperatively prior to near future foot surgery.

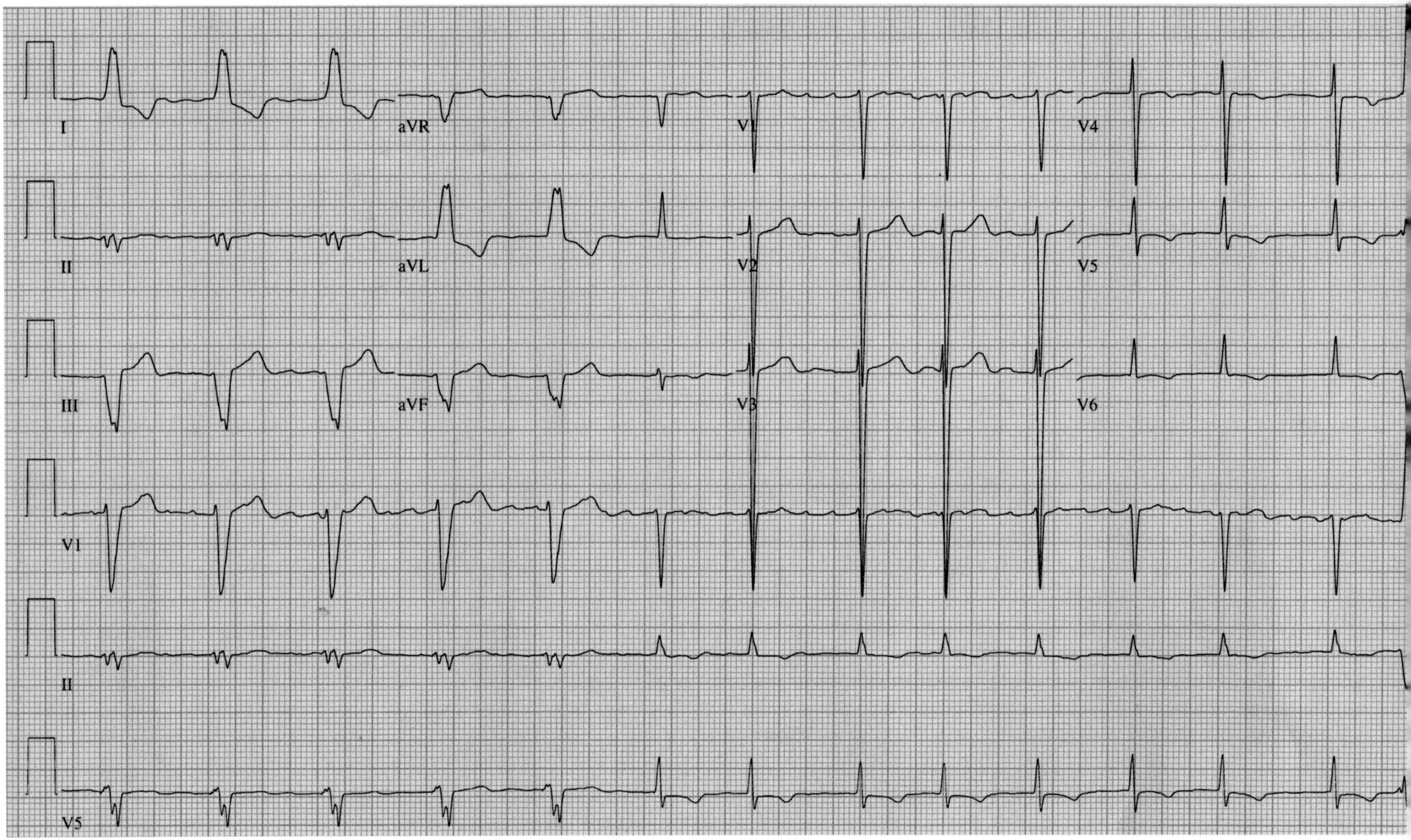

I aVR V1 V4
II aVL V2 V5
III aVF V3 V6
V1
II
V5

Interpretation Notes:

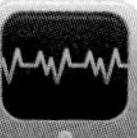

ELECTROCARDIOGRAM INTERPRETATION

This electrocardiogram demonstrates no discrete atrial activity. Instead, an undulating baseline rhythm is identified supporting atrial fibrillation. The ventricular response rate is approximately 80 per minute. On the right-hand portion of the electrocardiogram, prominent QRS complex voltage is seen, particularly in leads V2 and V3. This does not quite meet the diagnostic voltage criteria for left ventricular hypertrophy. Lateral nonspecific ST-T changes are seen. On the left-hand portion of the electrocardiogram, a widened QRS complex is noted. This demonstrates the morphology of complete left bundle branch block given the QRS complex duration >120 milliseconds coupled with the lack of septal Q waves in leads I and aVL. Additionally, during the period of complete left bundle branch block, QRS complex left-axis deviation is identified as the QRS complex vector is positive in lead I and negative in leads II, III, and aVF. In lead aVF, the complete left bundle branch block transitions to a narrower QRS complex supporting the presence of intermittent complete left bundle branch block. The R to R interval during the complete left bundle branch block is constant and therefore most consistent with an accelerated junctional rhythm.

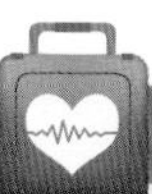

KEY DIAGNOSES

- Atrial fibrillation
- Accelerated junctional rhythm
- Nonspecific ST-T changes
- QRS complex left-axis deviation
- Complete left bundle branch block
- Aberrant conduction

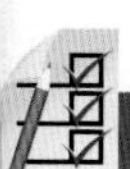

KEY TEACHING POINTS

- As demonstrated on this electrocardiogram, conduction abnormalities such as complete left bundle branch block can be intermittent. Most often, they are rate-related, associated with higher heart rates and resolving as the heart rate slows. In this case, the complete left bundle branch block is noted at a slightly slower heart rate compared to the narrow QRS complex.
- It is important not to diagnose an age-indeterminate myocardial infarction in the presence of complete left bundle branch block. Inferior Q waves are seen and this is due to the complete left bundle branch block and left-axis deviation. It is not diagnostic of a prior myocardial infarction and, in fact, this patient underwent echocardiography demonstrating vigorous and normal left ventricular systolic function. Note the absence of the q wave in lead aVF once the complete left bundle branch block abates.

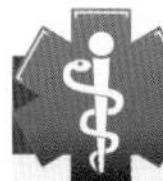

BOARD EXAMINATION ESSENTIALS

This is another example of aberrant conduction. On the right-hand portion of the electrocardiogram, board exam diagnostic codes include atrial fibrillation and nonspecific ST- and/or T-wave abnormalities. On the left-hand portion of the electrocardiogram, accelerated junctional rhythm, complete left bundle branch block and QRS complex left-axis deviation is demonstrated. This is a transient finding and, instead, coding aberrant conduction is most accurate. It is not recommended to code left bundle branch block complete or QRS complex-axis deviation in this transient setting for the board exam.

Electrocardiogram Case Study #58

CLINICAL HISTORY

An 82-year-old male with known coronary artery disease, status post a myocardial infarction 3 years prior to this electrocardiogram who returns for outpatient department follow-up. He feels well and has no cardiopulmonary symptoms at this time.

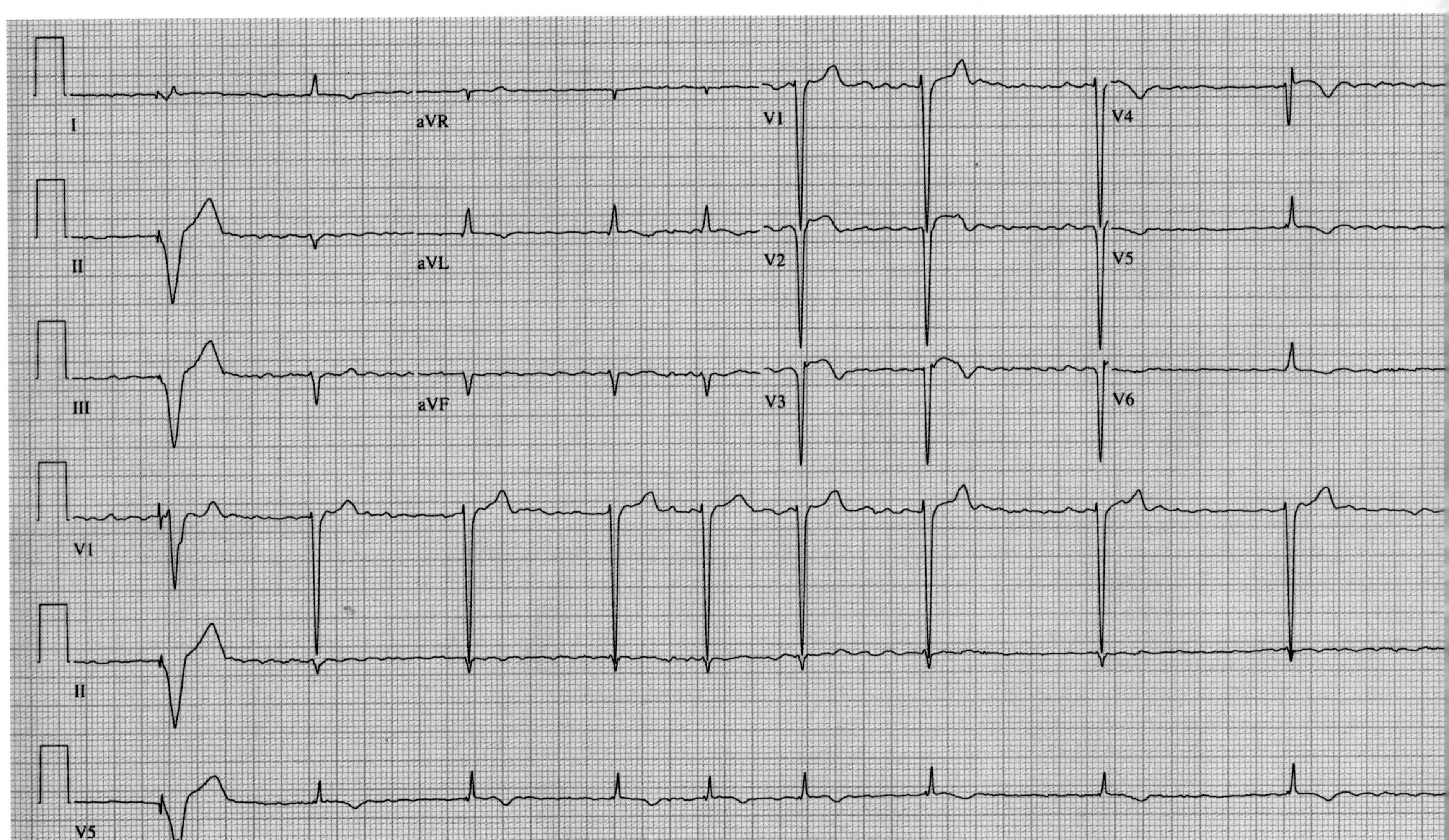

Interpretation Notes:

Electrocardiogram Case Study #58

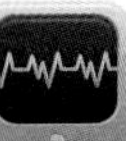

ELECTROCARDIOGRAM INTERPRETATION

This electrocardiogram demonstrates no discrete identifiable atrial activity. This confirms the presence of atrial fibrillation with an average ventricular response of approximately 60 per minute. The first QRS complex is widened with a discrete deflection preceding the QRS complex inscription indicative of one ventricular paced complex. In the limb leads, the QRS complexes are <0.5 mV in amplitude consistent with low-voltage QRS complex in the limb leads. The QRS complex vector is positive in lead I and negative in leads II, III, and aVF supporting left anterior fascicular block. An R wave is demonstrated in lead V1 with a Q wave in leads V2 and V3. A diminutive R wave is present in lead V4. This is consistent with an anteroseptal myocardial infarction, age indeterminate. The J point is elevated with upward coving and elevation of the ST segment suggesting, in the presence of Q waves, an acute myocardial infarction. Lateral nonspecific ST-T changes are also seen.

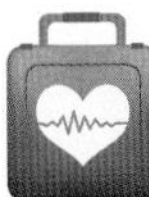

KEY DIAGNOSES

- Atrial fibrillation
- Ventricular pacemaker
- Low-voltage QRS complex limb leads
- Left anterior fascicular block
- Anteroseptal myocardial infarction, age indeterminate
- Left ventricular aneurysm

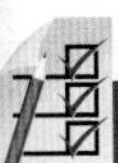

KEY TEACHING POINTS

- By history, the patient was being seen in the outpatient department and while not feeling well, was not having signs or symptoms of an acute coronary syndrome. A prior echocardiogram documented the presence of a left ventricular aneurysm in the left anterior descending coronary artery territory and this explains the persistent ST-segment elevation and ST-segment contour change.
- Left anterior fascicular block does not preclude the diagnosis of an anteroseptal myocardial infarction. A prominent and deep Q wave is seen in lead V3 and a very small R wave is seen in lead V4 with upward coving and ST-segment elevation. These collective findings confirm a prior left anterior descending coronary artery territory myocardial infarction.

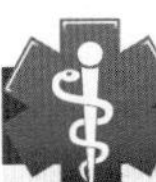

BOARD EXAMINATION ESSENTIALS

Appropriate diagnostic codes for the board exam include atrial fibrillation; left anterior fascicular block; low voltage; limb leads; anteroseptal myocardial infarction, age indeterminate; ventricular demand pacemaker (VVI), normally functioning. Given the patient's lack of symptoms consistent with an acute coronary syndrome, the J-point and the ST-segment elevation demonstrated in leads V1, V2, V3, and V4 support the presence of a left ventricular aneurysm. Since this diagnostic code does not appear on the board exam, it is a useful clinical indicator in terms of probable left ventricular systolic dysfunction but not directly applicable to board exam coding. This concept may appear in another format on the exam and it is important to keep this electrocardiogram pattern in mind.

Electrocardiogram Case Study #59

CLINICAL HISTORY

A 58-year-old female with a history of hypertrophic cardiomyopathy, status post open-heart surgery and myectomy.

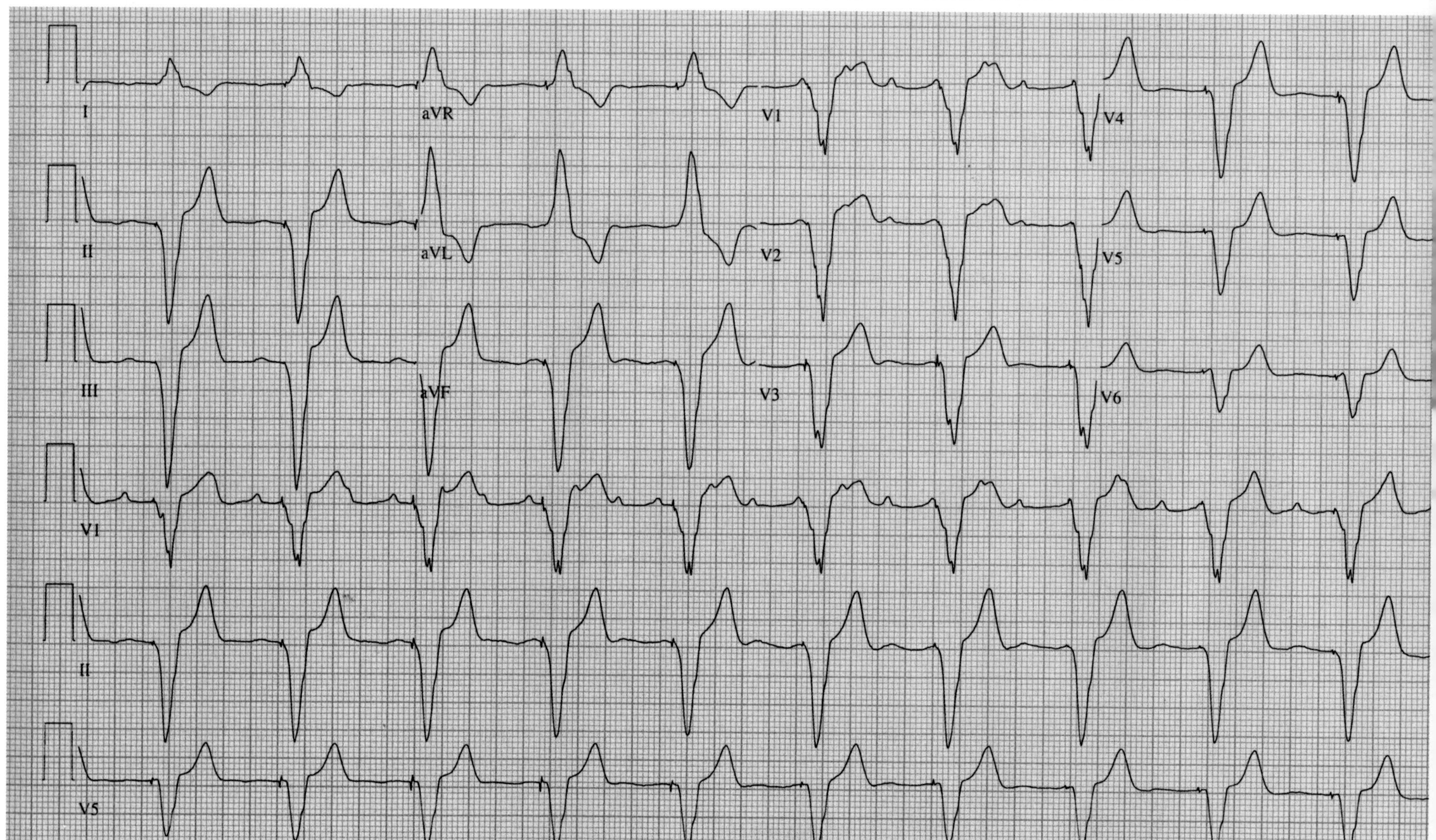

Interpretation Notes:

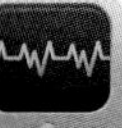

ELECTROCARDIOGRAM INTERPRETATION

This electrocardiogram demonstrates widened QRS complexes at a rate slightly >60 per minute with a narrow deflection preceding each QRS complex consistent with a ventricular pacemaker. P waves are readily identified occurring at regular intervals and demonstrate an abnormal P-wave axis given the negative P-wave vector in leads I, II, and aVL at an atrial rate of approximately 230 per minute. This is most consistent with an ectopic atrial tachycardia. The P waves demonstrate no relation to the QRS complexes reflecting the presence of complete heart block.

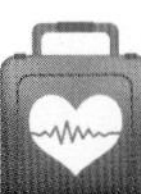

KEY DIAGNOSES

- Ectopic atrial tachycardia
- Ventricular pacemaker
- Complete heart block

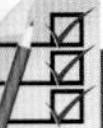

KEY TEACHING POINTS

- Complete heart block is accurately concluded given the lack of relationship between atrial depolarization and the ventricular paced complexes. Additionally, since the ventricular paced complexes occur at regular intervals, there is no evident atrioventricular conduction.
- The presence of QRS complex left-axis deviation is an expected finding given the location of the ventricular pacemaker lead in the right ventricular apex. Cardiac depolarization is reversed, occurring from the cardiac apex to base opposite the inferior leads II, III, and aVF.

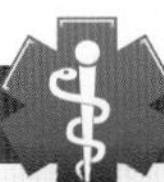

BOARD EXAMINATION ESSENTIALS

For board exam diagnostic coding, this is an example of a ventricular demand pacemaker (VVI) functioning normally. In addition, atrial tachycardia and complete heart block are present. In the presence of a ventricular pacemaker, do not code for QRS complex-axis deviation or conduction abnormalities such as complete left bundle branch block. Additionally, since this represents atrial tachycardia, the P-wave axis is not applicable as it pertains to assessing atrial abnormality/enlargement.

Electrocardiogram Case Study #60

CLINICAL HISTORY

An 82-year-old female with severe coronary artery disease including a left main coronary artery stenosis who is admitted urgently to the coronary intensive care unit with profound hypotension and intermittent wide-complex tachycardia.

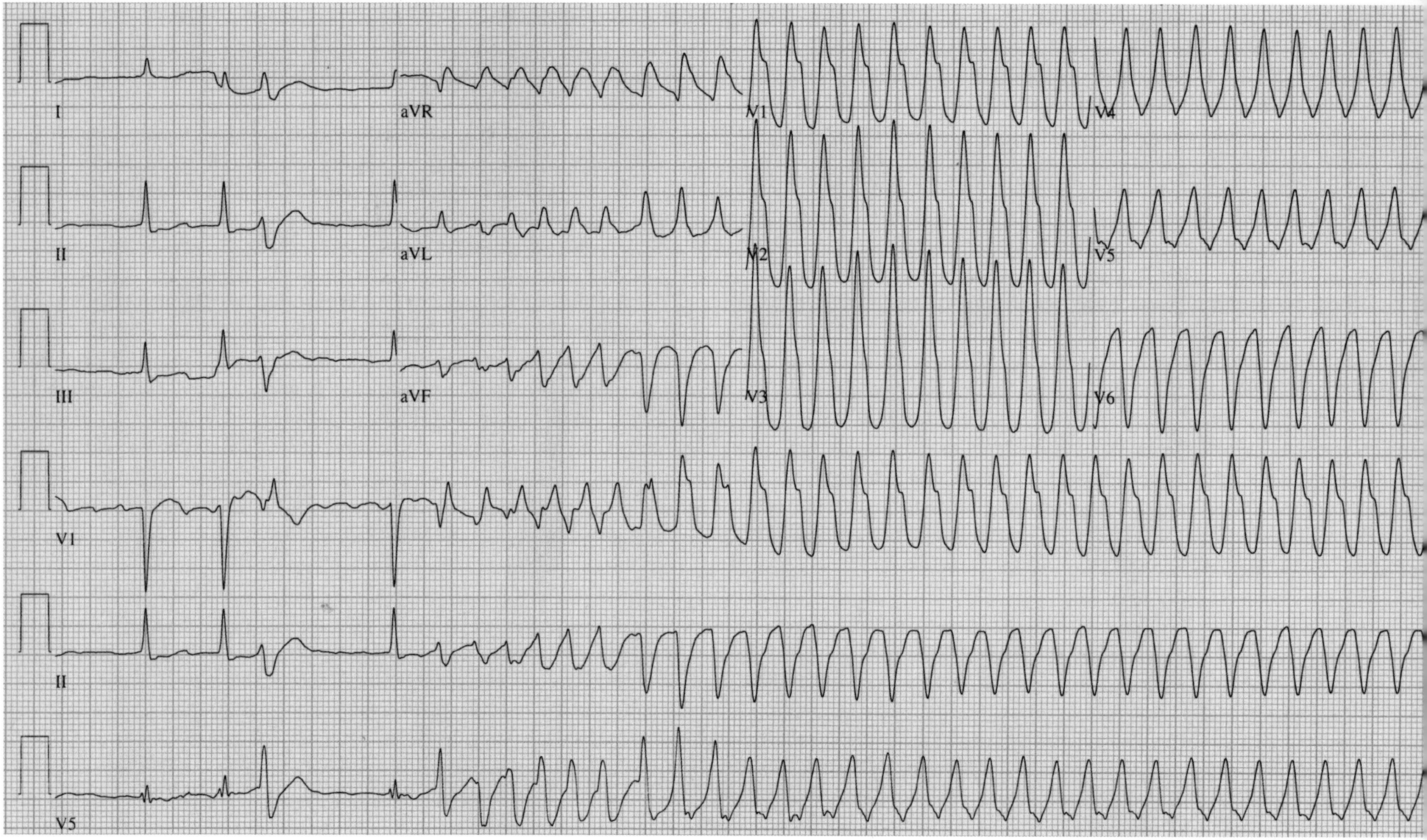

I aVR V1 V4
II aVL V2 V5
III aVF V3 V6
V1
II
V5

Interpretation Notes:

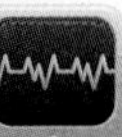

ELECTROCARDIOGRAM INTERPRETATION

On the left-hand portion, this electrocardiogram demonstrates no discernible organized atrial activity. This is consistent with atrial fibrillation. The third QRS complex represents a premature ventricular complex. Nonspecific ST-T changes are seen in leads I, II, and III. After the fourth QRS complex, a wide-complex tachycardic rhythm commences. The wide-complex tachycardia demonstrates monophasic R-wave morphology in lead V1 most consistent with ventricular tachycardia with a cycle length of approximately 250 milliseconds.

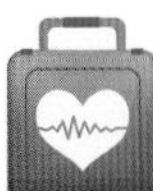

KEY DIAGNOSES

- Atrial fibrillation
- Premature ventricular complex
- Nonspecific ST-T changes
- Ventricular tachycardia

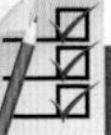

KEY TEACHING POINTS

- The paroxysm of ventricular tachycardia is initiated by a premature ventricular complex that is superimposed on the preceding T wave, best seen in leads aVL and aVF. A short period of torsade de pointes begins followed by a regular monomorphic tachycardia consistent with ventricular tachycardia.
- The ventricular tachycardia is extremely rapid in the presence of severe coronary artery disease likely resulting in profound myocardial ischemia, left ventricular systolic dysfunction, and hemodynamic compromise. The patient expired shortly after this electrocardiogram was obtained.

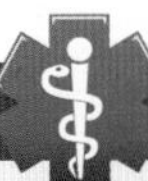

BOARD EXAMINATION ESSENTIALS

The first portion of this electrocardiogram demonstrates atrial fibrillation and nonspecific ST- and/or T-wave abnormalities. The third QRS complex is a ventricular premature complex. All three of these diagnoses should be coded for the board exam. What follows is a period of sustained ventricular tachycardia (three or more consecutive complexes). This should also be coded.

Electrocardiogram Case Study #61

CLINICAL HISTORY

A 29-year-old female with intermittent heart racing and associated lightheadedness who is referred to cardiovascular medicine for further evaluation.

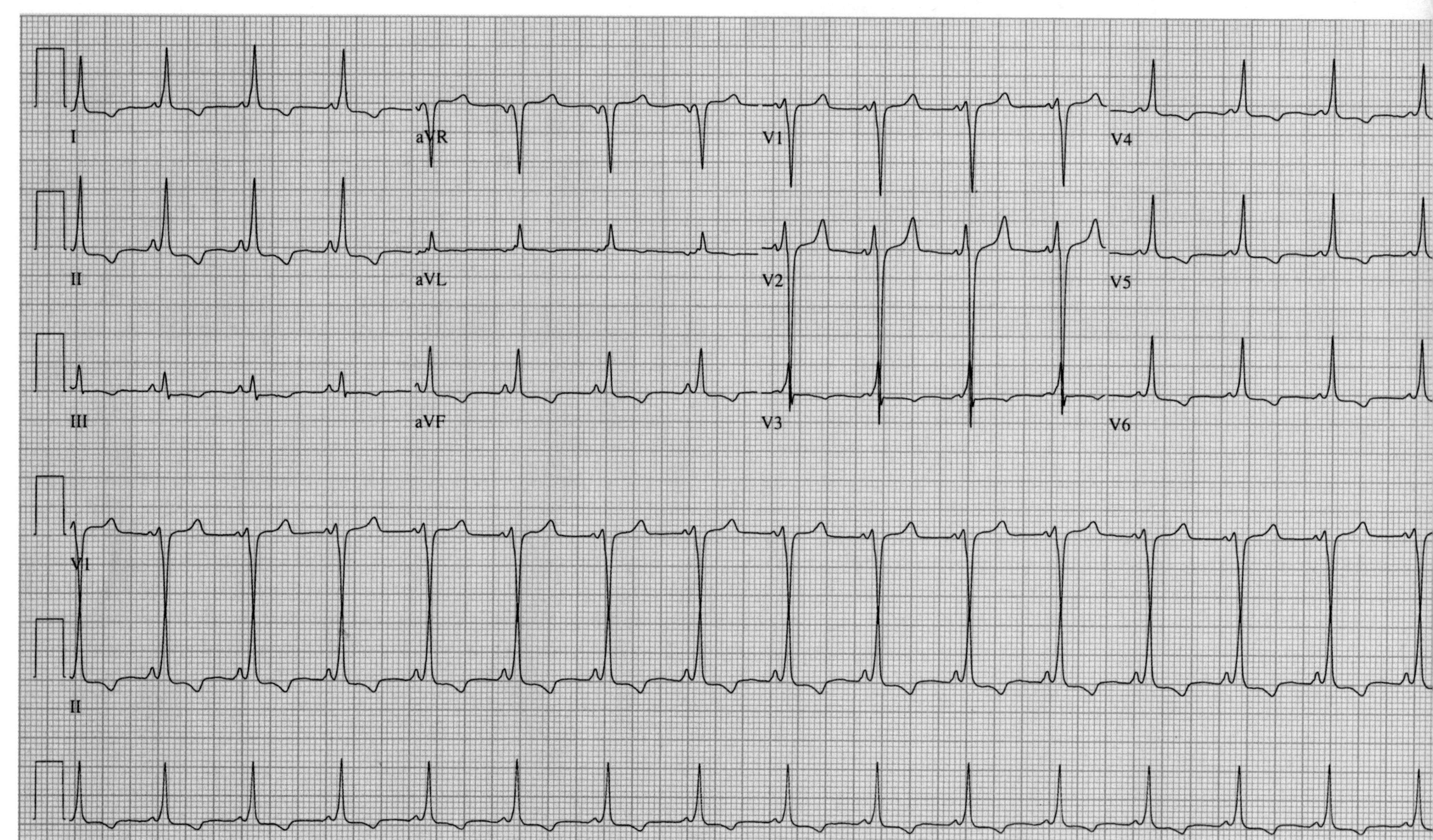

Interpretation Notes:

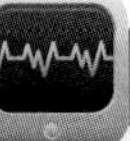

ELECTROCARDIOGRAM INTERPRETATION

This electrocardiogram demonstrates a normal P-wave axis at an atrial rate slightly <100 per minute consistent with normal sinus rhythm. In all leads, the PR interval is shortened and there is a slurred upstroke to the QRS complex consistent with ventricular pre-excitation and the Wolff-Parkinson-White syndrome. Diffuse nonspecific ST-T changes are also present.

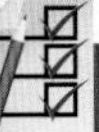

KEY TEACHING POINTS

- Ventricular pre-excitation in the Wolff-Parkinson-White syndrome is easily identified on this electrocardiogram given the short PR interval and slurred upstroke to the QRS complex. The repolarization changes identified in all leads is associated with abnormal ventricular activation via the accessory pathway.
- The repolarization changes suggest that the QRS complexes are fusion complexes reflecting simultaneous ventricular depolarization via normal antegrade conduction and also via the accessory pathway.

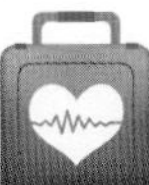

KEY DIAGNOSES

- Normal sinus rhythm
- Wolff-Parkinson-White syndrome

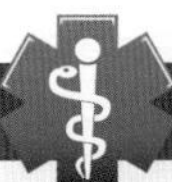

BOARD EXAMINATION ESSENTIALS

Expect to see a least one example of Wolff-Parkinson-White pattern on the board exam. This example demonstrates normal sinus rhythm and Wolff-Parkinson-White pattern. The ST segments and the T waves are abnormal and are due to ventricular pre-excitation. They do not necessitate additional coding. The PR interval is short as is expected with ventricular pre-excitation and no additional code is necessary.

Electrocardiogram Case Study #62

CLINICAL HISTORY

A 34-year-old female with sudden-onset palpitations and lightheadedness occurring intermittently over the past 12 months.

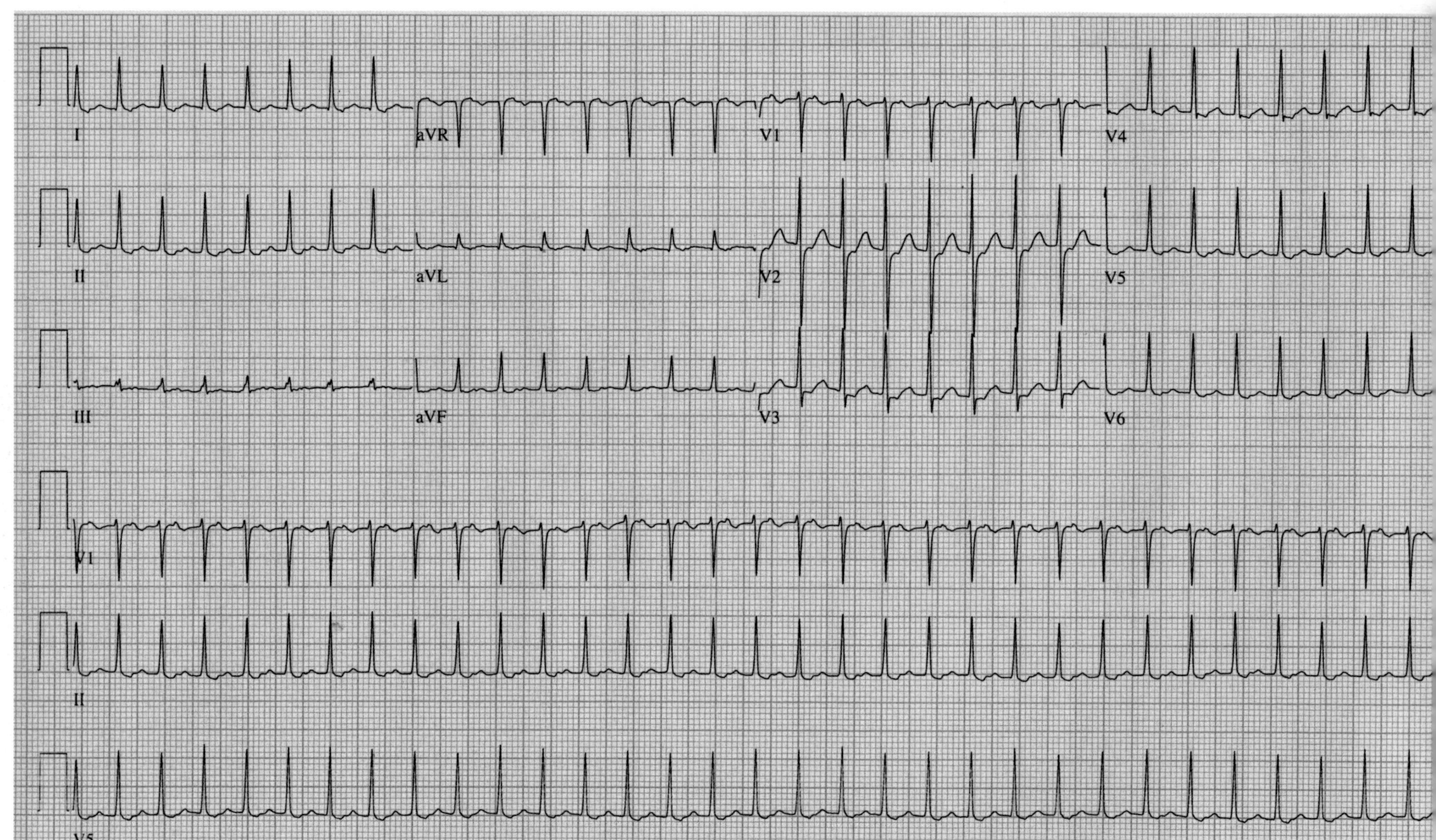

Interpretation Notes:

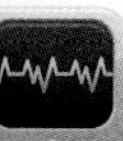

ELECTROCARDIOGRAM INTERPRETATION

This electrocardiogram demonstrates a narrow complex tachycardia with a cycle length of 310 milliseconds corresponding to an approximate heart rate of 190 per minute. P waves are identified perhaps best in lead V1 after the QRS complex. P waves are also seen within the ST segment of lead II and inverted P waves are seen within the ST segment of leads V4, V5, and V6.

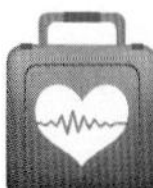

KEY DIAGNOSES

- Supraventricular tachycardia

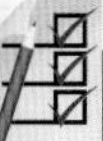

KEY TEACHING POINTS

- This narrow complex tachycardia demonstrates a short RP, long PR interval. Differential diagnostic possibilities include typical AV nodal re-entrant tachycardia, atrial tachycardia with first-degree atrioventricular block, and orthodromic atrioventricular reciprocating tachycardia as seen in the presence of an accessory bypass tract.
- This patient underwent electrophysiology study and an accessory bypass tract was confirmed. A successful intracardiac ablation of the accessory bypass tract was performed without symptomatic recurrence of her tachyarrhythmias.

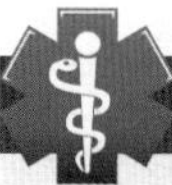

BOARD EXAMINATION ESSENTIALS

This electrocardiogram warrants a single diagnostic code, supraventricular tachycardia. Nonspecific ST- and T-wave changes are noted and they are secondary to the tachycardia. They do not necessitate an additional diagnostic code. No other abnormalities are identified on this electrocardiogram. An accessory pathway is not able to be diagnosed with certainty and is therefore not coded.

Electrocardiogram Case Study #63

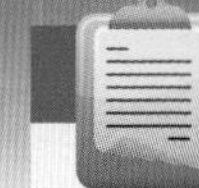

CLINICAL HISTORY

A 55-year-old female with recent-onset exertional shortness of breath and anterior chest pressure who presents to cardiovascular medicine after her primary care physician auscultated a systolic heart murmur.

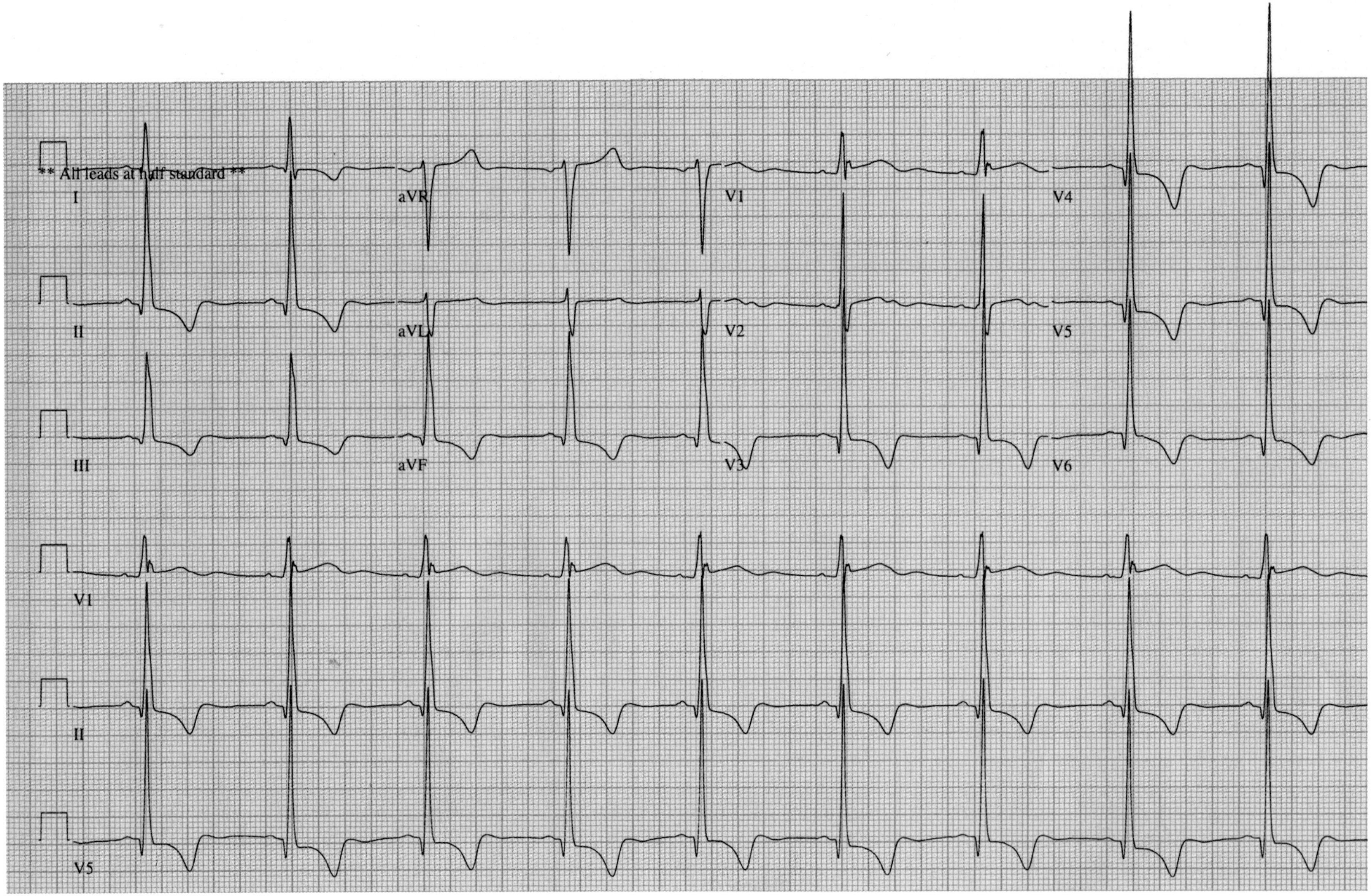

** All leads at half standard **

I aVR V1 V4

II aVL V2 V5

III aVF V3 V6

V1

II

V5

Interpretation Notes:

Electrocardiogram Case Study #63

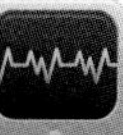

ELECTROCARDIOGRAM INTERPRETATION

This electrocardiogram demonstrates P waves with a normal axis at a rate slightly less than 60 per minute consistent with sinus bradycardia. The QRS complex is >100 milliseconds without a specific conduction morphology best described as a nonspecific intraventricular conduction delay. All leads are obtained at half standardization. Despite this, prominent QRS complex voltage is seen particularly in leads V4, V5, V6, II, and aVF. Asymmetric T-wave inversion is also seen in these leads supporting left ventricular hypertrophy with secondary ST-T changes. A prominent R wave is noted in leads V1 and V2 supporting right ventricular hypertrophy. This electrocardiogram is an example of biventricular hypertrophy as seen in a patient with hypertrophic cardiomyopathy.

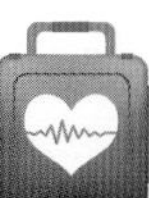

KEY DIAGNOSES

- Sinus bradycardia
- Nonspecific intraventricular conduction delay
- Left ventricular hypertrophy with secondary ST-T changes
- Right ventricular hypertrophy
- Biventricular hypertrophy
- Hypertrophic cardiomyopathy

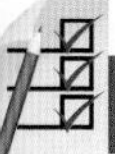

KEY TEACHING POINTS

- Q waves are noted in the inferior, anteroseptal, anterior, and lateral leads. The Q waves in this particular case do not reflect a myocardial infarction but instead represent depolarization of a markedly thickened interventricular septum.
- The Rsr′ QRS complex pattern in lead V1 suggests right ventricular conduction delay. Despite this, it is not typical for a right bundle branch block pattern and, thus, a nonspecific intraventricular conduction delay most accurately describes this finding.

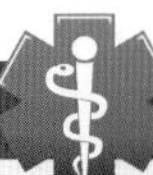

BOARD EXAMINATION ESSENTIALS

Appropriate board exam diagnostic codes for this electrocardiogram include the clinical disorder hypertrophic cardiomyopathy, sinus bradycardia, combined ventricular hypertrophy, ST- and/or T-wave abnormalities secondary to hypertrophy and intraventricular conduction disturbance, nonspecific type. Despite the common finding of atrial abnormality/enlargement with hypertrophy patterns, there is no clear evidence of atrial abnormality/enlargement on this electrocardiogram.

Electrocardiogram Case Study #64

CLINICAL HISTORY

A 43-year-old male with the acute onset of severe anterior chest pain. He drove himself immediately to the emergency room arriving within 30 minutes of chest pain onset. This electrocardiogram was obtained upon emergency room arrival and the patient was taken immediately to the cardiac catheterization laboratory.

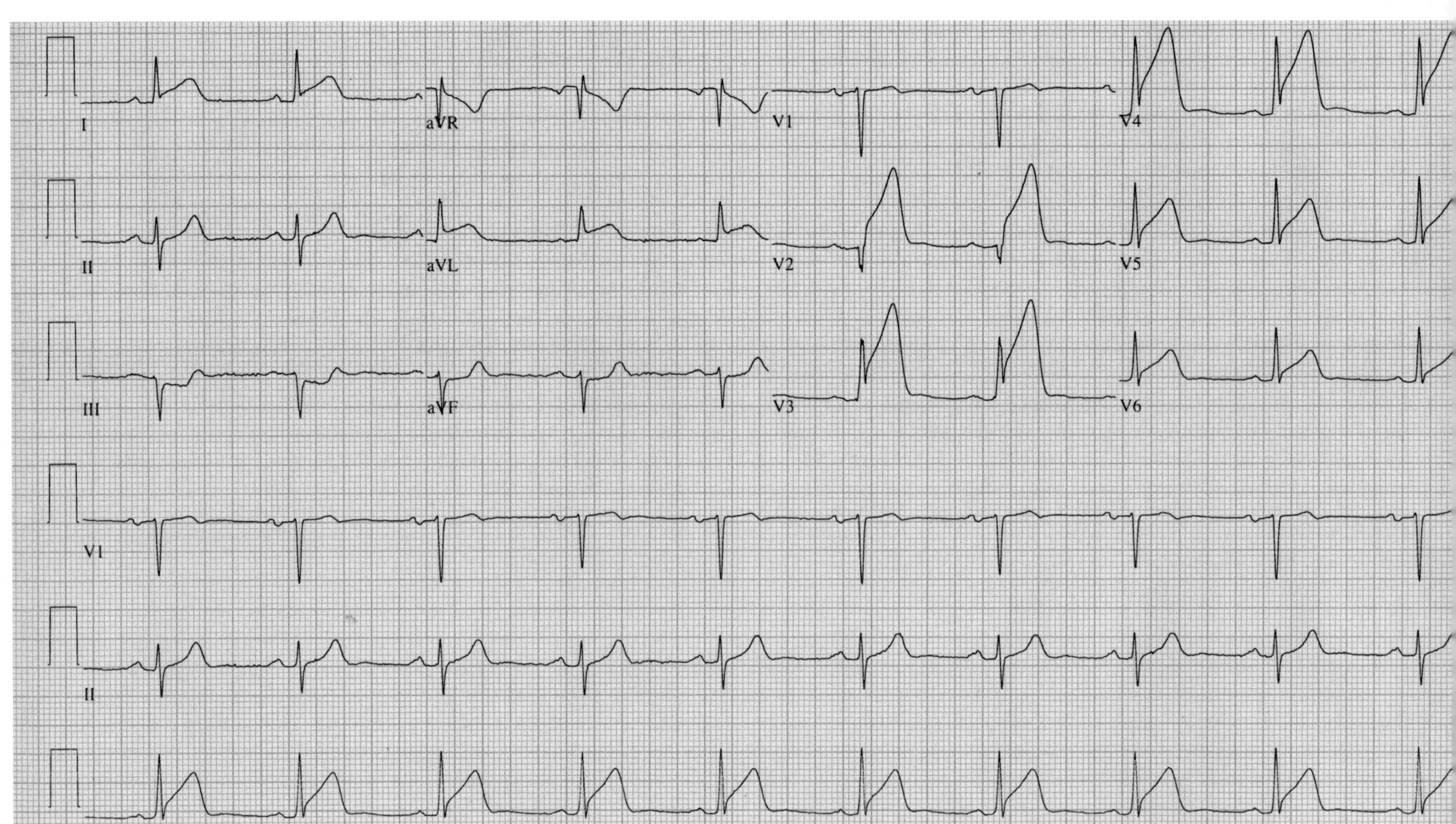

Interpretation Notes:

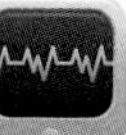

ELECTROCARDIOGRAM INTERPRETATION

This electrocardiogram demonstrates P waves with a normal axis at a rate of 60 per minute consistent with normal sinus rhythm. The QRS complex vector is positive in lead I, isoelectric in lead II and negative in leads III and aVF. This is consistent with QRS complex left-axis deviation. J-point elevation, ST-segment straightening and ST-segment elevation is identified in leads V2, V3, V4, V5, V6, I, and aVL. Reciprocal ST-segment depression is seen in lead III and less so in lead aVF. This is consistent with acute myocardial injury in the left anterior descending coronary artery distribution.

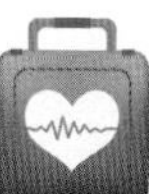

KEY DIAGNOSES

- Normal sinus rhythm
- Left-axis deviation
- Acute myocardial injury

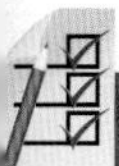

KEY TEACHING POINTS

- Note the lack of J-point and ST-segment elevation in lead V1. This supports a left anterior descending coronary artery occlusion after the first major septal perforator branch.
- The J-point and ST-segment elevation in leads I and aVL reflects a large diagonal branch that perfuses the high lateral myocardial territory.
- An urgent cardiac catheterization confirmed a left anterior descending coronary artery acute thrombosis just beyond the first septal perforator branch and also proximal to major diagonal branches in the setting of a nondominant left circumflex coronary artery.

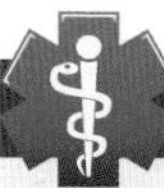

BOARD EXAMINATION ESSENTIALS

This electrocardiogram supports normal sinus rhythm. J-point and ST-segment elevation is demonstrated in leads V2 through V6, 1 and aVL consistent with ST- and/or T-wave abnormalities suggesting myocardial injury. Reciprocal ST- and T-wave findings are seen in leads III and aVF and do not merit diagnostic coding. Left-axis deviation (greater than –30 degrees) is identified and should be coded. There is no evidence of a Q-wave myocardial infarction and, therefore, an infarction pattern should not be coded for the board exam.

Electrocardiogram Case Study #65

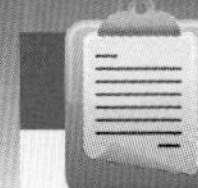

CLINICAL HISTORY

A 79-year-old male admitted to the hospital with mental status changes and urosepsis. The patient has a history of ischemic heart disease and an episode of decompensated congestive heart failure 6 months prior to this electrocardiogram being obtained.

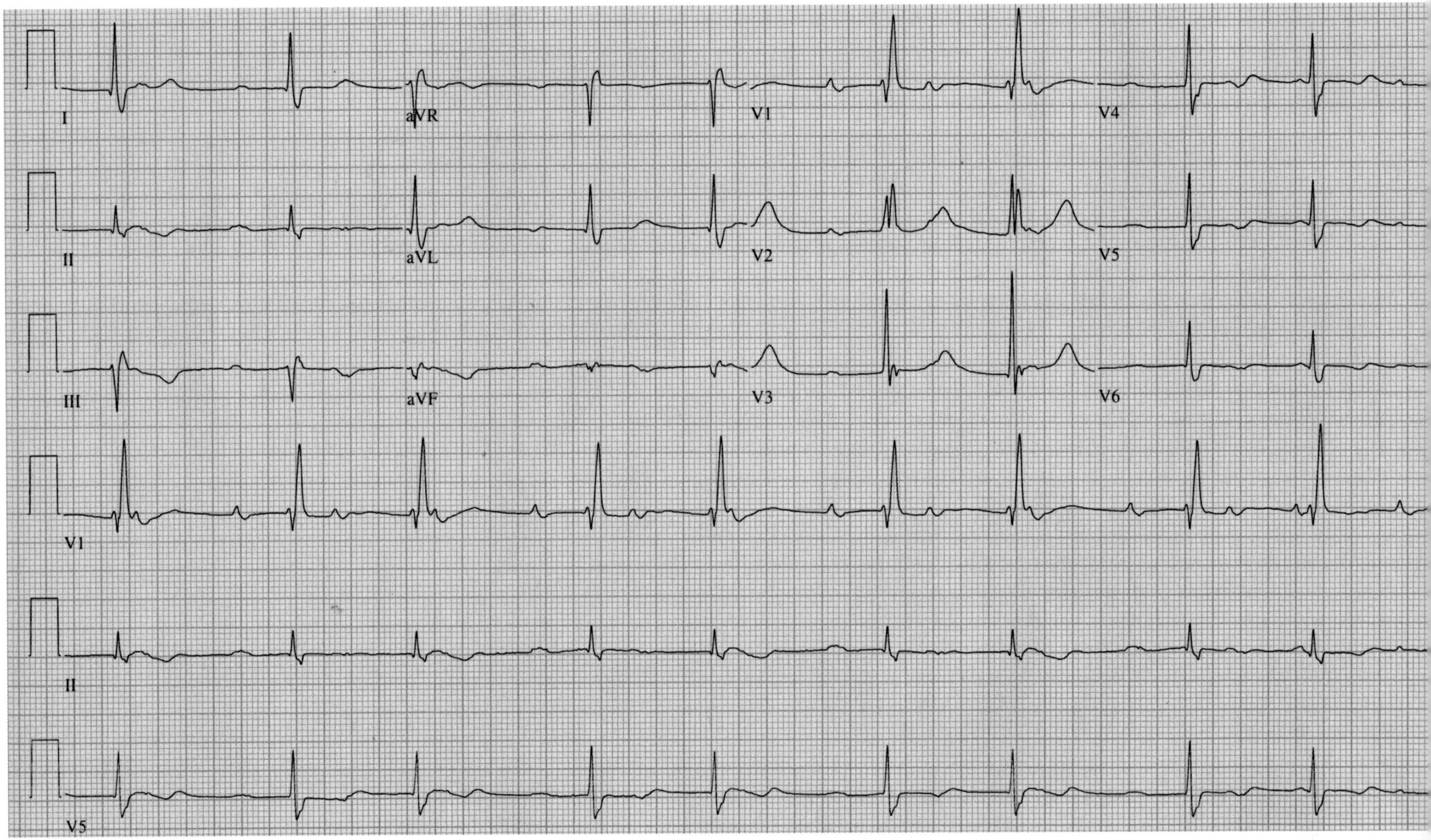

Interpretation Notes:

Electrocardiogram Case Study #65

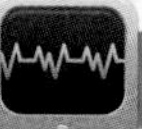

ELECTROCARDIOGRAM INTERPRETATION

This electrocardiogram demonstrates P waves occurring at a constant interval with a normal P-wave axis at a rate of 80 per minute consistent with normal sinus rhythm. Grouped QRS complexes are identified with a P wave to QRS complex ratio of 3:2 and progressive prolongation of the PR interval consistent with 3:2 Mobitz type I Wenckebach atrioventricular block. The third P wave of this sequence is located at the terminal aspect of the QRS complex followed by a nonconducted QRS complex. The P-wave morphology demonstrates terminal negativity in lead V1 and a prolonged duration of >110 milliseconds in lead II consistent with left atrial abnormality. Q waves >40-millisecond duration are present in the second QRS complex in lead III and also in lead aVF supporting the presence of an age-indeterminate inferior myocardial infarction. The QRS complex duration is prolonged at 120 milliseconds with an rsR′ QRS complex pattern in lead V1 and terminal S-wave conduction delay seen in leads I, aVL, V4, V5, and V6 consistent with complete right bundle-branch block. Lateral nonspecific ST-T changes that may be related to the inferior myocardial infarction are also seen.

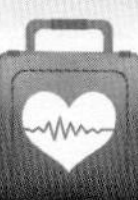

KEY DIAGNOSES

- Normal sinus rhythm
- Left atrial abnormality
- Mobitz I Wenckebach atrioventricular block
- Inferior myocardial infarction, age indeterminate
- Posterior myocardial infarction, age indeterminate
- Complete right bundle-branch block
- Primary T-wave changes

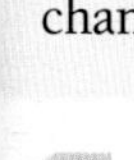

KEY TEACHING POINTS

- As for any electrocardiogram, identification of the heart rhythm is the most important first step. In this circumstance, the P to P interval is constant at a rate >60 per minute consistent with normal sinus rhythm. It is important to identify the P to P interval and define the P-wave relationship to the QRS complexes. Once the P to P interval is identified, the third nonconducted P wave within the Wenckebach sequence is more readily seen overlying the terminal aspect of the QRS complex. Wenckebach periodicity is thus more apparent following this algorithm.
- Lead aVF is the most important lead to assess for diagnostic Q waves in the right coronary artery or inferior myocardial distribution. Even in the absence of Q waves in leads II and III, Q waves of diagnostic duration solely identified in lead aVF are typically sufficient to meet the criteria of an age-indeterminate inferior myocardial infarction.
- Positive T waves are identified in leads V2 and V3 in the presence of complete right bundle-branch block. These represent primary T-wave changes and may reflect posterior involvement of the inferior myocardial infarction. Cardiac imaging such as echocardiography can confirm or refute this suspicion.

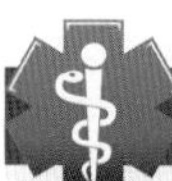

BOARD EXAMINATION ESSENTIALS

When considering the board exam, diagnostic codes include normal sinus rhythm; AV block, second degree—Mobitz type I (Wenckebach); left atrial abnormality/enlargement; inferior myocardial infarction, age indeterminate, based on the Q waves in lead aVF; possible posterior myocardial infarction, age indeterminate given the primary T-wave changes in leads V2 and V3 plus a prominent R wave in lead V2; and complete right bundle-branch block. This latter posterior myocardial infarction diagnosis is not conclusive and should not be coded. Should a posterior myocardial infarction appear on the board exam, anticipate the R-wave amplitude to be greater than the S-wave amplitude in lead V1 associated with either inferior or lateral Q waves of diagnostic duration.

Electrocardiogram Case Study #66

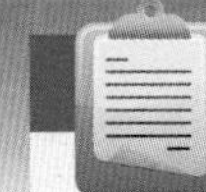

CLINICAL HISTORY

A 77-year-old male with a history of coronary artery disease admitted to the hospital anticipating near future abdominal aortic aneurysm reparative surgery.

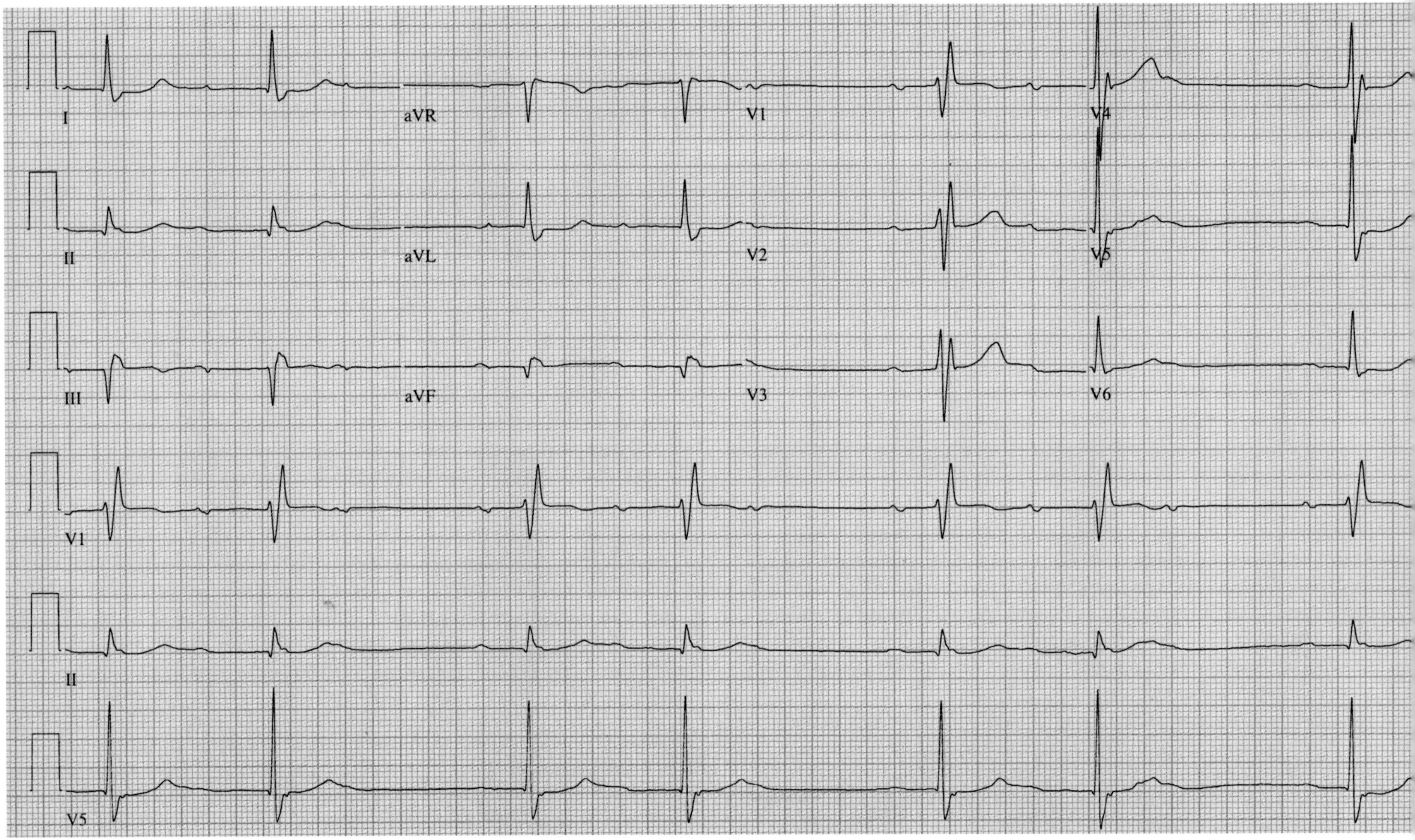

I aVR V1 V4

II aVL V2 V5

III aVF V3 V6

V1

II

V5

Interpretation Notes:

Electrocardiogram Case Study #66

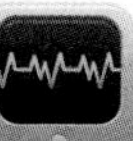

ELECTROCARDIOGRAM INTERPRETATION

This electrocardiogram demonstrates P waves of normal axis at a rate of 60 per minute. The P waves conduct to the ventricle with a progressively prolonging PR interval with a 3:2 atrial to ventricular conduction ratio consistent with Mobitz type I Wenckebach atrioventricular block. The P wave demonstrates terminal negativity in lead V1 consistent with left atrial abnormality. In leads II, III, and aVF, inferior Q waves of diagnostic duration are seen consistent with an age-indeterminate inferior myocardial infarction. Complete right bundle-branch block is also present as the QRS complex is approximately 150 milliseconds and demonstrates an rSR′ conduction pattern. Primary T-wave changes are present with upright T waves in leads V1, V2, and V3. This patient had undergone prior coronary arteriography and also transthoracic echocardiography. A complete right coronary artery occlusion was identified with minimal collateral flow. Additionally, both studies demonstrated an inferior basal left ventricular aneurysm. The ST-segment elevation that is demonstrated in leads III and aVF is consistent with the presence of an inferior basal left ventricular aneurysm.

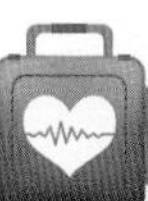

KEY DIAGNOSES

- Normal sinus rhythm
- Mobitz type I Wenckebach atrioventricular block
- Inferior myocardial infarction, age indeterminate
- Complete right bundle-branch block
- Primary T-wave changes
- Left ventricular aneurysm
- Left atrial abnormality

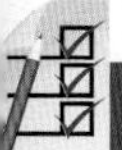

KEY TEACHING POINTS

- The electrocardiogram may be the first clinical manifestation of a left ventricular aneurysm. Persistent ST-segment elevation in an age-indeterminate myocardial infarction territory should raise left ventricular aneurysm as a diagnostic possibility. Further cardiac imaging to include echocardiography is the next best step.
- R-wave regression is seen transitioning from lead V5 to lead V6 and also, a small Q wave is seen in lead V6. The Q wave is not of diagnostic duration. R-wave regression coupled with a Q wave in lead V6 in the context of inferior Q waves suggests the possibility of lateral extension of the inferior myocardial infarction. Since the Q wave is not of diagnostic duration (40 milliseconds), this is not a diagnostic certainty.

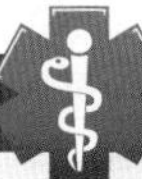

BOARD EXAMINATION ESSENTIALS

Appropriate board exam coding diagnoses include normal sinus rhythm; AV block, second degree—Mobitz type I (Wenckebach); inferior myocardial infarction, age indeterminate; complete right bundle-branch block. The diminutive Q wave in lead V6 is not of diagnostic duration to code a lateral myocardial infarction of indeterminate age. The terminal negativity of the P wave in lead V1 supports the presence of left atrial abnormality/enlargement. This would also be an appropriate diagnostic code for this electrocardiogram.

Electrocardiogram Case Study #67

CLINICAL HISTORY

A 55-year-old female with longstanding hypertension and severe bicuspid aortic valve stenosis.

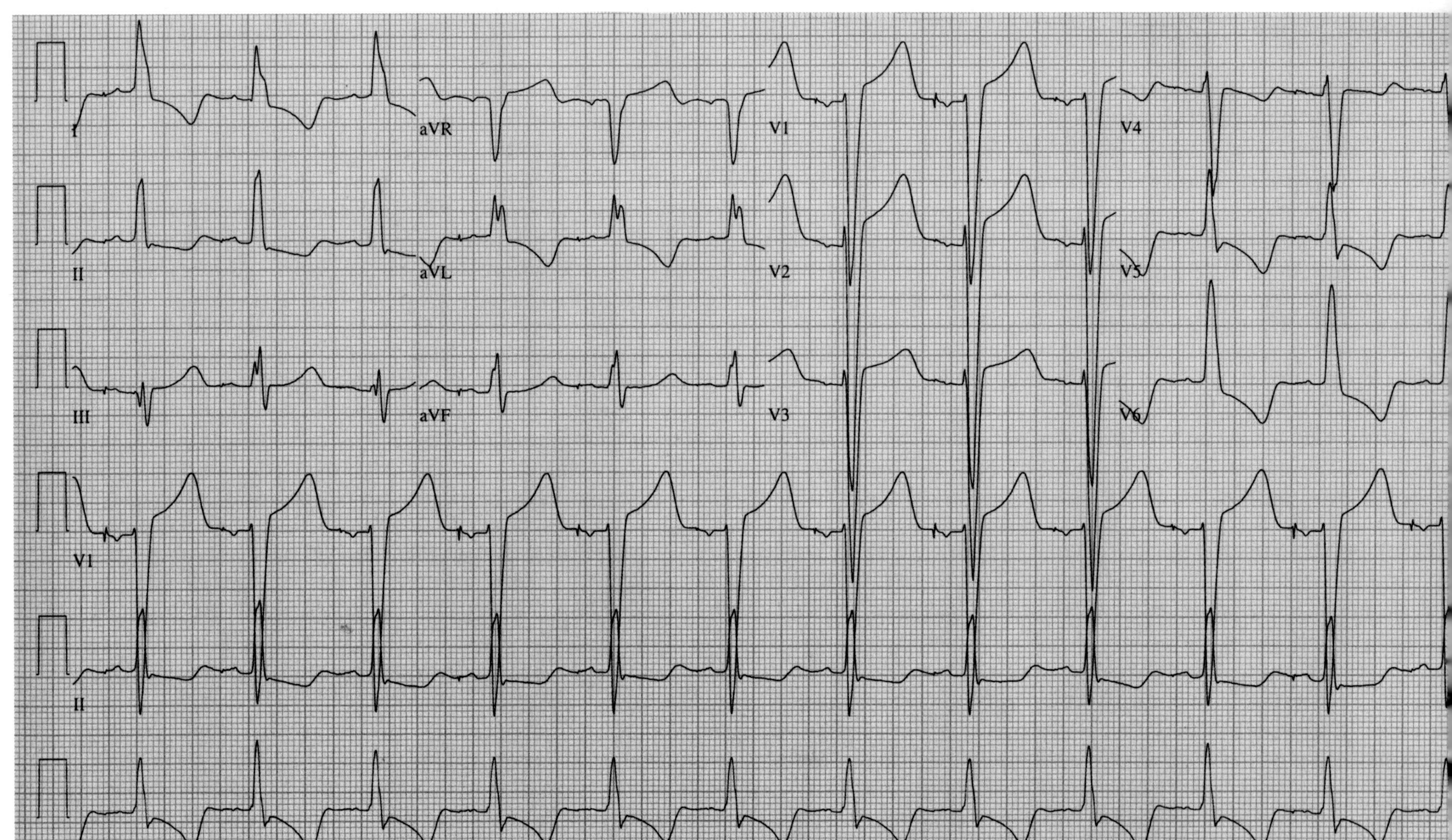

Interpretation Notes:

Electrocardiogram Case Study #67

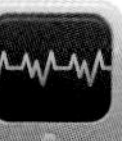

ELECTROCARDIOGRAM INTERPRETATION

This electrocardiogram demonstrates a discrete deflection preceding each P wave supporting the presence of an electronic atrial pacemaker. The QRS complex duration is prolonged measuring approximately 130 milliseconds with a morphology consistent with complete left bundle-branch block.

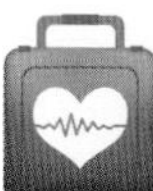

KEY DIAGNOSES

- Atrial pacemaker
- Complete left bundle-branch block

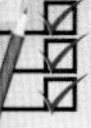

KEY TEACHING POINTS

- This electrocardiogram does not demonstrate atrioventricular pacing. Since the QRS complex demonstrates a complete left bundle-branch block morphology, in the presence of an atrial pacemaker, one might assume ventricular pacing is also present. That would be incorrect as a pacemaker deflection is not seen preceding the QRS complex.
- The QRS complex axis does not support the presence of ventricular pacing. In the presence of a ventricular pacemaker, typically the QRS complexes demonstrate a negative QRS complex vector in leads II, III, and aVF. On this electrocardiogram, the QRS complex vector is positive in leads II and aVF.
- In lead III, the QRS complex axis varies with the second QRS complex being positive and the first and the third QRS complexes being negative. This is likely due to respiratory variation and a slight change of cardiac position.

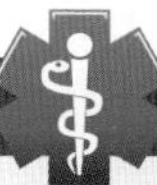

BOARD EXAMINATION ESSENTIALS

Board exam diagnostic codes for this electrocardiogram include atrial or coronary sinus pacing and complete left bundle-branch block. Be careful not to code for atrial morphology such as left atrial abnormality/enlargement in the presence of atrial pacing. Additionally, when complete left bundle-branch block QRS complex morphology is identified, carefully inspect the beginning or proximal portion of the QRS complex to assess for the possibility of diminutive ventricular pacemaker spikes. These are not identified on this electrocardiogram. Do not code for ST- or T-wave changes in the presence of complete left bundle-branch block as they reflect secondary repolarization findings. Lastly, do not code for ventricular hypertrophy patterns in the presence of left bundle-branch block as left ventricular depolarization is abnormal with unopposed vectors that contribute to increased QRS complex voltage of uncertain significance.

Electrocardiogram Case Study #68

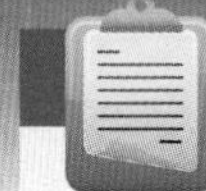

CLINICAL HISTORY

A 54-year-old female with nonischemic left ventricular systolic dysfunction and severe mitral regurgitation who is status post recent mitral valve reparative surgery.

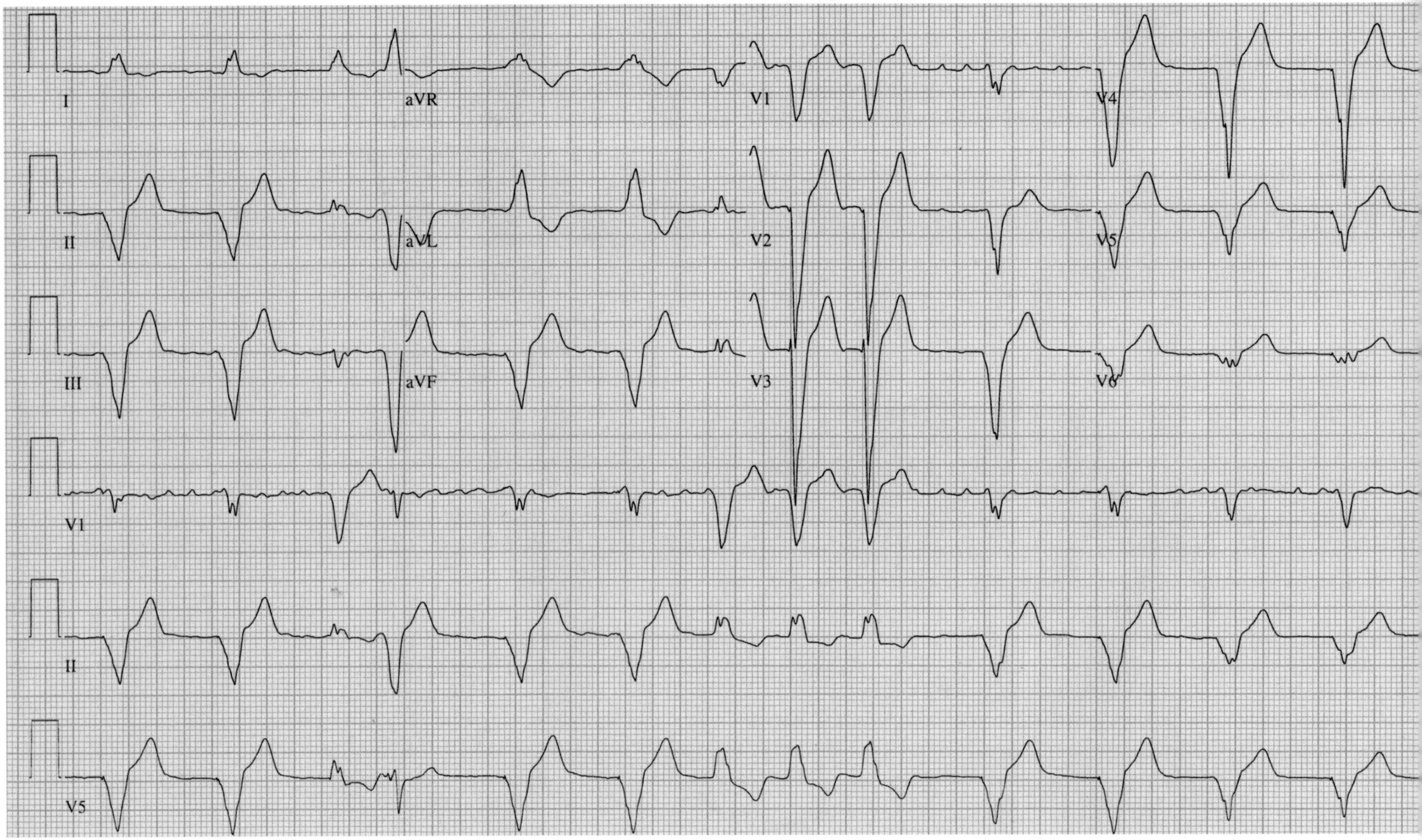

Interpretation Notes:

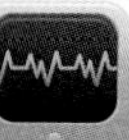

ELECTROCARDIOGRAM INTERPRETATION

This electrocardiogram demonstrates an undulating electrocardiogram baseline without identifiable atrial activity consistent with atrial fibrillation. The 1st, 2nd, 5th, 6th, 10th 11th, 12th, and 13th QRS complexes represent ventricular pacing. The seventh, eighth, and ninth QRS complexes demonstrate a prolonged QRS complex duration with a complete left bundle-branch block morphology. This is consistent with complete left bundle-branch block. The 3rd and the 4th QRS complexes represent intermediate complexes between the native complete left bundle branch block QRS complex morphology and the ventricular paced complexes. These are best classified as pacemaker fusion complexes.

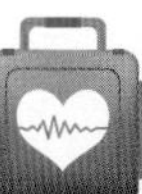

KEY DIAGNOSES

- Atrial fibrillation
- Complete left bundle-branch block
- Ventricular pacemaker
- Pacemaker fusion complexes

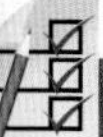

KEY TEACHING POINTS

- It is important to distinguish the native QRS complex morphology from ventricular paced complexes if the electrocardiogram provides the opportunity. On this electrocardiogram, ventricular pacing is intermittent thus permitting the additional diagnosis and identification of complete left bundle branch block.
- This electrocardiogram demonstrates atrial fibrillation. In the lead V1 rhythm strip, the undulating baseline suggests the possibility of atrial flutter. This is an inconsistent finding across the entirety of the electrocardiogram with atrial fibrillation remaining the preferred diagnosis.

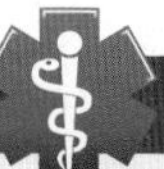

BOARD EXAMINATION ESSENTIALS

Diagnostic codes for the board exam include atrial fibrillation, complete left bundle-branch block, and ventricular demand pacemaker (VVI), normally functioning. Be careful not to code for ventricular tachycardia (three or more consecutive complexes) or myocardial infarction patterns. The Q waves on his electrocardiogram are secondary to ventricular pacing and not diagnostic of a prior myocardial infarction. The QRS complex axis is normal.

Electrocardiogram Case Study #69

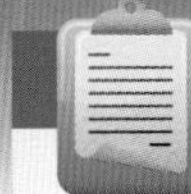

CLINICAL HISTORY

A 50-year-old male who has been experiencing exertional lightheadedness, chest discomfort, and presyncope for the past month. This electrocardiogram was obtained at the time of the initial cardiovascular medicine appointment.

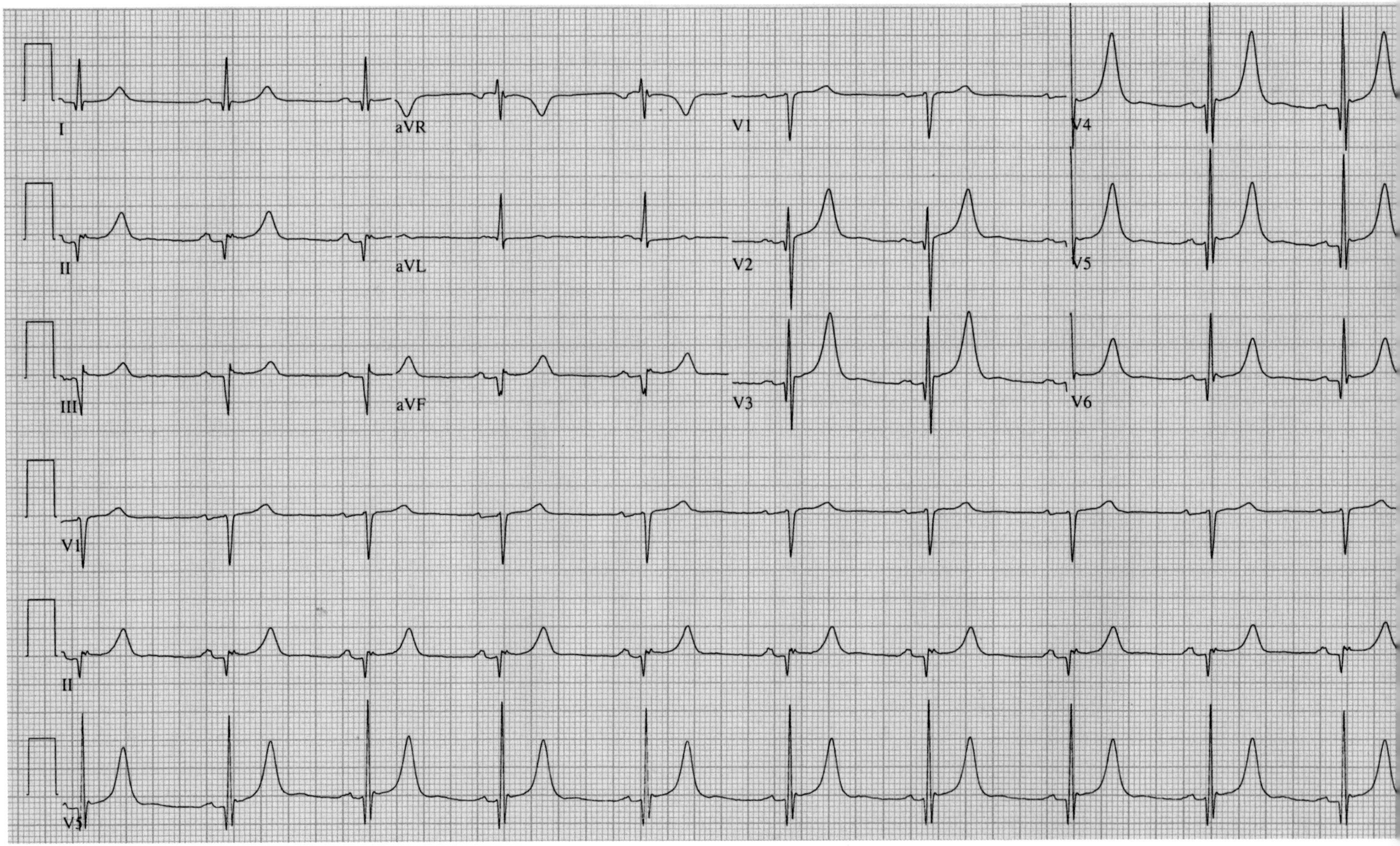

I aVR V1 V4
II aVL V2 V5
III aVF V3 V6
V1
II
V5

Interpretation Notes:

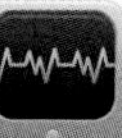

ELECTROCARDIOGRAM INTERPRETATION

This electrocardiogram demonstrates P waves of normal axis occurring at a regular rate slightly less than 60 per minute consistent with sinus bradycardia. Q waves are present in leads V2, V3, V4, V5, and V6. These Q waves are narrow and are not of diagnostic duration to conclude a myocardial infarction with certainty. Q waves are also present in leads II, III, and aVF. In lead aVF, the Q wave is 40 milliseconds in duration suggesting an age-indeterminate inferior myocardial infarction.

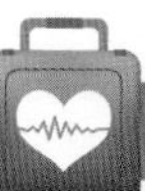

KEY DIAGNOSES

- Sinus bradycardia
- Hypertrophic cardiomyopathy
- Pseudoinfarction pattern

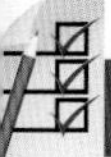

KEY TEACHING POINTS

- This patient was known to suffer from hypertrophic cardiomyopathy. An echocardiogram was performed and the interventricular septal measurement was 2.2 cm and the posterior wall thickness was 1.4 cm confirming asymmetric septal hypertrophy. Regional wall motion was normal without evidence of a prior inferior myocardial infarction.
- The Q waves in leads V2, V3, V4, V5, and V6 reflect septal depolarization of the hypertrophied interventricular septum.
- The inferior Q waves, while suggestive of an inferior myocardial infarction of indeterminate age, are also related to hypertrophic cardiomyopathy. This was corroborated by the echocardiogram finding of normal wall motion in the right coronary artery distribution.
- Hypertrophic cardiomyopathy often demonstrates Q waves spanning coronary artery distributions. Additionally, repolarization abnormalities can be present although they are not seen on this electrocardiogram. Another finding frequently present is left atrial abnormality due to diastolic dysfunction and increased intracardiac pressures.

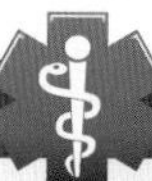

BOARD EXAMINATION ESSENTIALS

With a clinical history supporting the presence of hypertrophic cardiomyopathy, the electrocardiogram findings become readily apparent. Hypertrophic cardiomyopathy is supported and should be coded for on the board exam under the clinical disorder category given the prominent and short duration Q waves that appear in virtually all electrocardiogram leads. Appropriate diagnostic codes thus include sinus bradycardia and hypertrophic cardiomyopathy.

Electrocardiogram Case Study #70

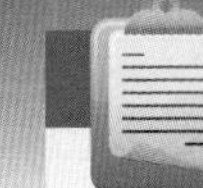

CLINICAL HISTORY

A 73-year-old male with multiple myeloma who underwent this electrocardiogram as part of a routine follow-up evaluation. The patient was not previously diagnosed with heart disease.

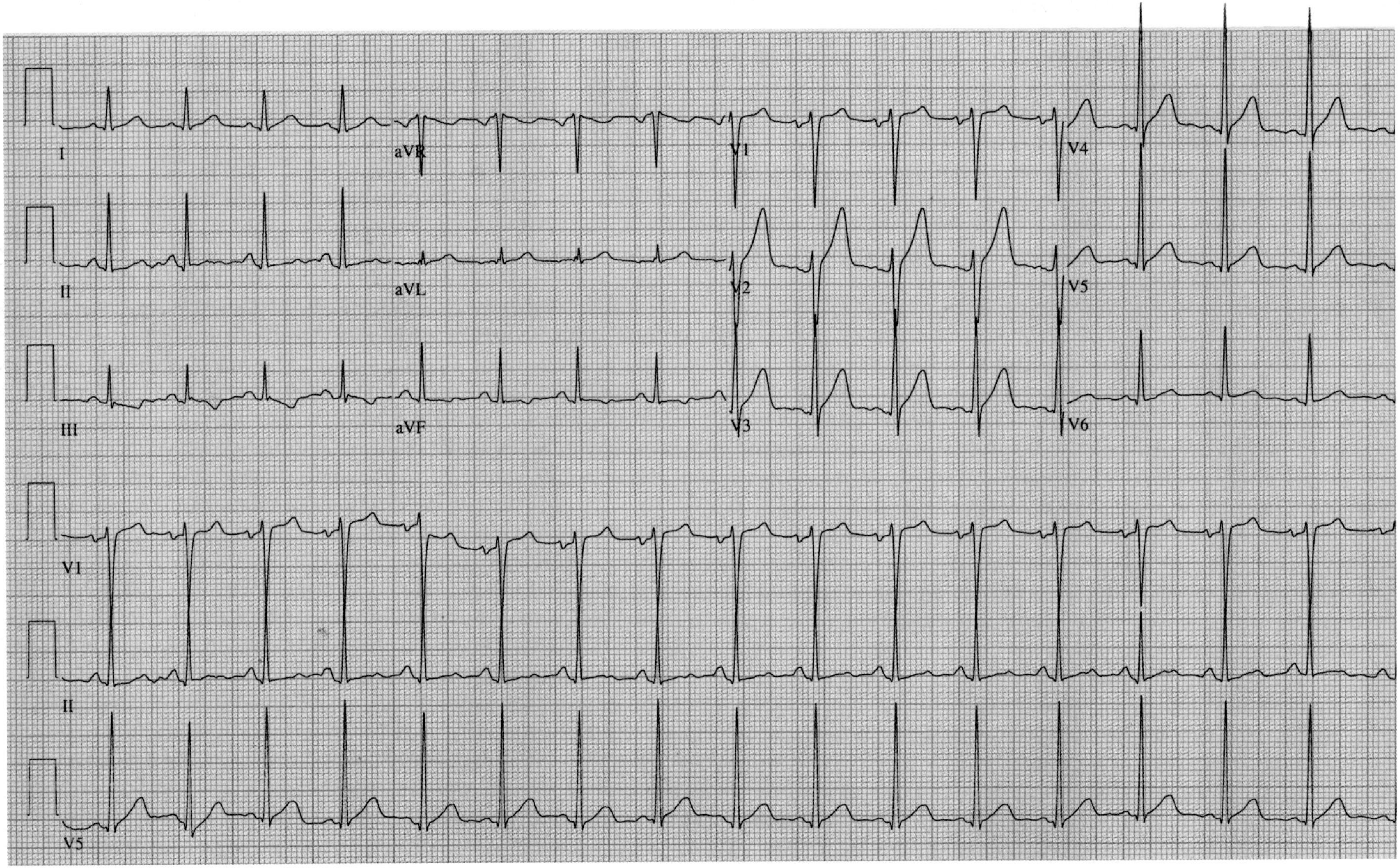

I aVR V1 V4
II aVL V2 V5
III aVF V3 V6
V1
II
V5

Interpretation Notes:

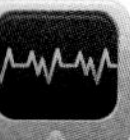

ELECTROCARDIOGRAM INTERPRETATION

This electrocardiogram demonstrates a normal P-wave axis at a rate of 100 per minute consistent with normal sinus rhythm. Nonspecific T-wave flattening and slight T-wave inversion is seen in leads II, III, and aVF. Slight J-point elevation is seen in leads V2, V3, and V4 of uncertain significance, likely reflecting early repolarization. Most importantly, this electrocardiogram demonstrates a truncated ST segment and a shortened QT interval. This is best seen in leads V4 and V5. This patient was known to suffer from hypercalcemia and at the time of this electrocardiogram, the patient's serum calcium level was 12.2 mEq per L.

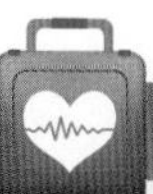

KEY DIAGNOSES

- Normal sinus rhythm
- Short QT interval
- Nonspecific ST-T changes
- Hypercalcemia
- Early repolarization

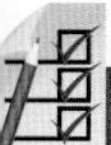

KEY TEACHING POINTS

- Calcium disorders affect the ST segments, not the T wave. In the presence of hypercalcemia, the ST segment is shortened and there is an abrupt transition from the QRS complex to the T wave with a minimal or an absent ST segment.
- The inferior nonspecific ST-T changes are of uncertain diagnostic significance. There is no myocardial infarction pattern on this electrocardiogram and there is no clear evidence of pericarditis.

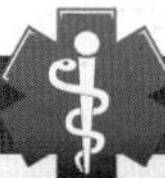

BOARD EXAMINATION ESSENTIALS

This electrocardiogram demonstrates the subtle clinical finding of hypercalcemia. In addition to coding for hypercalcemia on the board exam, other appropriate diagnostic codes include normal sinus rhythm and ST- and/or T-wave abnormalities suggesting electrolyte disturbances. The slight J-point elevation suggests early repolarization and this should be coded. There is no PR segment elevation in lead aVR to support pericarditis.

Electrocardiogram Case Study #71

CLINICAL HISTORY

A 74-year-old female with symptomatically severe palpitations, fatigue, and lightheadedness for the past 24 hours. The patient presented to the emergency room and was subsequently admitted to the hospital.

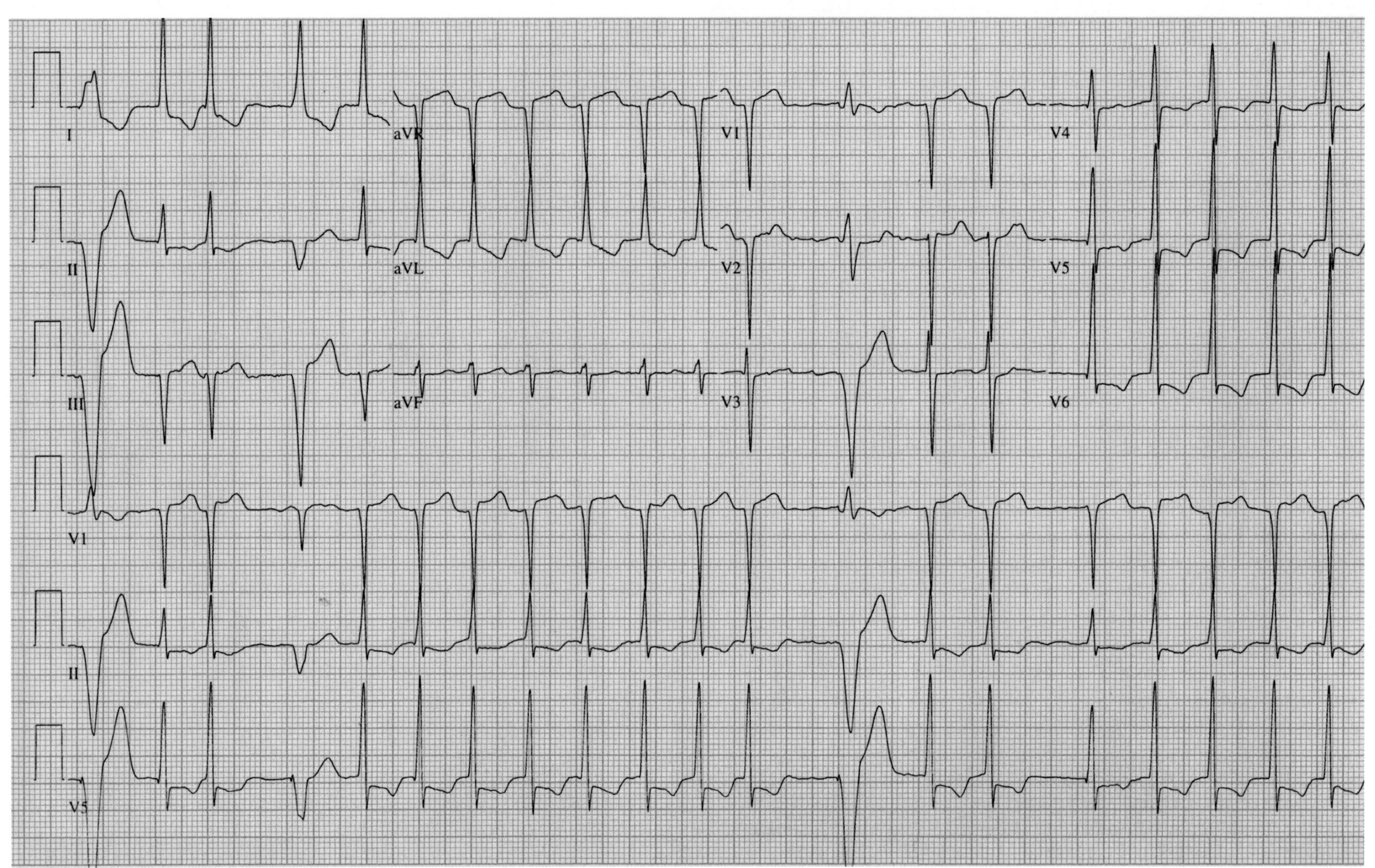

Interpretation Notes:

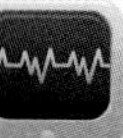

ELECTROCARDIOGRAM INTERPRETATION

This electrocardiogram demonstrates no identifiable atrial depolarizations. The atrial rhythm is consistent with atrial fibrillation. A lack of atrial activity is best seen in the rhythm strips on the bottom of the electrocardiogram in leads V1, II, and V5. This patient demonstrates a rapid ventricular response. Diffuse nonspecific ST-T changes are seen. J-point depression is noted particularly in leads V5, V6, I, and aVL. The downsloping ST-segment depression is suspicious for myocardial ischemia or a non–ST segment elevation myocardial infarction. Periodic pauses are seen. The 1st, 4th, and 13th QRS complexes are widened. Preceding each of the QRS complexes is a discrete diminutive deflection indicating a ventricular pacemaker. The fourth QRS complex is a fusion or a hybrid complex with simultaneous ventricular depolarization via the atrioventricular node and the ventricular pacemaker.

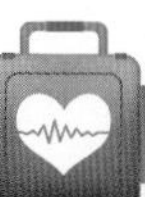

KEY DIAGNOSES

- Atrial fibrillation
- Rapid ventricular response
- Nonspecific ST-T changes
- Ventricular pacemaker
- Pacemaker fusion complex

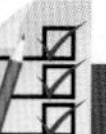

KEY TEACHING POINTS

- This patient was diagnosed with an acute non–ST segment elevation myocardial infarction based on a transient rise in serum cardiac isoenzymes. A left heart catheterization identified severe multivessel coronary artery disease prompting coronary artery bypass grafting.
- This patient's pacemaker was placed 2 years prior to this clinical presentation. It appears to be functioning normally during periods of prolonged R to R intervals in the presence of atrial fibrillation with a rapid ventricular response.

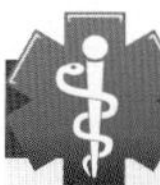

BOARD EXAMINATION ESSENTIALS

Diagnostic codes for the board exam include atrial fibrillation, left ventricular hypertrophy (lead aVL), ST- and/or T-wave abnormalities secondary to hypertrophy and ventricular demand pacemaker (VVI), normally functioning. Be careful not to mistakenly code the ventricular paced complexes as either ventricular escape complexes (note the pacemaker deflection) or premature ventricular complexes as the complexes are not premature. Also, make sure to use your calipers when assessing the ventricular response and R to R intervals. As the ventricular rate increases, the differences in the R to R cycle length are less apparent.

Electrocardiogram Case Study #72

CLINICAL HISTORY

A 78-year-old male postoperative day 3 status post multivessel coronary artery bypass grafting and aortic valve replacement for severe aortic stenosis. The patient was demonstrating a satisfactory recovery however experienced new-onset shortness of breath shortly before this electrocardiogram was obtained.

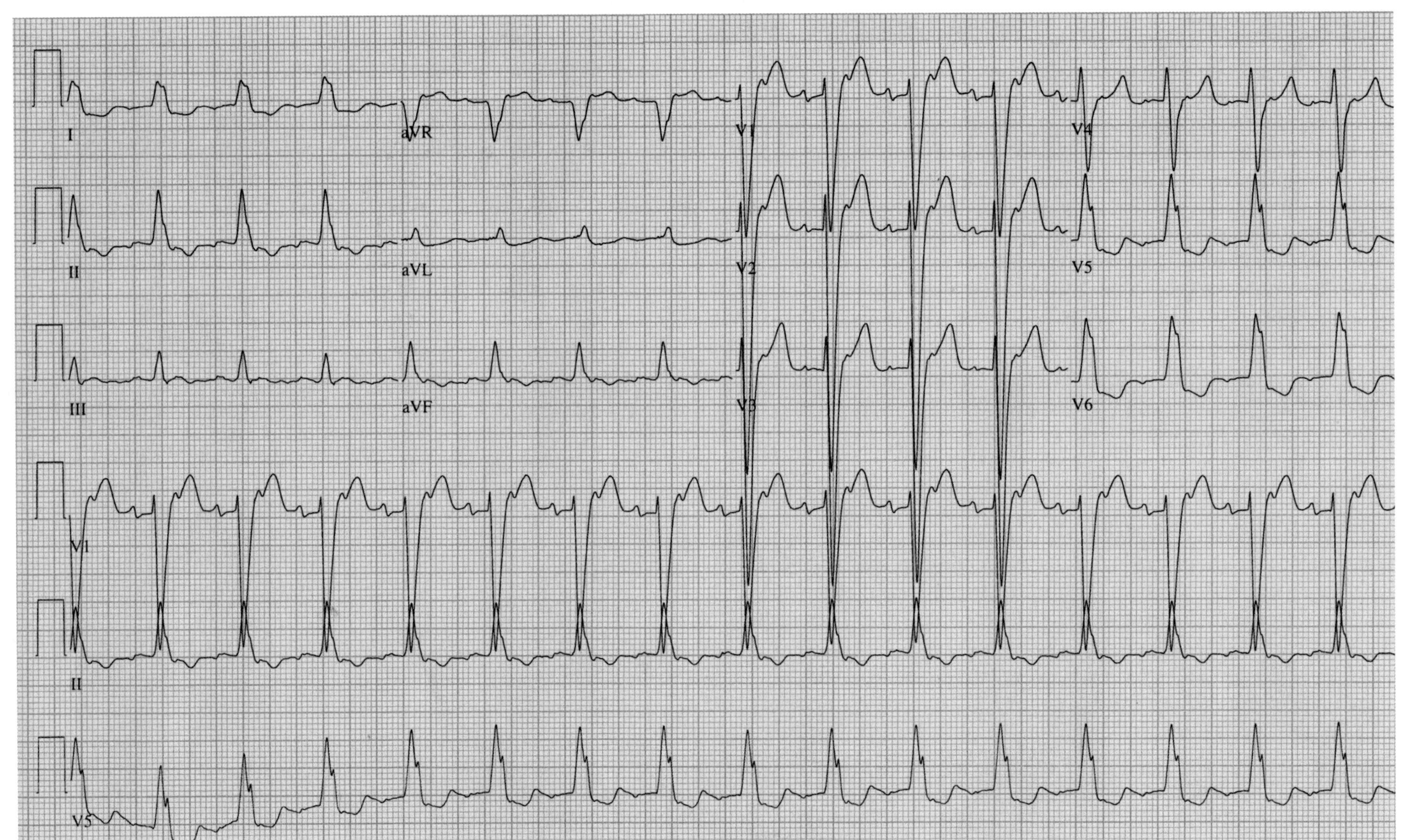

Interpretation Notes:

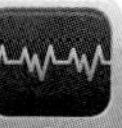

ELECTROCARDIOGRAM INTERPRETATION

This electrocardiogram demonstrates regular atrial depolarizations at a rate of approximately 190 per minute best identified in the lead V1 rhythm strip. The atrial depolarization axis is abnormal, inverted in leads I and II. This is consistent with an ectopic atrial tachycardia. Two atrial depolarizations are seen for each QRS complex confirming the presence of 2:1 atrioventricular conduction. The second atrial depolarization is just after the QRS complex within the very proximal portion of the ST-segment/T wave. The QRS complex is widened >120 milliseconds without identifiable septal Q waves. This confirms the presence of complete left bundle-branch block.

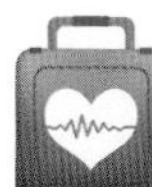

KEY DIAGNOSES

- Ectopic atrial tachycardia
- 2:1 atrioventricular conduction
- Complete left bundle-branch block

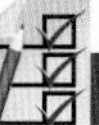

KEY TEACHING POINTS

- In the presence of an abnormal P-wave axis, it is of importance to confirm the atrioventricular conduction ratio. Using calipers, two P waves per each QRS complex occur at regular intervals per QRS complex confirming 2:1 atrioventricular conduction. This does not reflect conduction block but instead, the atrioventricular node exerts its normal gatekeeper function with every other ectopic atrial depolarization reaching the ventricle.
- The presence of complete left bundle-branch block is not a normal finding and suggests myocardial disease, almost certainly present given the multivessel coronary artery disease and severe aortic stenosis.

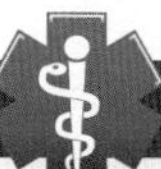

BOARD EXAMINATION ESSENTIALS

For the board exam, this electrocardiogram emphasizes coding both atrial rhythm and atrioventricular conduction. The P-wave axis is abnormal and atrial rate approaches 200 per minute. Each atrial depolarization is discrete and supports an ectopic atrial tachycardia. AV block, 2:1 is present as is complete left bundle-branch block. Do not code AV dissociation as the atrial tachycardic P waves demonstrate a constant interval and therefore possess a temporal relationship with the QRS complexes. No ventricular pacemaker deflections are identified. The QRS complex axis is normal.

Electrocardiogram Case Study #73

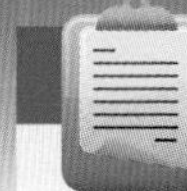

CLINICAL HISTORY

A 29-year-old female with a known malignancy undergoing intensive chemotherapy. The patient's serum potassium level at the time of this electrocardiogram was 2.6 mEq per L.

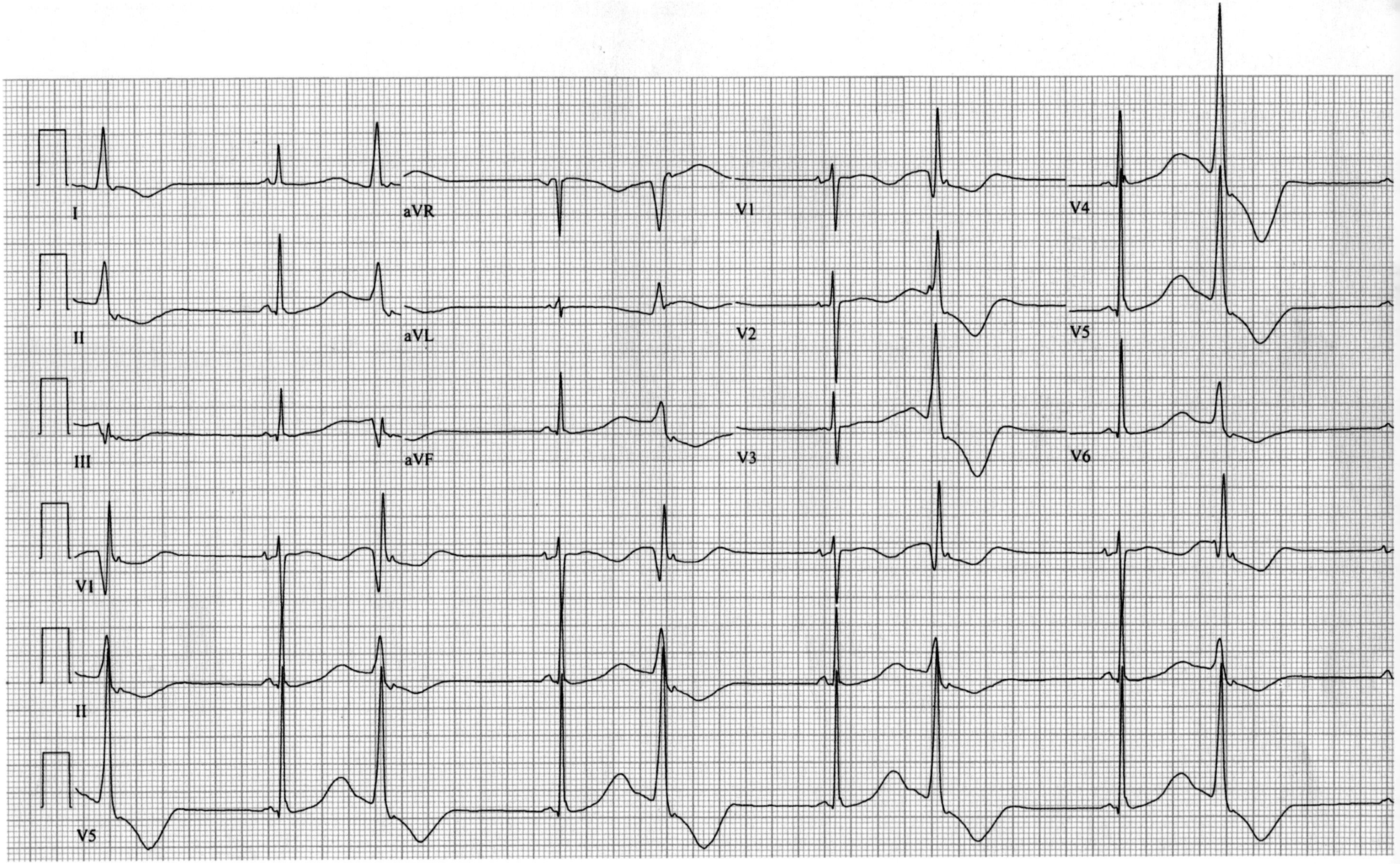

I aVR V1 V4

II aVL V2 V5

III aVF V3 V6

V1

II

V5

Interpretation Notes:

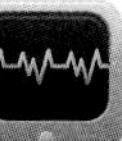

ELECTROCARDIOGRAM INTERPRETATION

This electrocardiogram demonstrates sinus bradycardia with an atrial rate slightly <60 per minute in the presence of a normal P wave axis. Frequent premature ventricular complexes are seen in a bigeminal pattern. The QT interval is markedly prolonged. In fact, this represents a prolonged QT-U interval as positive U waves are seen in leads V2, V3, and V4. The T wave is somewhat diminutive in leads V2 and V3 compared with a markedly positive U wave. This is commonly seen in advanced forms of hypokalemia.

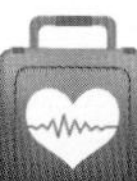

KEY DIAGNOSES

- Sinus bradycardia
- Premature ventricular complexes
- Prolonged QT-U interval
- Hypokalemia
- R-on-T phenomenon

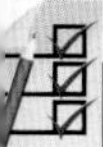

KEY TEACHING POINTS

- Shortly after this electrocardiogram was obtained, the patient became hemodynamically unstable developing paroxysms of torsade de pointes. This was ascribed to the premature ventricular complexes occurring within the vulnerable period, the so-called R-on-T phenomenon.
- Evidence of the R-on-T phenomenon is seen on this electrocardiogram, particularly in leads V2 and V3 where the premature ventricular complex is noted within the terminal aspect of the U wave.
- Keep in mind that the QT-U interval duration is inversely proportional to the heart rate. Given the sinus bradycardia as seen on this electrocardiogram, the QT-U interval demonstrates even greater prolongation.
- This patient demonstrates a short PR interval. There is no evidence of ventricular pre-excitation.

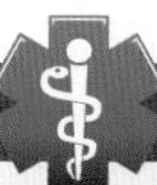

BOARD EXAMINATION ESSENTIALS

This electrocardiogram reinforces the need for a systematic assessment. Frequent premature ventricular complexes are documented. Accounting for the premature ventricular complexes, the average atrial rate is slightly <60 per minute supporting sinus bradycardia. Marked QT interval prolongation is present as are prominent U waves. This supports hypokalemia. For the board exam, diagnostic codes include sinus bradycardia, prolonged QT interval, prominent U waves, ST- and/or T-wave abnormalities suggesting electrolyte disturbances, ventricular premature complexes, and under clinical disorders, hypokalemia.

Electrocardiogram Case Study #74

CLINICAL HISTORY

A 78-year-old male with recent-onset intermittent palpitations and lightheadedness. The patient is seen in cardiovascular medicine consultation at the request of his internal medicine physician.

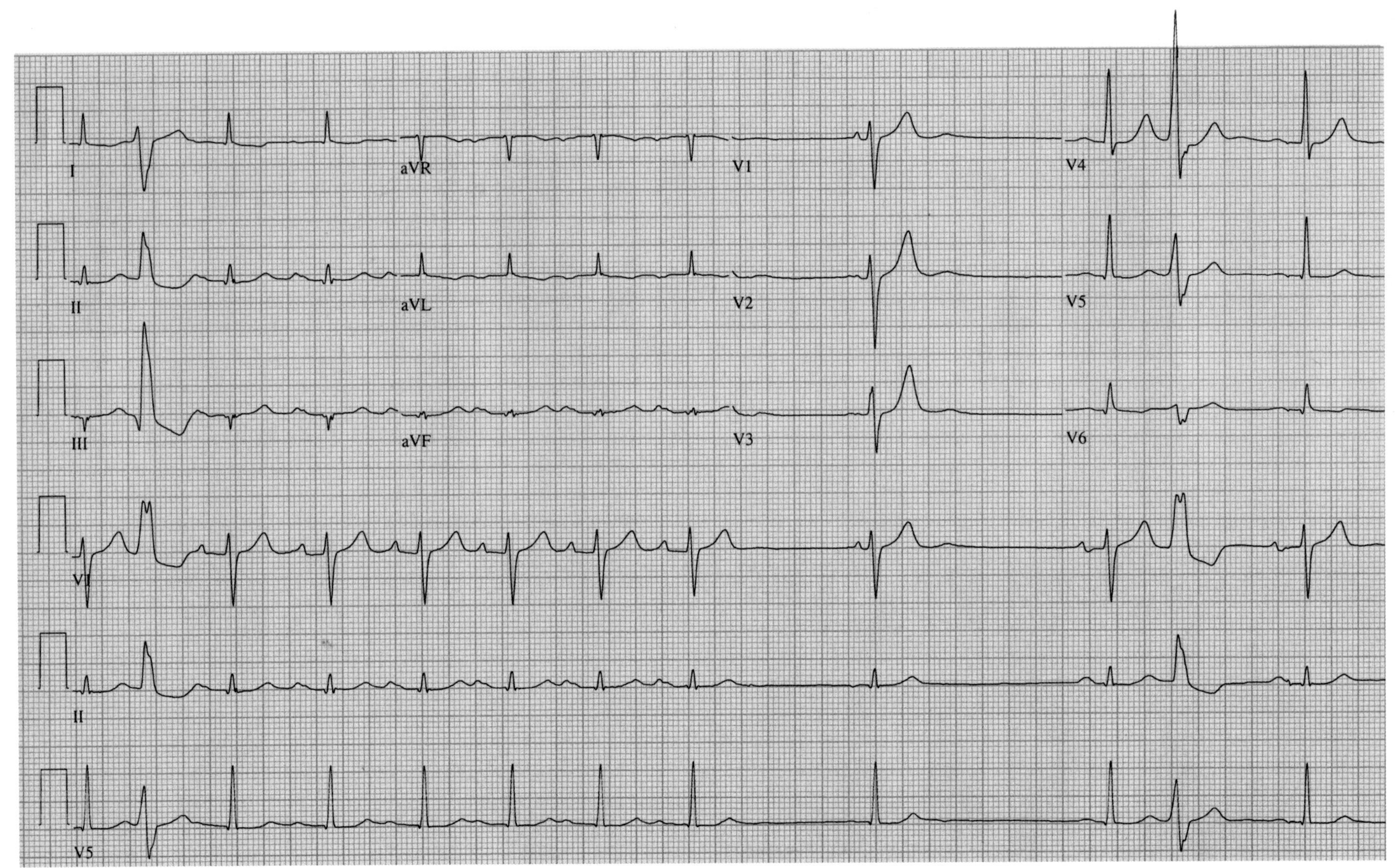

Interpretation Notes:

Electrocardiogram Case Study #74

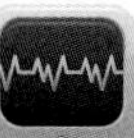

ELECTROCARDIOGRAM INTERPRETATION

This electrocardiogram demonstrates normal sinus rhythm at a rate of approximately 80 per minute. The P wave preceding the 9th and the 11th QRS complex toward the right-hand portion of the electrocardiogram demonstrates a normal P-wave axis and confirms the presence of normal sinus rhythm. Two wide QRS complexes are seen, occurring on the left- and the right-hand portions of the electrocardiogram consistent with premature ventricular complexes of left ventricular origin given the RsR′ QRS complex pattern in lead V1. Preceding the third through the seventh QRS complexes is a P wave of differing axis from the sinus rhythm P wave. It is more upright and monophasic in lead V1 without terminal negativity. This is consistent with an ectopic atrial rhythm. In the middle of the electrocardiogram best seen in the lead V1 rhythm strip, a pause occurs and the P wave preceding the eighth QRS complex is different from the sinus P wave and the P wave reflecting the paroxysmal ectopic atrial rhythm. This represents an atrial escape complex. Diminutive Q waves are seen in leads II, III, aVF, V5, and V6. These Q waves are not of diagnostic duration and therefore it is not possible to conclude with certainty that a myocardial infarction is present. Nonspecific ST-T changes are seen in leads I and aVL. The sinus P waves suggest left atrial abnormality.

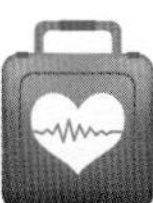

KEY DIAGNOSES

- Normal sinus rhythm
- Ectopic atrial rhythm
- Atrial escape complex
- Premature ventricular complex
- Nonspecific ST-T changes
- Sinus pause or arrest
- Sick sinus syndrome
- Left atrial abnormality

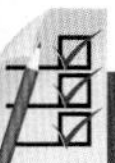

KEY TEACHING POINTS

- While a myocardial infarction cannot be diagnosed with certainty, suspicion exists. R-wave regression is seen from leads V5 to V6. This, with the presence of a Q-wave and T-wave inversion in lead V6, raises ischemic heart disease as a distinct possibility.
- This patient actually demonstrated elevated cardiac enzymes and underwent a left heart catheterization. An acute occlusion of the left circumflex coronary artery was seen and an intracoronary stent was successfully implanted. The patient was discharged 2 days later without incident.
- An atrial escape complex represents a subsidiary atrial focus, most often seen after a pause in atrial depolarization. This electrocardiogram is of particular interest as three separate atrial foci are demonstrated given the three morphologically distinct P waves.

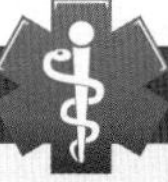

BOARD EXAMINATION ESSENTIALS

This electrocardiogram is complex as three separate P-wave morphologies are identifiable. The last two P waves represent normal sinus rhythm. The initial portion of the electrocardiogram reflects an ectopic atrial rhythm. Be sure to code for a sinus pause. Premature ventricular complexes are present. Diminutive inferior and lateral Q waves are present, not of diagnostic width to confidently code an inferior and lateral myocardial infarction of indeterminate age. In summary, diagnostic codes for the board exam include normal sinus rhythm, ventricular premature complex, sinus pause or arrest, and left atrial abnormality/enlargement. The lateral and the high lateral ST- and T-wave changes support the additional diagnostic code of nonspecific ST- and/or T-wave abnormalities.

Electrocardiogram Case Study #75

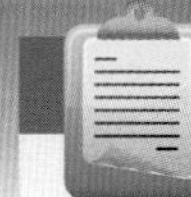

CLINICAL HISTORY

A 68-year-old male who presents for an annual physical examination. He has no known cardiac history and is not experiencing any symptoms referable to his heart.

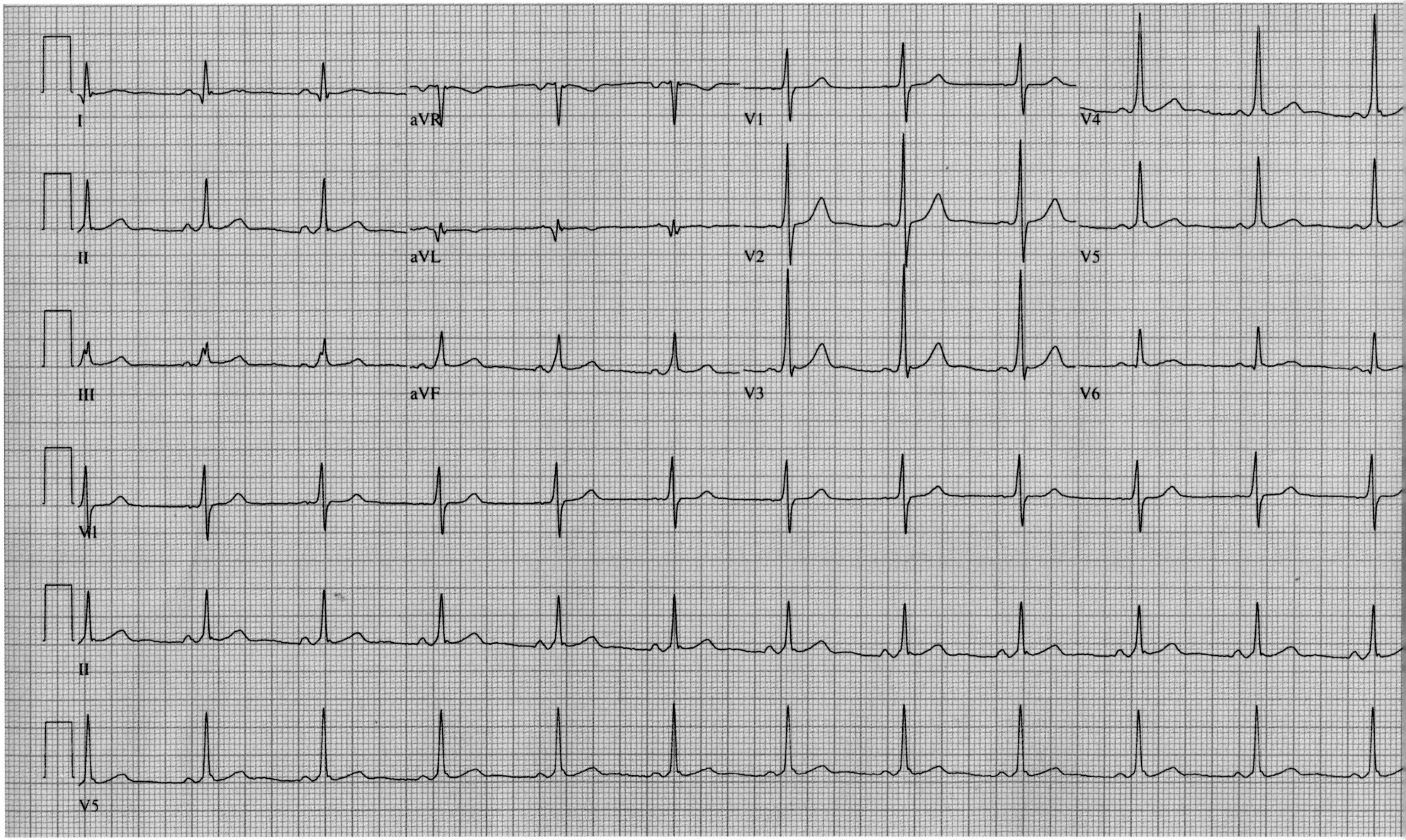

I aVR V1 V4

II aVL V2 V5

III aVF V3 V6

V1

II

V5

Interpretation Notes:

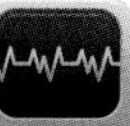

ELECTROCARDIOGRAM INTERPRETATION

This electrocardiogram demonstrates normal sinus rhythm at a rate slightly <70 per minute. The P waves are upright in leads I, II, and aVF confirming a normal P-wave axis. Q waves are seen in leads I and aVL raising the possibility of a high lateral myocardial infarction. These Q waves represent a pseudoinfarction and not true ischemic heart disease. They are due to ventricular pre-excitation and the Wolff-Parkinson-White syndrome. A delta wave is seen reflecting ventricular pre-excitation in leads II, III, aVF, V1, V2, V3, V4, and V5. The PR interval is short consistent with Wolff-Parkinson-White syndrome. A prominent R wave in leads V1 and V2 is also commonly identified in Wolff-Parkinson-White syndrome and not indicative of a posterior myocardial infarction, instead reflecting left to right ventricular activation.

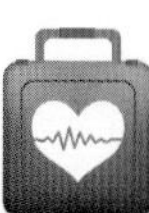

KEY DIAGNOSES

- Normal sinus rhythm
- Wolff-Parkinson-White syndrome
- Pseudoinfarction pattern

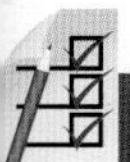

KEY TEACHING POINTS

- In this case, the diagnosis of Wolff-Parkinson-White syndrome is most evident based upon the shortened PR interval. This is easily overlooked.
- This electrocardiogram suggests a posterior lateral myocardial infarction. When this electrocardiogram pattern is present, make sure to exclude the possibility of a short PR interval and delta waves. On this electrocardiogram, the myocardial infarction pattern does not represent true ischemic heart disease.

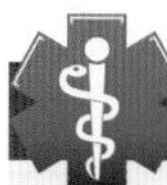

BOARD EXAMINATION ESSENTIALS

Diagnostic codes for the board exam include normal sinus rhythm and Wolff-Parkinson-White pattern. Several important board exam relevant concepts are present. The high-amplitude R waves in lead V1 raise the possibility of ventricular pre-excitation. Q waves in leads I and aVL in conjunction with the high-amplitude R waves in lead V1 initially support a posterior and lateral myocardial infarction of indeterminate age. A subtle shortening of the PR interval with a slurred upstroke to the QRS complex supersedes any suspicion of ischemic heart disease and solidifies the diagnosis of normal sinus rhythm and Wolff-Parkinson-White pattern as the sole appropriate board exam diagnostic codes.

Electrocardiogram Case Study #76

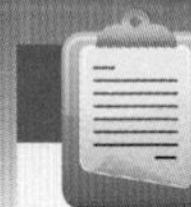

CLINICAL HISTORY

A 66-year-old female who was found unconscious at home and brought to the emergency room by ambulance. The patient expired a short time after this electrocardiogram was obtained.

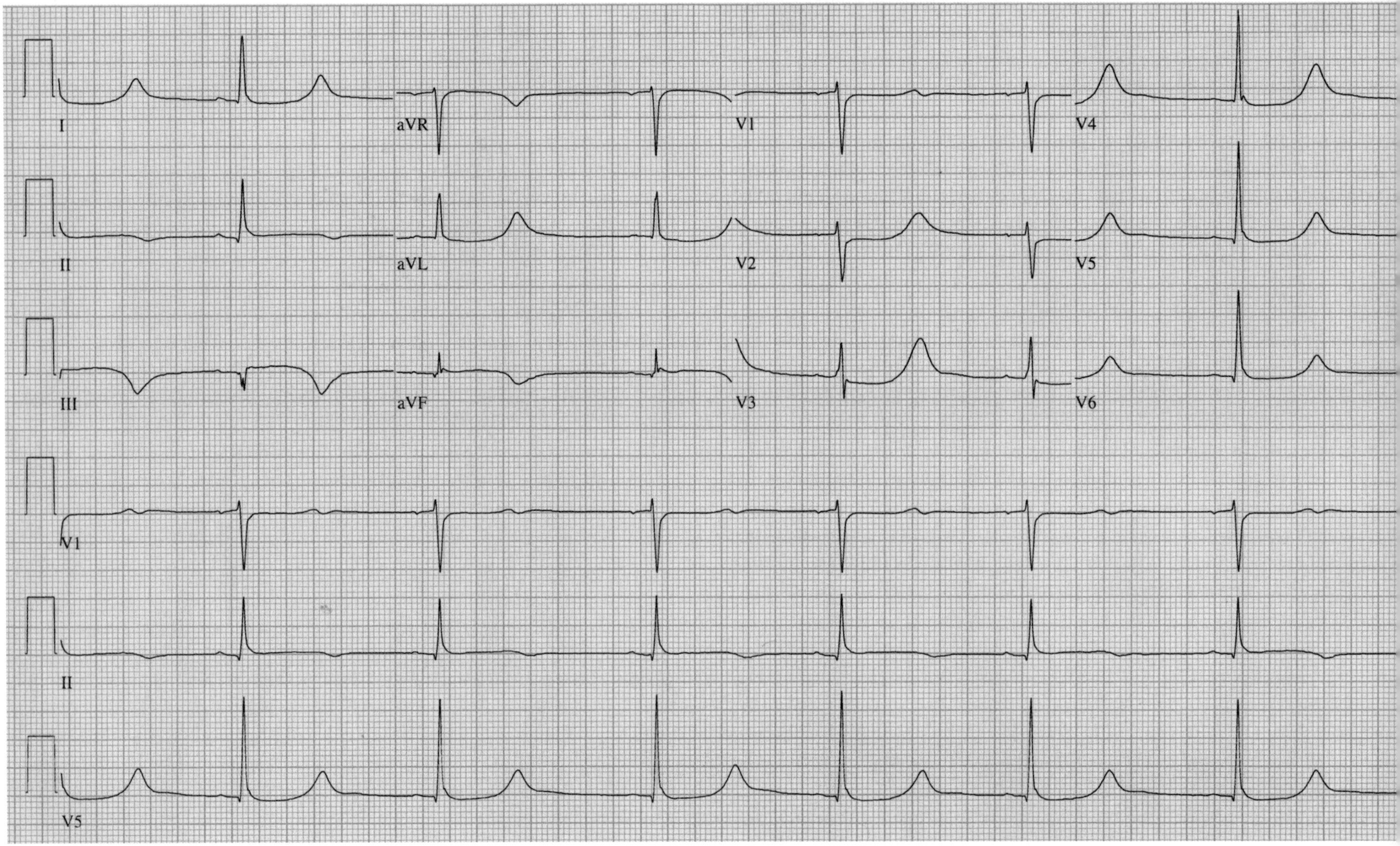

I aVR V1 V4
II aVL V2 V5
III aVF V3 V6
V1
II
V5

Interpretation Notes:

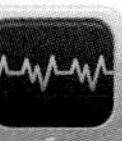

ELECTROCARDIOGRAM INTERPRETATION

This electrocardiogram demonstrates upright P waves in leads I and II and a diminutive P wave in lead aVF at a sinus rate of approximately 40 per minute most consistent with sinus bradycardia. Most impressive on this electrocardiogram is a markedly prolonged ST segment, broadened T wave, and lengthened QT interval. Both sinus bradycardia and QT interval prolongation are often seen in the presence of an acute increase in intracranial pressure. Inferior ST-T changes are also seen. ST-segment elevation is noted in lead III. Initial cardiac enzymes did not support the presence of acute myocardial injury.

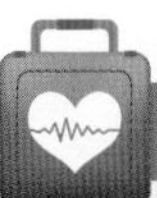

KEY DIAGNOSES

- Sinus bradycardia
- Prolonged QT interval
- Nonspecific ST-T changes
- Central nervous system event

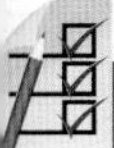

KEY TEACHING POINTS

- Oftentimes, it is difficult to electrocardiographically distinguish an acute increase in intracranial pressure from myocardial ischemia. In the presence of an acute rise in intracranial pressure, QT interval prolongation is frequently seen as is bradycardia.
- Symmetric T-wave inversion can also be present in the presence of an acute increase in intracranial pressure. This finding can also be seen in the presence of myocardial ischemia and non–ST segment elevation myocardial infarction. Blood sampling of serial cardiac enzymes, echocardiography to assess left ventricular wall motion and function and serial electrocardiograms can assist in distinguishing between these two diagnostic possibilities.

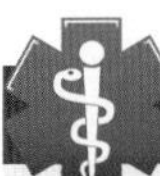

BOARD EXAMINATION ESSENTIALS

With a consistent clinical history, this electrocardiogram supports board exam diagnostic coding for a central nervous system disorder. Appropriate board exam diagnostic codes in addition to the clinical diagnosis of a central nervous system disorder include sinus bradycardia and a prolonged QT interval. An optional diagnostic code is nonspecific ST-and/or T-wave abnormalities.

Electrocardiogram Case Study #77

CLINICAL HISTORY

A 49-year-old male with profound shortness of breath with minimal exertion in the setting of previously diagnosed severe mitral stenosis and severe pulmonary hypertension. The patient is being evaluated for mitral valve replacement surgery.

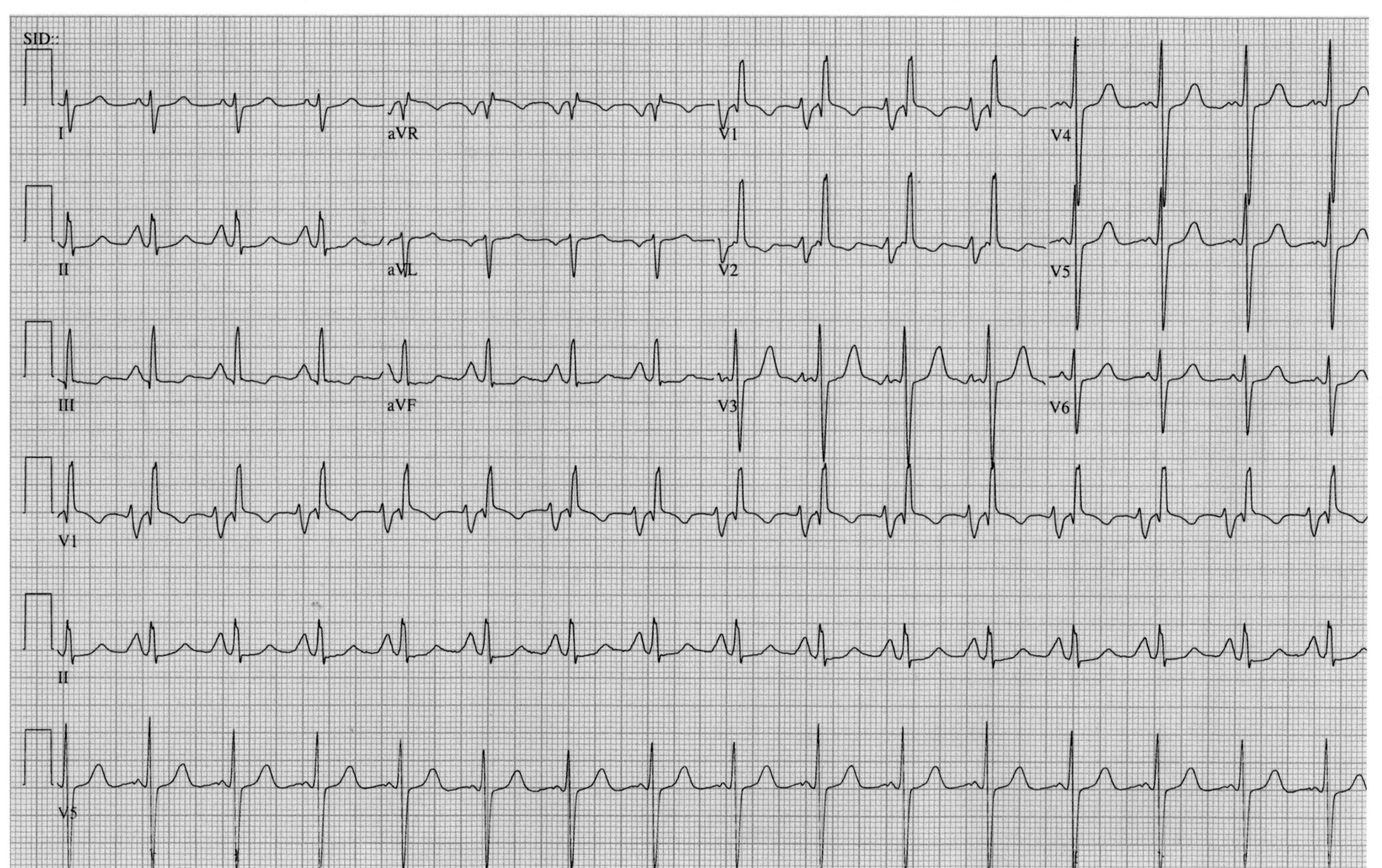

Interpretation Notes:

Electrocardiogram Case Study #77

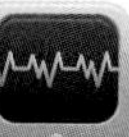

ELECTROCARDIOGRAM INTERPRETATION

This electrocardiogram demonstrates upright P waves in leads I, II, III, and aVF at an atrial rate slightly <100 per minute consistent with normal sinus rhythm. In lead II, the P wave is between 0.4 mV and 0.5 mV in amplitude supporting right atrial abnormality, also known as "P. Pulmonale." In lead V1, the P wave demonstrates a deep terminal negativity supporting left atrial abnormality, also known as "P. Mitrale." Left atrial abnormality is further supported given the P-wave duration in lead II being >110 milliseconds. Right-axis QRS complex deviation is present given the negative QRS complex vector in lead I and positive QRS complex vectors in leads II, III, and aVF. The QRS complex duration is normal. A qR QRS complex pattern is seen in leads V1 and V2 with terminal T-wave inversion. There is poor R-wave progression with the R to S ratio being <1 in lead V6. This is consistent with right ventricular hypertrophy with secondary ST-T changes.

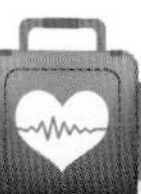

KEY DIAGNOSES

- Normal sinus rhythm
- Left atrial abnormality
- Right atrial abnormality
- QRS complex right-axis deviation
- Right ventricular hypertrophy with secondary ST-T changes

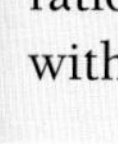

KEY TEACHING POINTS

- This electrocardiogram demonstrates the classic findings of severe, unoperated longstanding mitral stenosis. Both left and right atrial abnormalities are present as is right ventricular hypertrophy supporting markedly elevated pulmonary arterial pressures.
- Be careful not to confuse this electrocardiogram with primary pulmonary hypertension. In the presence of primary pulmonary hypertension, right atrial abnormality would be expected to be present. Left atrial abnormality would be absent. The absence of left atrial abnormality distinguishes primary pulmonary hypertension from mitral stenosis.

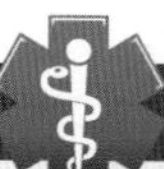

BOARD EXAMINATION ESSENTIALS

This electrocardiogram is classic for severe longstanding mitral stenosis. Board exam diagnostic codes include normal sinus rhythm, left atrial abnormality/enlargement, right atrial abnormality/enlargement, right-axis deviation (greater than + 100 degrees), right ventricular hypertrophy, and ST- and/or T-wave abnormalities secondary to hypertrophy.

Electrocardiogram Case Study #78

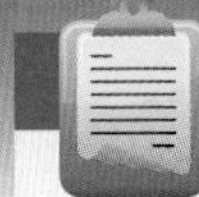

CLINICAL HISTORY

A 63-year-old female with dialysis-dependent end-stage renal disease. She is currently admitted to the hospital due to a catheter-associated bloodstream infection.

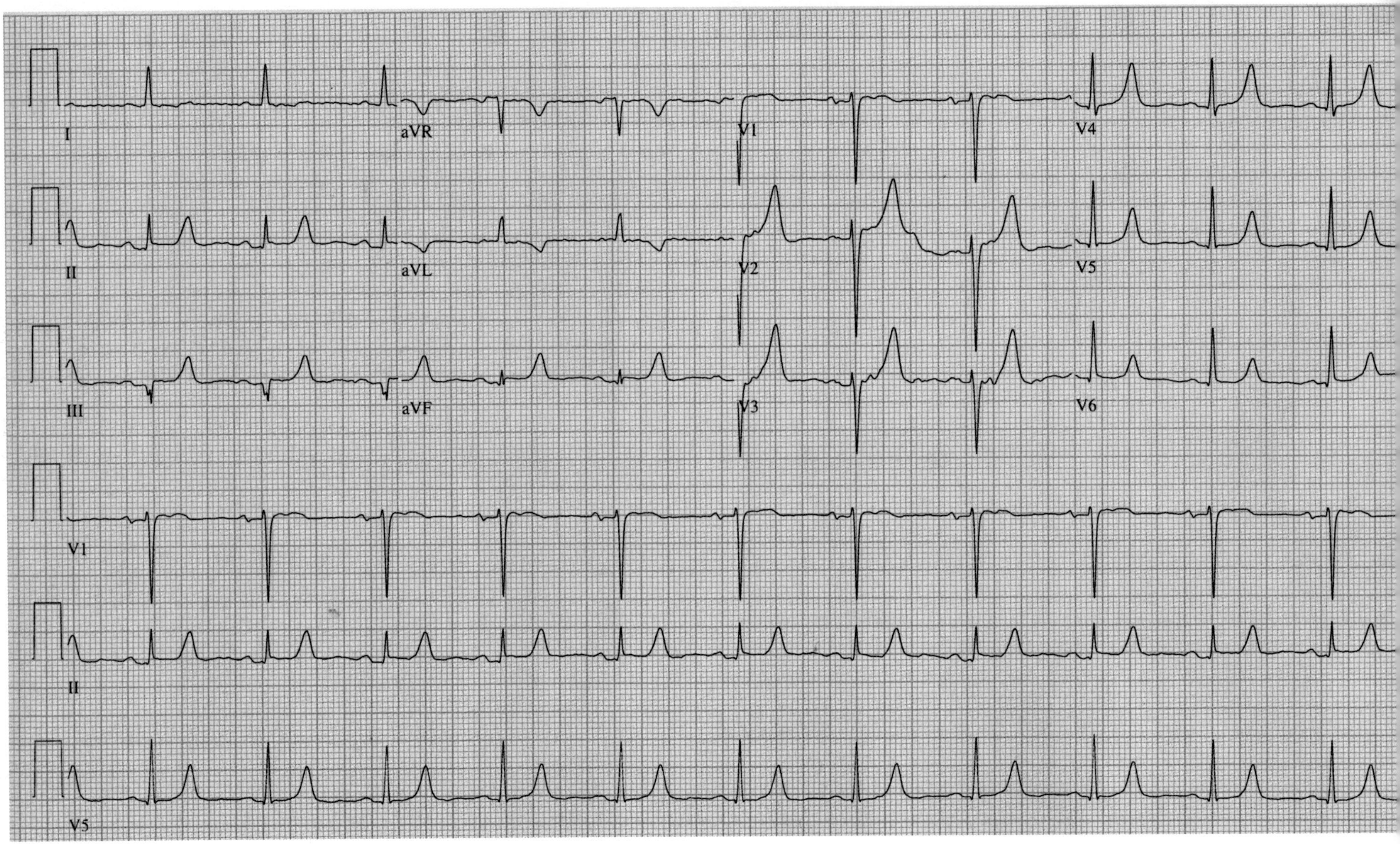

I aVR V1 V4
II aVL V2 V5
III aVF V3 V6
V1
II
V5

Interpretation Notes:

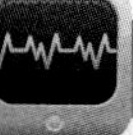

ELECTROCARDIOGRAM INTERPRETATION

This electrocardiogram demonstrates upright P waves in leads I, II, III, and aVF at an atrial rate slightly less than 70 per minute supporting normal sinus rhythm. J-point and ST-segment elevation is seen in leads II, III, aVF, V4, V5, and V6. In addition, PR-segment elevation is seen in lead aVR all supporting pericarditis in this uremic patient. Additionally, the T waves are symmetric and somewhat peaked best seen in leads V4, V5, and V6. This supports hyperkalemia. Nonspecific ST-T changes are seen in lead I and T-wave inversion is present in lead aVL.

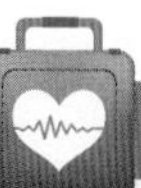

KEY DIAGNOSES

- Normal sinus rhythm
- Pericarditis
- Hyperkalemia
- Nonspecific ST-T changes

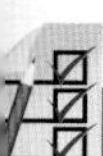

KEY TEACHING POINTS

- This electrocardiogram is classic for an end-stage renal disease patient who is uremic. Both hyperkalemia and pericarditis are observed.
- When assessing the electrocardiogram for the presence of hyperkalemia, the T-wave amplitude is one component. Equally important is the presence of narrow-based symmetric T waves as are demonstrated on this electrocardiogram. In the absence of a significant increase in T-wave amplitude, the symmetric and the narrow-based component can be overlooked.

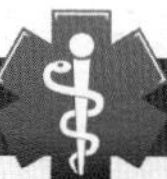

BOARD EXAMINATION ESSENTIALS

This electrocardiogram is an example of uremic pericarditis. Relevant board exam diagnostic codes include normal sinus rhythm, pericarditis, and hyperkalemia. Artifact is also present. Be sure to code ST- and/or T-wave abnormalities suggesting electrolyte disturbances. The lack of QT interval prolongation does not support the presence of hypocalcemia.

Electrocardiogram Case Study #79

CLINICAL HISTORY

A 65-year-old male who presents for outpatient cardiovascular medicine follow-up in the setting of known coronary artery disease, status post a myocardial infarction 4 years prior to this electrocardiogram.

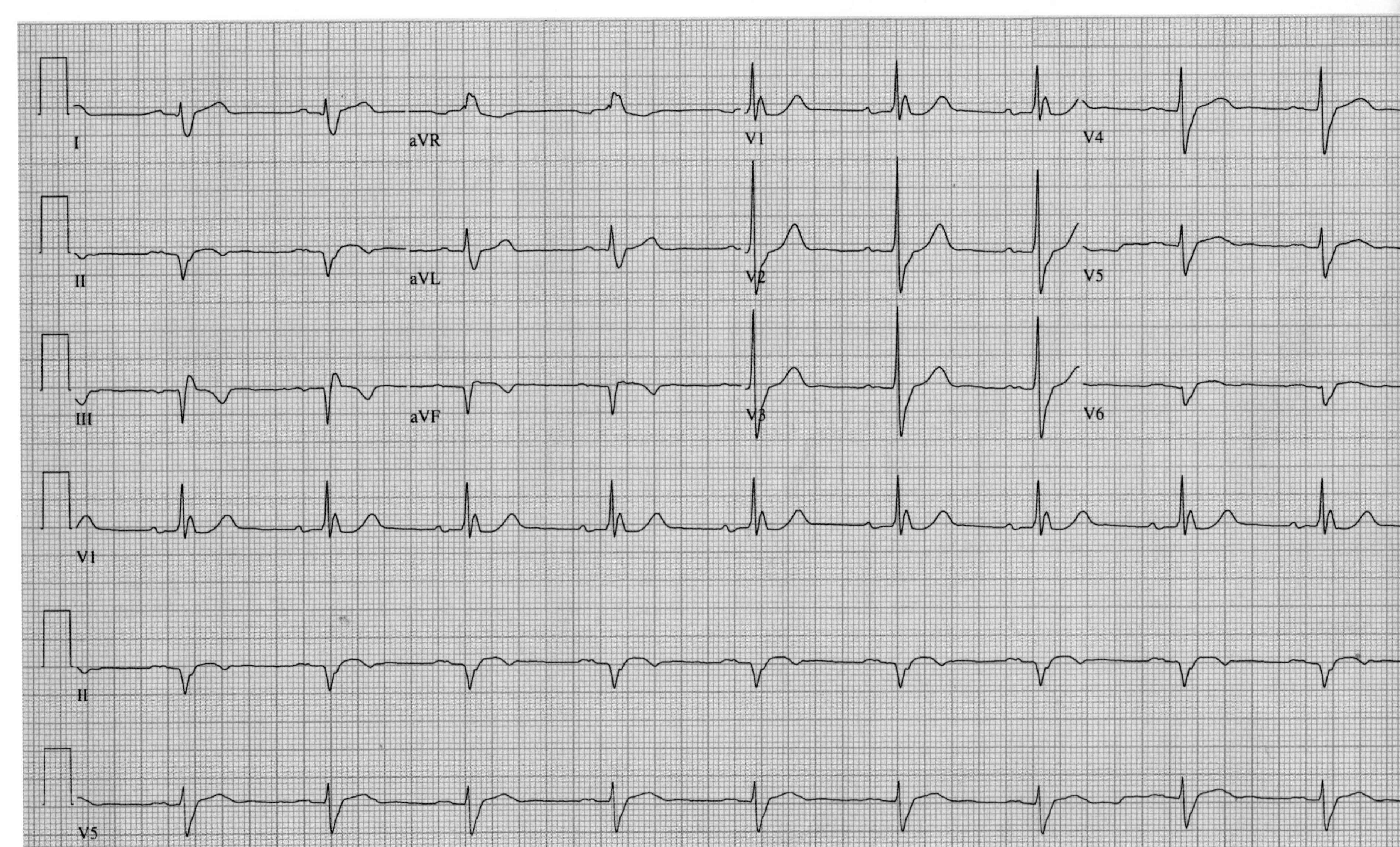

Interpretation Notes:

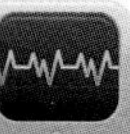

ELECTROCARDIOGRAM INTERPRETATION

This electrocardiogram demonstrates upright P waves in leads I, II, and aVF at a rate slightly <60 per minute supporting sinus bradycardia. The PR interval is slightly >200 milliseconds consistent with first-degree atrioventricular block. Left atrial abnormality is present given the bifid P wave best seen in lead II. Inferior Q waves >40 milliseconds in duration are present as is a Q wave in lead V6. This is consistent with age-indeterminate inferior and lateral myocardial infarctions. ST-segment elevation is seen in the inferior leads and in this patient with a confirmed myocardial infarction 4 years previously, this supports the presence of a left ventricular aneurysm. The QRS complex is prolonged to greater than 120 milliseconds with an Rsr′ morphological pattern seen in leads V1 and V2 supporting complete right bundle-branch block. A prominent R wave is seen in leads V1, V2, and V3 and in the presence of an inferior and lateral age-indeterminate myocardial infarction confirms the presence of a posterior myocardial infarction, age indeterminate. These three myocardial territories are contiguous and likely reflective of a single myocardial event. Upright T waves are seen in leads V1, V2, and V3 supporting a primary T-wave change due to underlying ischemic heart disease.

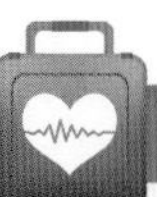

KEY DIAGNOSES

- Sinus bradycardia
- First-degree atrioventricular block
- Left atrial abnormality
- Complete right bundle-branch block
- Primary T-wave changes
- Inferior myocardial infarction, age indeterminate
- Lateral myocardial infarction, age indeterminate
- Posterior myocardial infarction, age indeterminate
- Left ventricular aneurysm

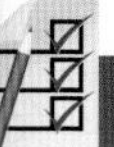

KEY TEACHING POINTS

- This patient underwent a heart catheterization shortly after their myocardial infarction demonstrating an acute proximal occlusion of a dominant right coronary artery that perfused the inferoposterolateral myocardial territories.
- The presence of an inferior left ventricular aneurysm was confirmed by echocardiography.

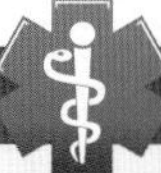

BOARD EXAMINATION ESSENTIALS

For the board exam, electrocardiogram patterns of ischemic heart disease are typically well represented. This electrocardiogram demonstrates an important pattern of findings emphasizing the concept of contiguous electrocardiogram territories. Diagnostic codes for the board exam include sinus bradycardia; inferior myocardial infarction, age indeterminate; posterior myocardial infarction, age indeterminate; lateral myocardial infarction, age indeterminate; and complete right bundle-branch block. ST-segment elevation is present inferiorly. An inferior myocardial infarction pattern should be coded as acute only if supported by the clinical history. In this case, this patient was known to suffer from an inferior wall left ventricular aneurysm. This electrocardiogram does not represent an acute coronary syndrome.

Electrocardiogram Case Study #80

CLINICAL HISTORY

A 57-year-old female with nonischemic left ventricular systolic dysfunction who returns for outpatient cardiovascular medicine follow-up evaluation. The patient underwent implantable cardiac defibrillator placement 3 weeks prior to this electrocardiogram.

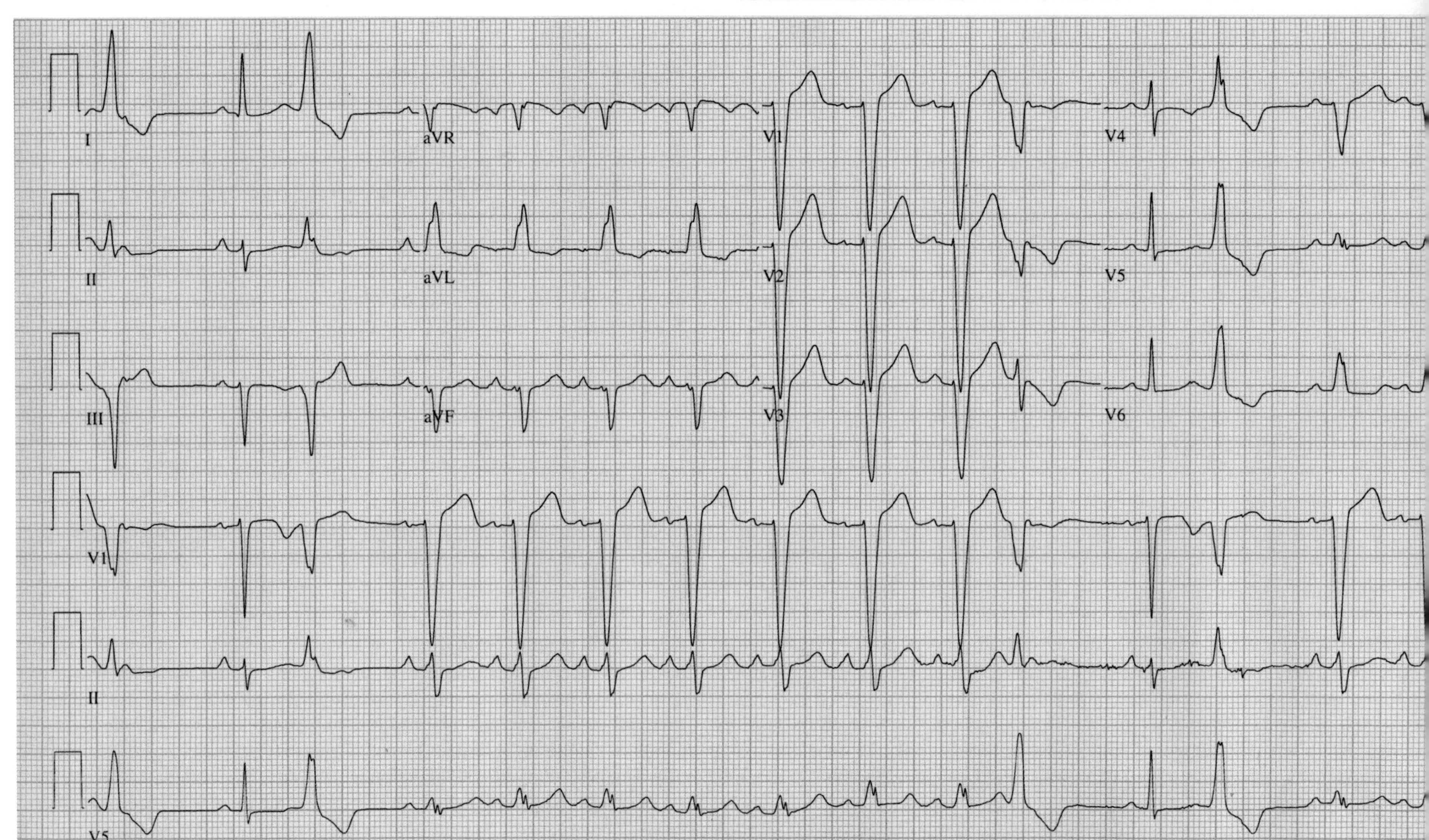

Interpretation Notes:____

____

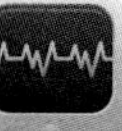

ELECTROCARDIOGRAM INTERPRETATION

This electrocardiogram demonstrates upright P waves in leads I, II, III, and aVF at an atrial rate slightly <100 per minute confirming normal sinus rhythm. Left anterior hemiblock is present given the positive QRS complex vector in lead I and negative QRS complex vectors in leads II and III. The 1st, 3rd, 11th, and 14th QRS complexes are widened with a complete left bundle-branch block morphology consistent with premature ventricular complexes of right ventricular origin. Following the third premature ventricular complex, normal sinus rhythm continues with a complete left bundle-branch block QRS complex morphology. After the 11th QRS complex that represents a premature ventricular complex, a normal QRS complex duration is seen. Following the last premature ventricular complex, complete left bundle-branch block reappears. In leads V4 and V5, the QRS complex with a normal duration demonstrates nonspecific T-wave inversion and T-wave flattening, respectively.

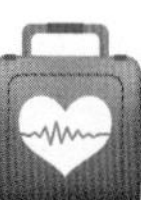

KEY DIAGNOSES

- Normal sinus rhythm
- Left anterior fascicular block
- Rate-dependent complete left bundle-branch block
- Premature ventricular complexes
- Nonspecific ST-T changes

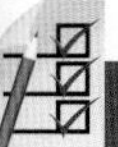

KEY TEACHING POINTS

- At a slightly higher heart rate, the left bundle-branch demonstrates absolute refractoriness in the form of complete left bundle-branch block. This is not a normal finding. This conduction abnormality masks nonspecific ST-T changes as evidenced in leads V4 and V5.
- Complete left bundle-branch block is not a normal finding and is consistent with structural heart disease such as left ventricular systolic dysfunction, left ventricular hypertrophy, valvular heart disease, or ischemic heart disease.

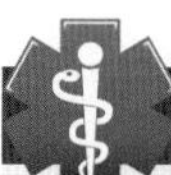

BOARD EXAMINATION ESSENTIALS

This is another example of functional (rate-related) aberrancy, a concept often emphasized on the board exam. Board exam diagnostic codes found on this electrocardiogram include normal sinus rhythm, ventricular premature complexes, left anterior fascicular block, nonspecific ST- and/or T-wave abnormalities (best identified in leads V4 and V5), and functional (rate-related) aberrancy.

Electrocardiogram Case Study #81

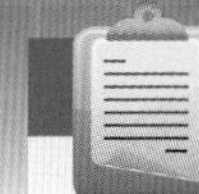

CLINICAL HISTORY

A 55-year-old female with mitral valve prolapse and severe mitral regurgitation. The patient underwent mitral valve reparative surgery and is currently resting in the intensive care unit on postoperative day 1.

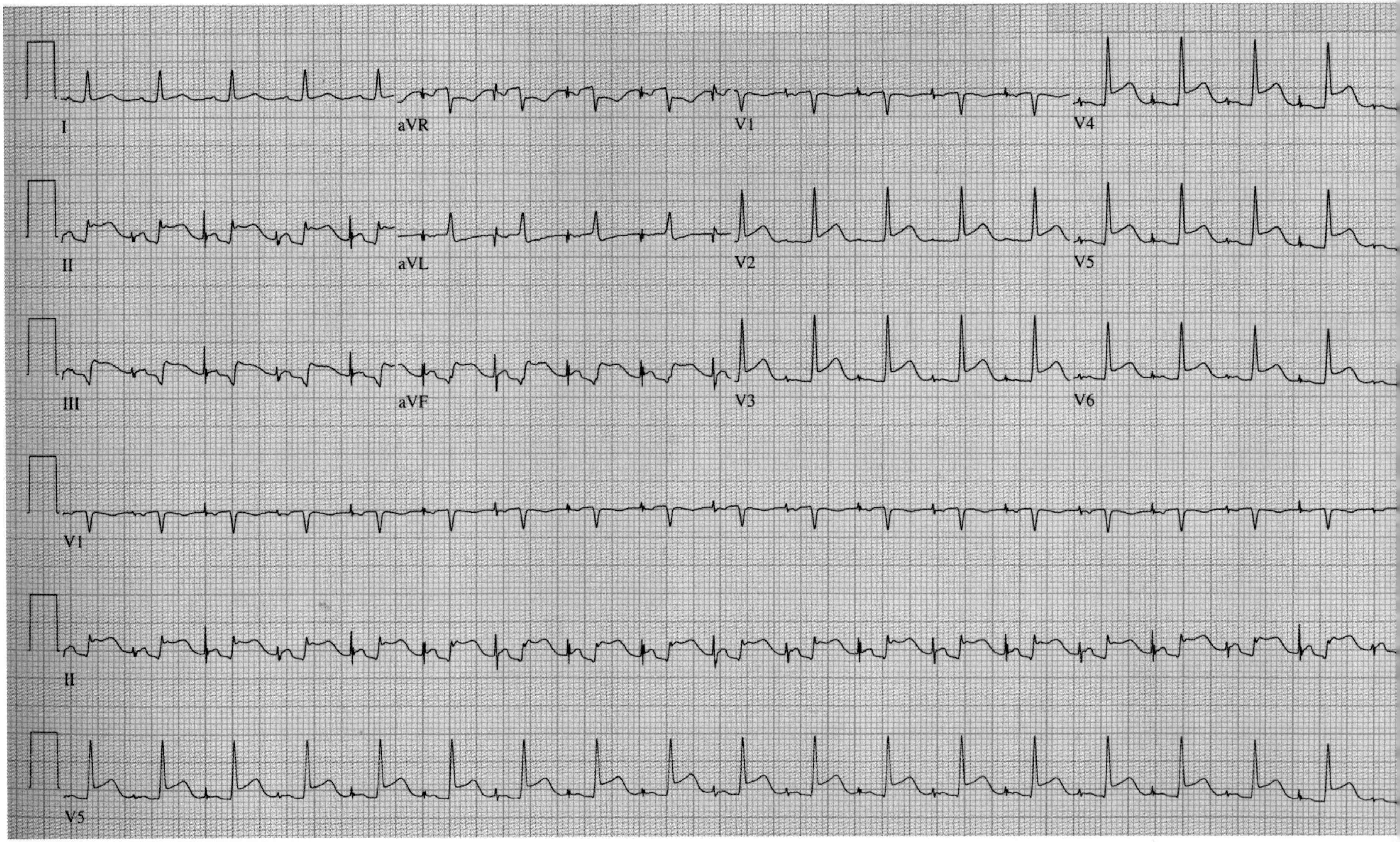

I aVR V1 V4
II aVL V2 V5
III aVF V3 V6
V1
II
V5

Interpretation Notes:

Electrocardiogram Case Study #81

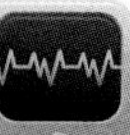

ELECTROCARDIOGRAM INTERPRETATION

This electrocardiogram demonstrates electronic atrial pacing at a rate of approximately 110 per minute. An upright P wave is demonstrated in leads II, III, and aVF following the pacemaker deflection. Diffuse J point and ST-segment elevation is present as is PR segment elevation in lead aVR. These findings collectively support the presence of postoperative pericarditis. Diminutive Q waves are seen in leads III and aVF. These are not of diagnostic duration to support the presence of an age-indeterminate myocardial infarction, particularly the Q wave in lead aVF.

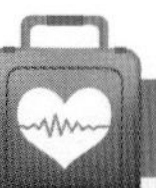

KEY DIAGNOSES

- Atrial pacemaker
- Pericarditis

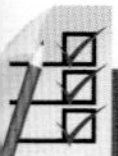

KEY TEACHING POINTS

- In this patient, obtaining serial electrocardiograms is important. Acute myocardial injury remains in the differential diagnosis as the inferior ST-segment elevation appears out of proportion to that seen in the other electrocardiogram leads.
- An echocardiogram was performed shortly after this electrocardiogram was obtained. A small circumferential pericardial effusion was seen with a hypercontractile left ventricle without evidence of regional systolic dysfunction. Follow-up evaluation confirmed resolution of the elevated ST segments and the patient was discharged on postoperative day 5 without complication.

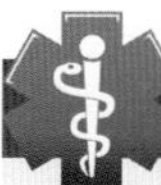

BOARD EXAMINATION ESSENTIALS

For the board exam, diagnostic codes include atrial or coronary sinus pacing and acute pericarditis. Equivocal codes include inferior myocardial infarction acute and ST and/or T-wave abnormalities suggesting myocardial injury. For the board exam, anticipate electrocardiograms where the findings are reasonably indisputable, unlike this tracing where an acute infarction may be present as well as acute pericarditis. In the setting of acute pericarditis, coding for ST- and/or T-wave abnormalities suggesting myocardial injury is not routinely favored. Acute pericarditis typically represents epicardial, not myocardial injury.

Electrocardiogram Case Study #82

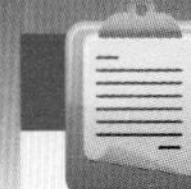

CLINICAL HISTORY

A 58-year-old male postoperative day 3 mitral and tricuspid valve reparative surgery. The patient is resting comfortably on a telemetry ward. Shortly before this electrocardiogram was obtained, a narrow complex tachycardia was noted by the nursing staff.

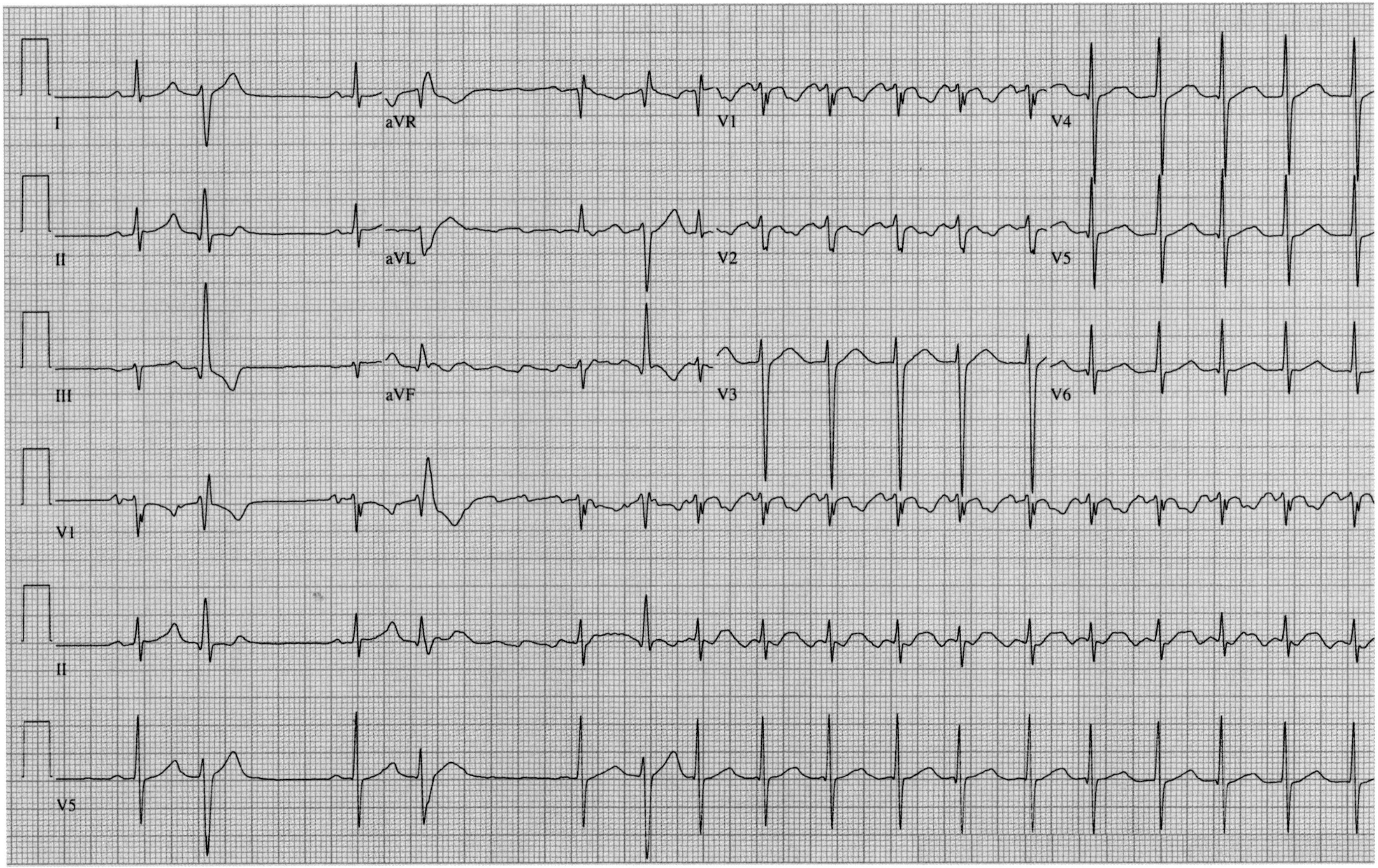

I aVR V1 V4
II aVL V2 V5
III aVF V3 V6
V1
II
V5

Interpretation Notes:

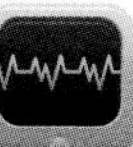

ELECTROCARDIOGRAM INTERPRETATION

On the left hand portion of the tracing, this electrocardiogram demonstrates an upright P wave in leads I and II supporting normal sinus rhythm. The second QRS complex is preceded by a P wave that deforms the terminal T wave supporting the presence of a premature atrial complex conducted with complete right bundle-branch block aberrancy. The fourth QRS complex also represents an aberrantly conducted premature atrial complex. After the fourth QRS complex, atrial flutter waves are seen best in lead aVF, the lead II rhythm strip, and the lead V1 rhythm strip. Three atrial flutter waves are seen followed by a paroxysm of atrial flutter with 2:1 atrioventricular conduction with a ventricular response of approximately 135 per minute.

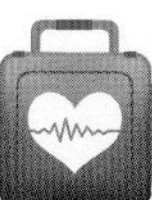

KEY DIAGNOSES

- Normal sinus rhythm
- Premature atrial complex
- Complete right bundle-branch block aberrancy
- Atrial flutter
- 2:1 atrioventricular conduction

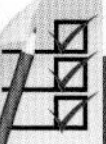

KEY TEACHING POINTS

- Premature atrial complexes are a frequent trigger of supraventricular dysrhythmias including atrial flutter as demonstrated on this electrocardiogram.
- The prolonged QRS complexes represent premature atrial complexes with complete right bundle-branch aberration, potentially misinterpreted as premature ventricular complexes. To avoid this error, it is important to inspect the preceding ST segment and T wave that may be deformed by the presence of a superimposed P wave. That is the case for this electrocardiogram, especially after analysis of the rhythm strip leads.

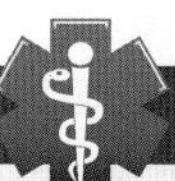

BOARD EXAMINATION ESSENTIALS

This electrocardiogram demonstrates several important board exam coding concepts. Diagnostic codes include normal sinus rhythm, atrial premature complexes, functional (rate-related) aberrancy, atrial flutter, and AV block, 2:1. Be sure not to code for right bundle-branch block, complete as the aberrant conduction is due to a long-short R to R interval and an atrial premature complex with rate-related aberrancy.

Electrocardiogram Case Study #83

CLINICAL HISTORY

A 38-year-old male with sudden-onset palpitations and near-syncope. The patient was rushed to the hospital, admitted to the coronary intensive care unit, and sedated. Emergent electrical cardioversion was performed.

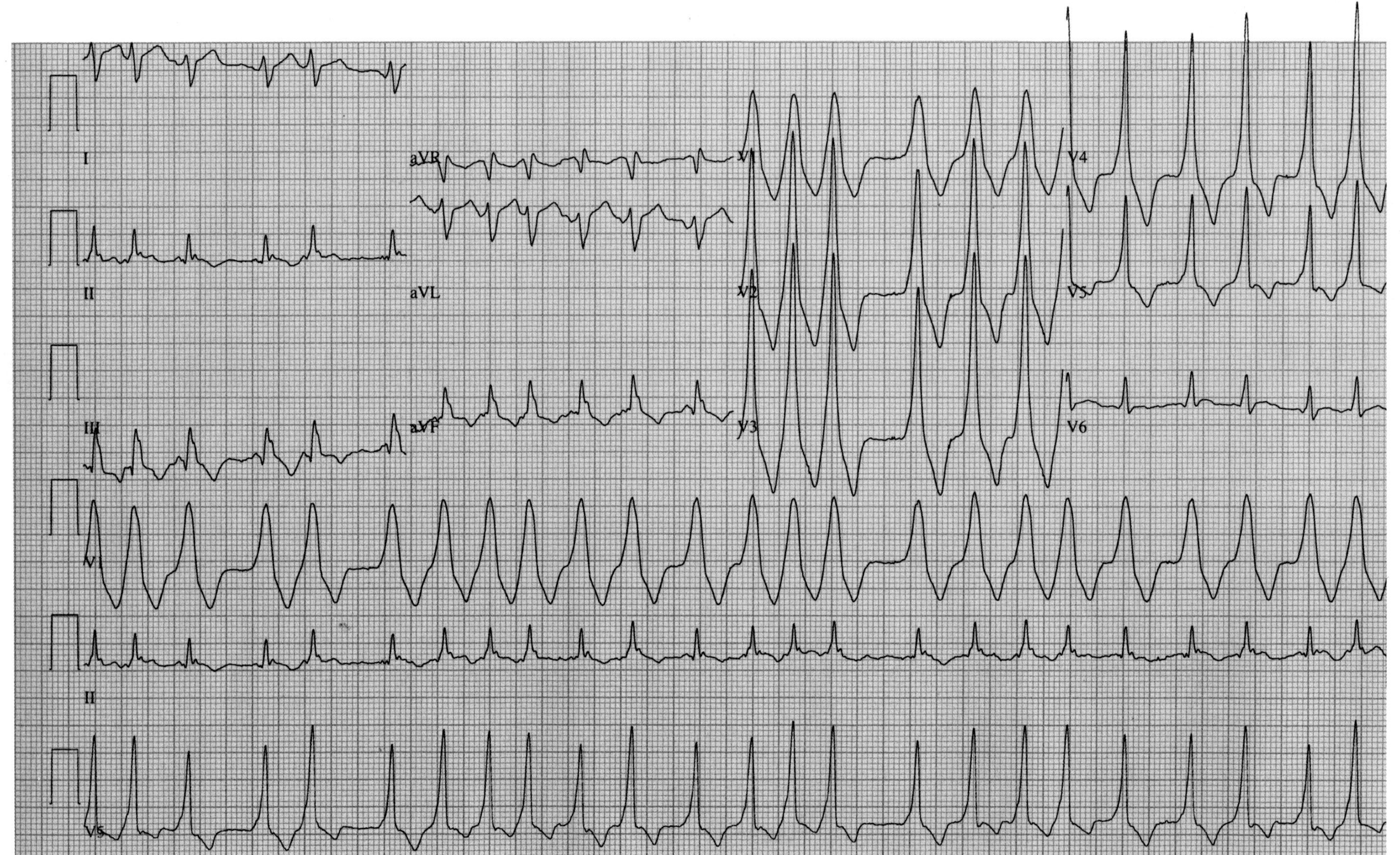

Interpretation Notes:

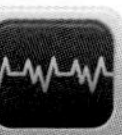

ELECTROCARDIOGRAM INTERPRETATION

This electrocardiogram demonstrates widened QRS complexes at a tachycardic rate approaching an average of 150 per minute. No discrete atrial depolarizations are seen supporting atrial fibrillation. The ventricular response is irregularly irregular with ventricular pre-excitation seen best in leads V2, V3, V4 in the form of a delta wave. This electrocardiogram represents antidromic atrioventricular tachycardia and antegrade conduction via the accessory pathway in the presence of atrial fibrillation and a rapid ventricular response.

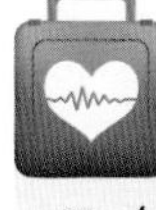

KEY DIAGNOSES

- Atrial fibrillation
- Wolff-Parkinson-White syndrome

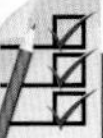

KEY TEACHING POINTS

- This electrocardiogram depicts a potentially life-threatening situation where potential exists for exceedingly fast antegrade atrioventricular conduction via the accessory pathway in the presence of atrial fibrillation. As this patient demonstrated, significant hemodynamic compromise can occur and shortly after this electrocardiogram was obtained, he underwent successful intracardiac ablation of the accessory pathway.
- In symptomatic patients with evidence of ventricular pre-excitation on the surface electrocardiogram, the current standard of care is intracardiac ablation.
- This patient's accessory pathway was left sided, suggested by the monophasic R wave as seen in lead V1.

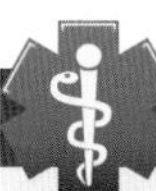

BOARD EXAMINATION ESSENTIALS

This is an essential electrocardiogram to be familiar with in preparation for the board exam. Board exam diagnostic codes include atrial fibrillation and Wolff-Parkinson-White pattern. Do not code right-axis deviation (greater than +100 degrees) as the axis deviation is not intrinsic to the QRS but instead due to altered ventricular depolarization via the accessory pathway. Make certain that you avoid coding ventricular tachycardia (three or more consecutive complexes) as the underlying rhythm is highly irregular, more so than one would expect with a ventricular tachycardic rhythm.

Electrocardiogram Case Study #84

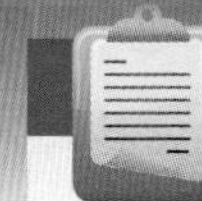

CLINICAL HISTORY

A 73-year-old male with hypertension who is seen in internal medicine follow-up after experiencing recent-onset shortness of breath.

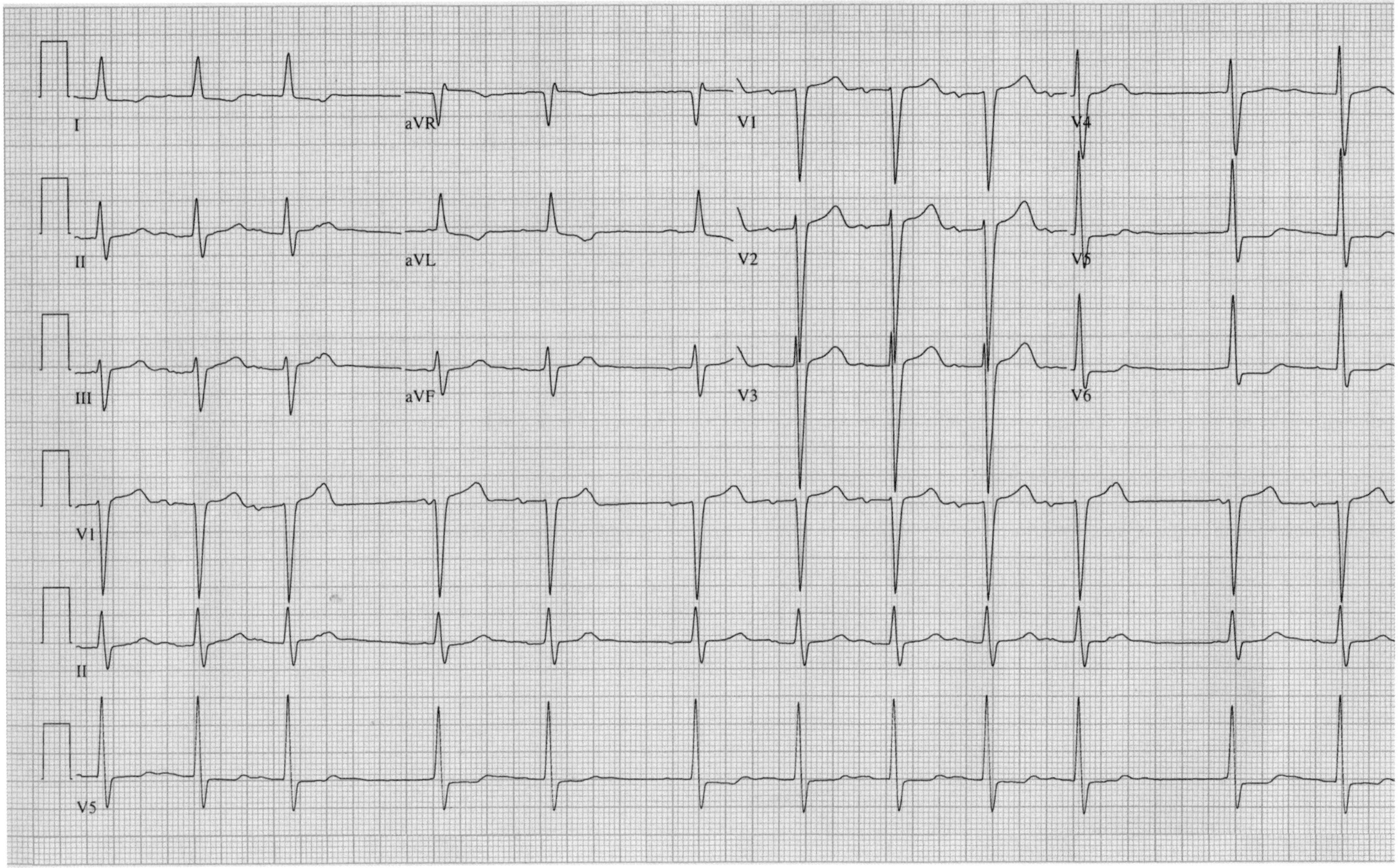

Interpretation Notes:

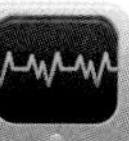

ELECTROCARDIOGRAM INTERPRETATION

On the left-hand side of this electrocardiogram, P waves precede each QRS complex with an isoelectric P wave noted in leads I and aVF consistent with an ectopic atrial rhythm at an atrial rate of approximately 70 per minute. First-degree atrioventricular block is present as the PR interval is >200 milliseconds. The third QRS complex demonstrates a superimposed P wave within the ST segment supporting a nonconducted premature atrial complex. The fourth QRS complex is preceded by a P wave with an extremely short PR interval, too short to conduct to the ventricle. This represents a junctional escape complex. The P wave preceding the fifth QRS complex conducts to the ventricle. The P wave preceding the sixth QRS complex possesses a different morphology and reflects an atrial escape complex. On the right-hand portion of the electrocardiogram, a pause is present secondary to a nonconducted premature atrial complex followed once again by a junctional escape complex. The QRS complex is widened >100 milliseconds supporting a nonspecific intraventricular conduction delay. Lateral and high lateral nonspecific ST-T changes are also seen.

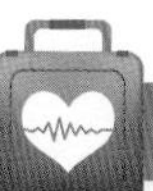

KEY DIAGNOSES

- Ectopic atrial rhythm
- First-degree atrioventricular block
- Nonconducted premature atrial complex
- Junctional escape complex
- Atrial escape complex
- Nonspecific intraventricular conduction delay
- Nonspecific ST-T changes
- Sick sinus syndrome

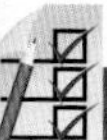

KEY TEACHING POINTS

- This patient demonstrates sinoatrial node disease given the presence of an ectopic atrial rhythm, junctional escape complexes, and an atrial escape complex.

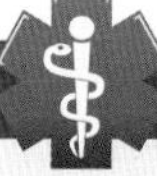

BOARD EXAMINATION ESSENTIALS

An ectopic atrial rhythm is present. For the purposes of the board exam, code normal sinus rhythm as ectopic atrial rhythm is not an available code. AV block, first degree, is present as are atrial premature complexes and AV junctional escape complexes. The QRS complex duration is >100 milliseconds consistent with an intraventricular conduction disturbance, nonspecific type. Lateral and high lateral nonspecific ST- and/or T-wave abnormalities are also demonstrated.

Electrocardiogram Case Study #85

CLINICAL HISTORY

An 83-year-old male with known coronary artery disease who returns for outpatient follow-up evaluation. The patient has a history of ischemic left ventricular systolic dysfunction with an estimated left ventricular ejection fraction of 30%.

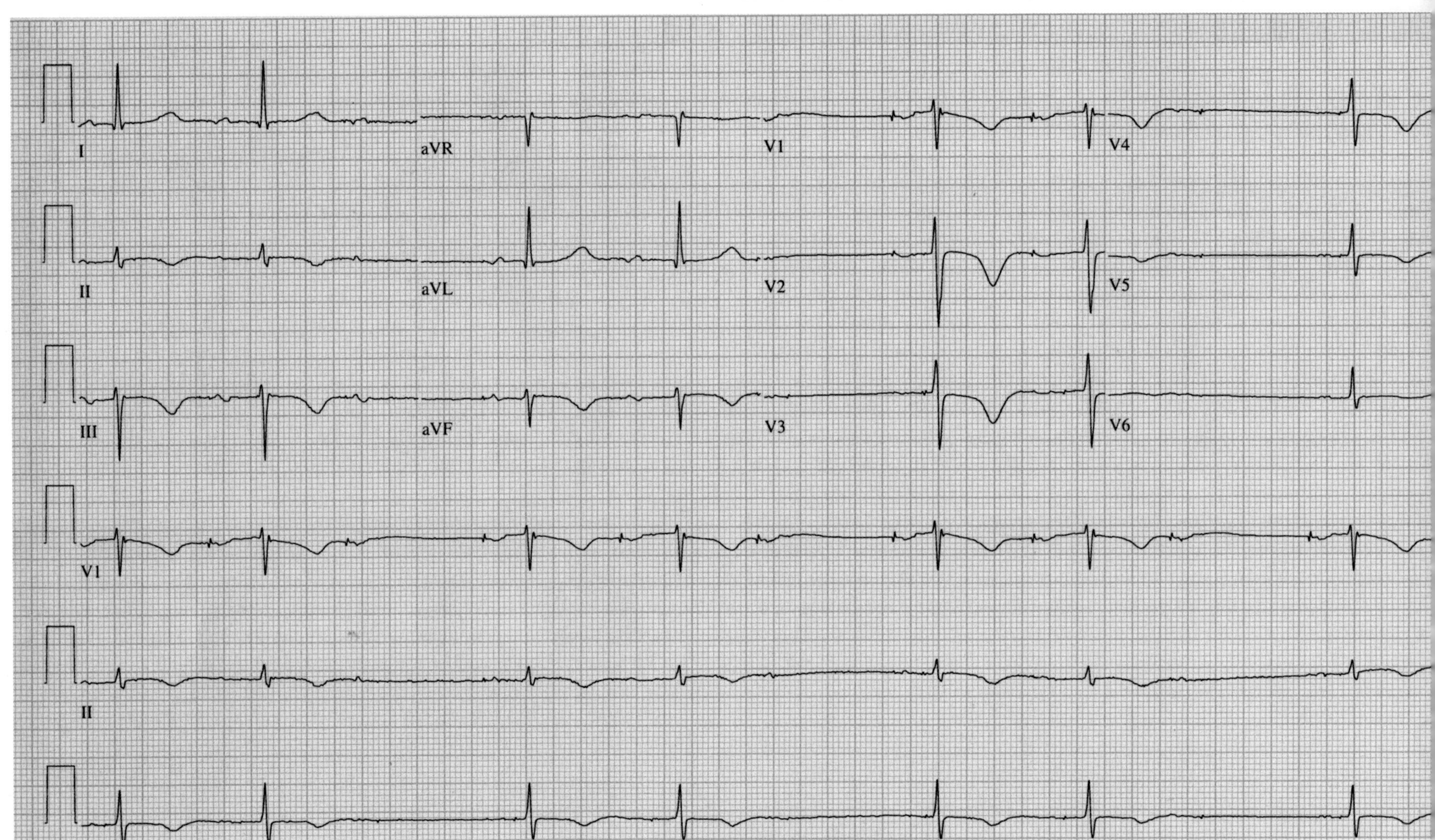

Interpretation Notes:

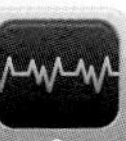

ELECTROCARDIOGRAM INTERPRETATION

This electrocardiogram demonstrates a discrete deflection prior to each P wave at a rate of 60 per minute consistent with an atrial pacemaker. The atrial pacemaker to QRS complex interval is prolonged to >200 milliseconds. This interval progressively prolongs. Three atrial pacemaker complexes are identified and grouped with two QRS complexes consistent with 3:2 Mobitz 1 Wenckebach atrioventricular block. Diffuse nonspecific ST-T changes predominantly in the form of T-wave inversion are identified in the anterolateral and the inferior leads.

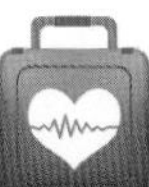

KEY DIAGNOSES

- Atrial pacemaker
- Mobitz I Wenckebach atrioventricular block
- Nonspecific ST-T changes

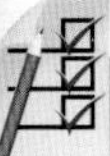

KEY TEACHING POINTS

- As evidenced on this electrocardiogram, atrioventricular conduction abnormalities are easily identified in the presence of atrial pacing.
- Despite the ischemic left ventricular systolic dysfunction, no discrete Q waves are seen diagnostic of an age-indeterminate myocardial infarction.
- A small rsr′ QRS complex morphology is seen in lead V1. The r′ is <30 milliseconds in duration not satisfying the criteria for incomplete right bundle-branch block.

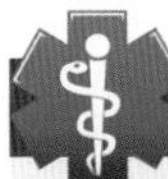

BOARD EXAMINATION ESSENTIALS

In the presence of pacemaker rhythms, it is equally important to assess for conduction system abnormalities pertaining to both atrioventricular and ventricular conduction. For this electrocardiogram, board exam diagnostic codes include atrial or coronary sinus pacing; AV block, second degree—Mobitz type I (Wenckebach); and nonspecific ST- and/or T-wave abnormalities. The deep T-wave inversion is likely secondary to the known ischemic heart disease. For the purpose of the board exam, in the absence of a clinical history suggesting an acute coronary syndrome coding for a less specific finding such as nonspecific ST-T changes is recommended.

Electrocardiogram Case Study #86

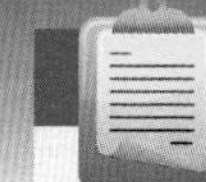

CLINICAL HISTORY

A 71-year-old male immediately postoperative pancreatic mass resection who developed acute blood loss and profound hypotension. This electrocardiogram was obtained in the immediate postoperative period.

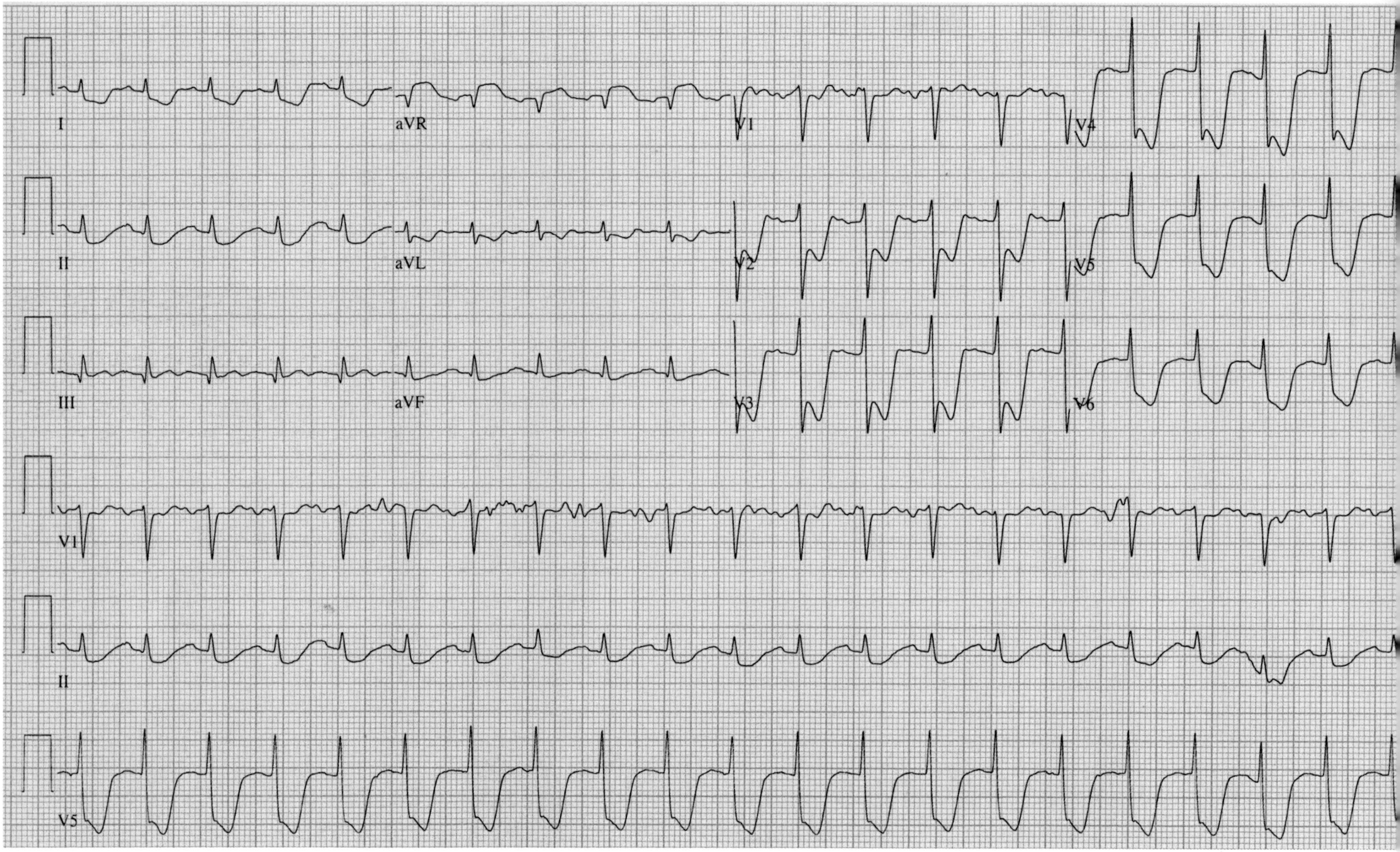

Interpretation Notes:

Electrocardiogram Case Study #86

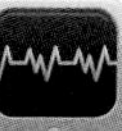

ELECTROCARDIOGRAM INTERPRETATION

This electrocardiogram demonstrates P waves at a constant interval with a normal P-wave axis at a rate of 125 per minute consistent with sinus tachycardia. Profound downsloping ST-segment depression is present in leads V2, V3, V4, V5, and V6. Downsloping ST-segment depression is also seen in leads I and II. Reciprocal ST-segment elevation is noted in lead aVR. This electrocardiogram is consistent with profound myocardial ischemia during an acutely hypotensive event.

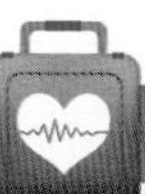

KEY DIAGNOSES

- Sinus tachycardia
- Myocardial ischemia

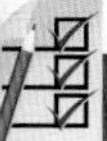

KEY TEACHING POINTS

- The combination of acute blood loss and hypotension resulted in advanced myocardial ischemia, left ventricular systolic dysfunction, and elevated serum cardiac enzymes confirming acute myocardial injury.
- Perfusion pressure to the subendocardium was significantly reduced resulting in severe left ventricular systolic dysfunction and myocardial injury. The patient expired shortly after this electrocardiogram was obtained.

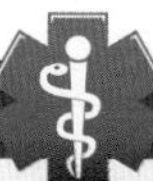

BOARD EXAMINATION ESSENTIALS

This electrocardiogram is straightforward from a diagnostic coding perspective. Sinus tachycardia and ST- and/or T-wave abnormalities suggesting myocardial ischemia completes the assessment. This electrocardiogram in some ways parallels a markedly positive exercise stress test with profound downsloping ST-segment depression as one might see in the presence of severe multivessel /left main coronary artery disease at peak exercise.

Electrocardiogram Case Study #87

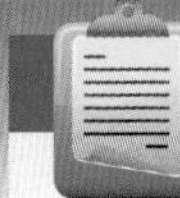

CLINICAL HISTORY

A 73-year-old male with previously diagnosed coronary artery disease who returns for an outpatient cardiovascular medicine check-up. The patient feels well at the present time.

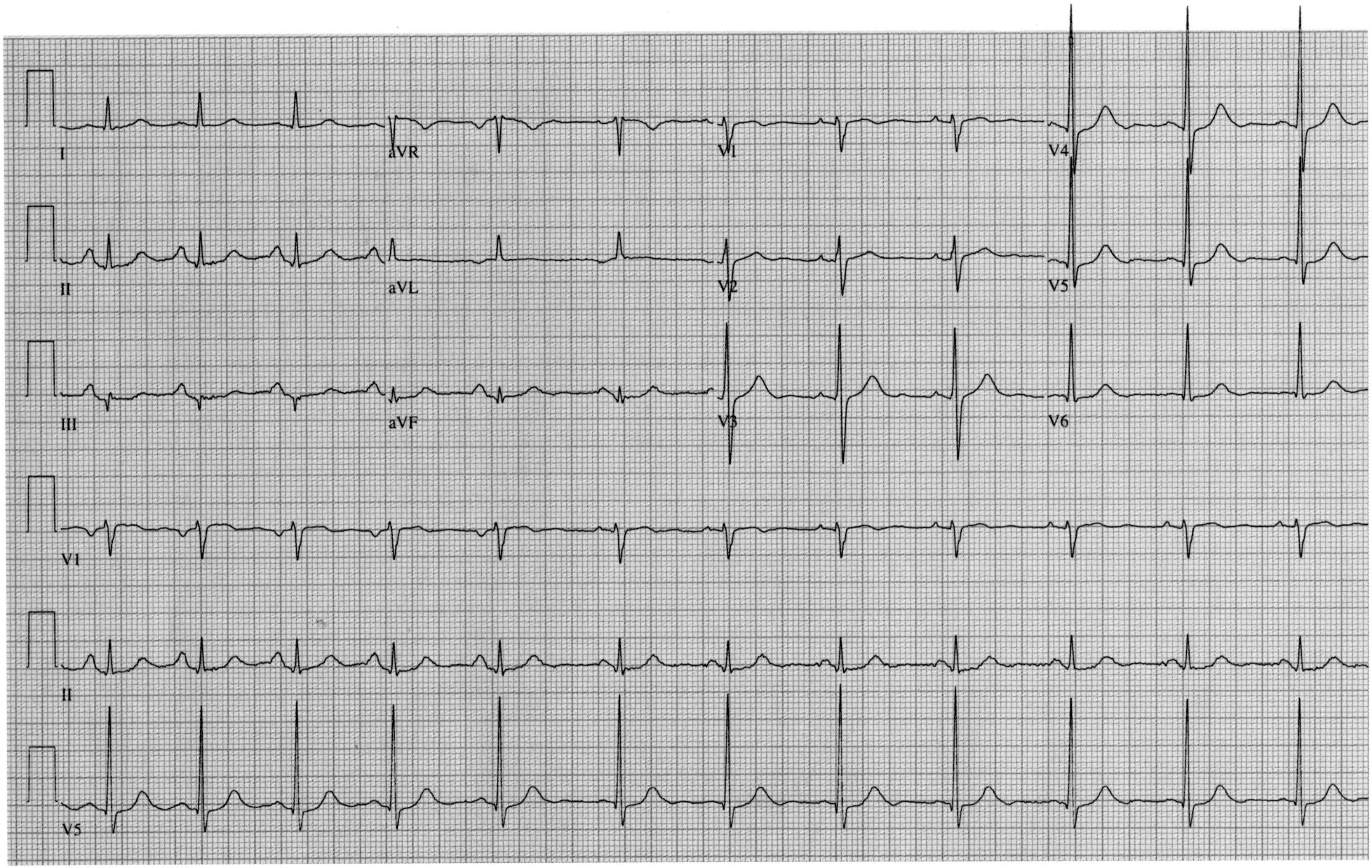

I aVR V1 V4

II aVL V2 V5

III aVF V3 V6

V1

II

V5

Interpretation Notes:

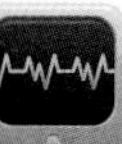

ELECTROCARDIOGRAM INTERPRETATION

This electrocardiogram demonstrates P waves of similar morphology preceding the initial five QRS complexes with a normal P-wave axis and an atrial rate of 85 per minute supporting normal sinus rhythm. In lead II, the P-wave amplitude is increased supporting right atrial abnormality. Immediately preceding the sixth QRS complex, the P-wave morphology shifts after a slight pause and continues for the remainder of the electrocardiogram. This reflects an ectopic atrial rhythm at a rate of approximately 70 per minute. Q waves are seen in leads II, III, and aVF but are not of diagnostic duration to conclude an age-indeterminate myocardial infarction. Negative U waves just after the T wave are seen in leads V4, V5, and V6 most likely indicative of the patient's coronary artery disease.

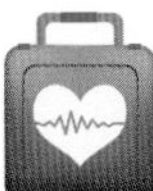

KEY DIAGNOSES

- Normal sinus rhythm
- Ectopic atrial rhythm
- Negative U waves
- Right atrial abnormality

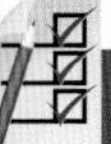

KEY TEACHING POINTS

- Negative U waves are an important electrocardiogram finding to identify. Most often, they are best seen in leads V4, V5, and V6. They can reflect increased left ventricular mass such as in patients with longstanding poorly controlled hypertension. Negative U waves are also seen in patients with underlying coronary artery disease and may be the first clinical indicator of structural heart disease.
- It is important to identify the P-wave axis and also ensure that the P-wave axis remains constant throughout the electrocardiogram. In this circumstance, the P-wave axis shifts due to the presence of a paroxysmal ectopic atrial rhythm.

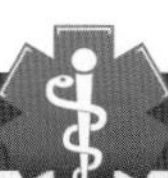

BOARD EXAMINATION ESSENTIALS

Several P-wave morphologies are identified on this electrocardiogram. For the purpose of the board exam, code normal sinus rhythm. This is not strictly sinus arrhythmia as the P-wave morphology should remain constant with sinus arrhythmia. Borderline criteria for left atrial abnormality/enlargement are present. For the board exam, expect a more pronounced and less equivocal abnormality. Right atrial abnormality/enlargement is present given the high-amplitude P wave in lead II. The negative U waves are an important clinical observation but not relevant to the diagnostic electrocardiogram coding section of the board exam. No definitive atrial prematurity is identified.

Electrocardiogram Case Study #88

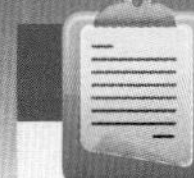

CLINICAL HISTORY

A 71-year-old female postoperative day 2 status post large abdominal sarcoma resection. The patient acutely developed an accelerated heart rate, confusion, and labored breathing. This electrocardiogram was obtained immediately after her telemetry monitoring reflected an abrupt elevation of heart rate.

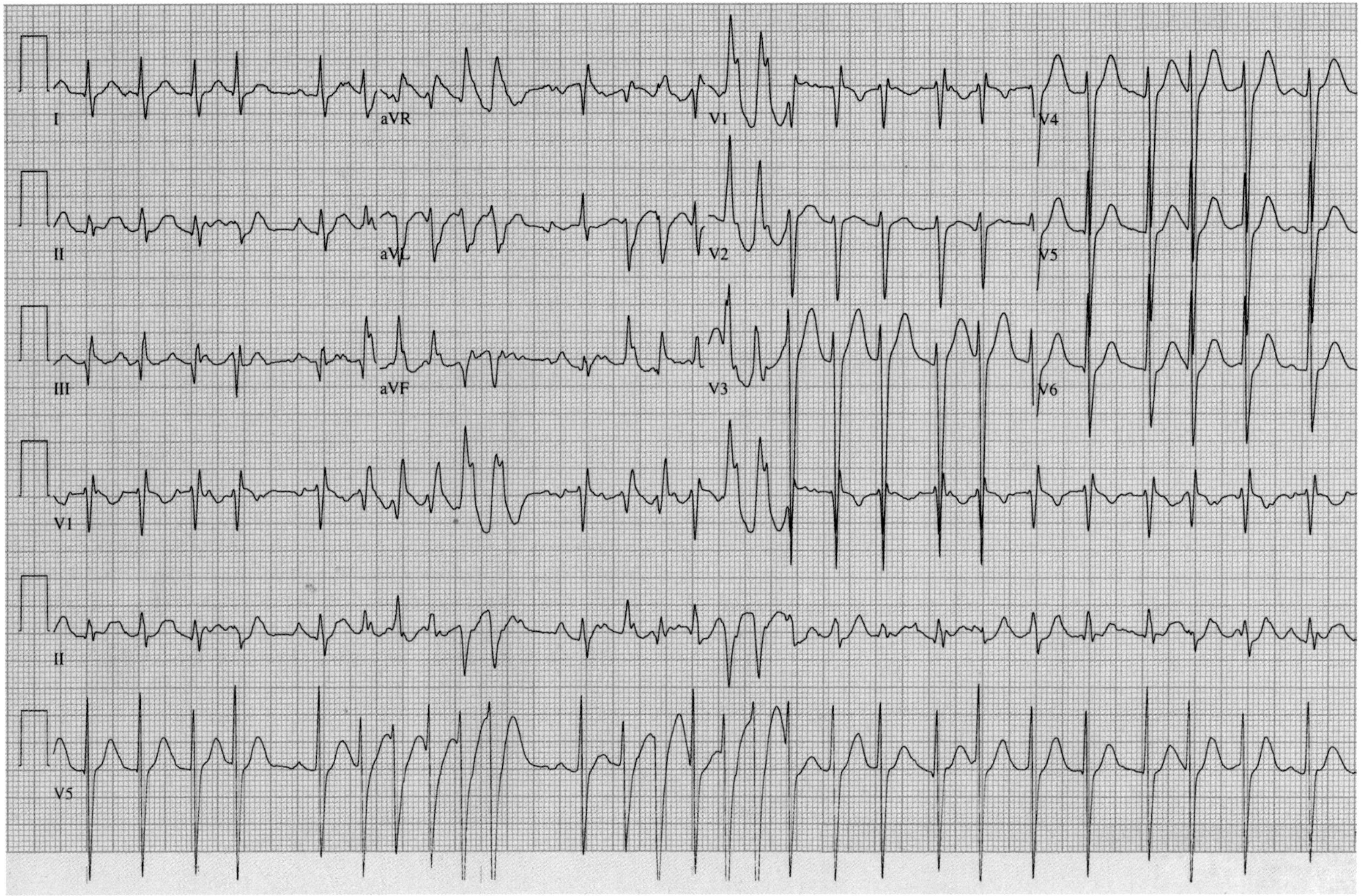

I aVR V1 V4
II aVL V2 V5
III aVF V3 V6
V1
II
V5

Interpretation Notes:

Electrocardiogram Case Study #88

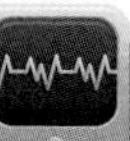

ELECTROCARDIOGRAM INTERPRETATION

This electrocardiogram demonstrates a rapid heart rhythm without clearly identifiable P waves most consistent with atrial fibrillation with a rapid ventricular response. Before the 5th and the 11th QRS complexes, P waves are seen with a normal P-wave axis. This supports the presence of normal sinus rhythm and paroxysms of atrial fibrillation with a rapid ventricular response. In lead V1, an rSr′ QRS complex is identified denoting ventricular aberration during the period of atrial fibrillation with a rapid ventricular response.

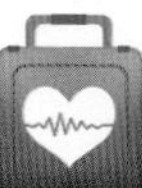

KEY DIAGNOSES

- Normal sinus rhythm
- Atrial fibrillation
- Rapid ventricular response
- Incomplete right bundle-branch block
- Aberrant conduction

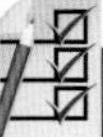

KEY TEACHING POINTS

- Aberrant ventricular conduction is commonly seen in the presence of tachycardic atrial arrhythmias with a rapid ventricular response. It often follows a longer R to R interval where the absolute refractory period of the ventricular conduction system is typically proportional to the preceding R to R interval.

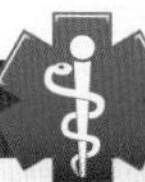

BOARD EXAMINATION ESSENTIALS

This electrocardiogram demonstrates several important diagnostic codes for the board exam. The tachycardic heart rate contributes to the complexity of this tracing. For starters, code baseline artifact. Next, code normal sinus rhythm and atrial fibrillation. Aberrant conduction is identified with a right ventricular conduction delay QRS complex pattern. Be certain not to code for ventricular tachycardia (three or more consecutive complexes) or ventricular premature complexes. Right bundle-branch block, incomplete, is present as well, best assessed in lead V1. Make sure to assess each electrocardiogram for technical adequacy including baseline artifact, limb lead or precordial lead incorrect electrode placement, one half or double standardization, right-sided precordial leads, and low voltage. Each of these potential findings should be embedded in your electrocardiogram interpretation algorithm.

Electrocardiogram Case Study **#89**

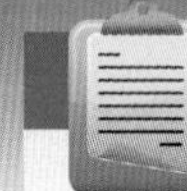

CLINICAL HISTORY

A 67-year-old female with longstanding systemic hypertension, known increased left ventricular mass, and coronary artery disease. The patient returns for an outpatient cardiovascular medicine follow-up evaluation.

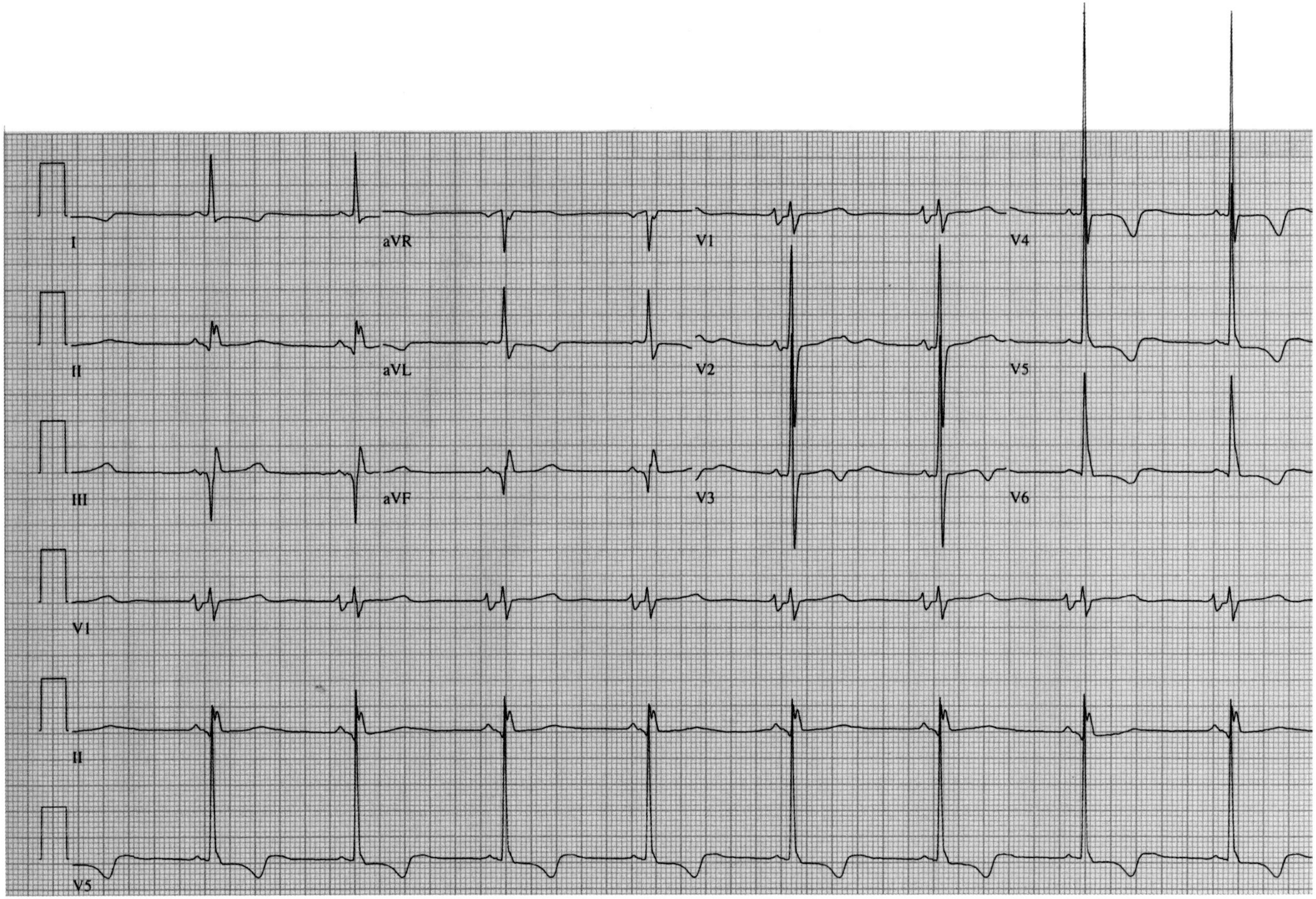

Interpretation Notes:____

____

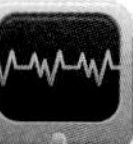

ELECTROCARDIOGRAM INTERPRETATION

This electrocardiogram demonstrates P waves occurring at regular intervals preceding each QRS complex possessing a normal P-wave axis at a rate of 50 per minute consistent with sinus bradycardia. The P wave demonstrates prominent terminal negativity in lead V1 and a bifid appearance in lead II supporting left atrial abnormality. The QRS complex voltage is markedly increased with asymmetric T-wave inversion in the lateral precordial leads supporting left ventricular hypertrophy with secondary ST-T changes and the so-called pressure overload pattern. Prominent inferior Q waves are seen with terminal conduction delay and a widened QRS complex. This is consistent with an age-indeterminate inferior myocardial infarction with peri-infarction block. Prominent R waves are demonstrated in leads V1, V2, and V3 supporting a posterior myocardial infarction, age indeterminate

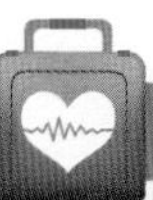

KEY DIAGNOSES

- Sinus bradycardia
- Left atrial abnormality
- Left ventricular hypertrophy with secondary ST-T changes
- Inferior myocardial infarction, age indeterminate
- Posterior myocardial infarction, age indeterminate
- Peri-infarction block

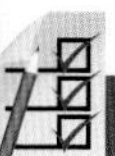

KEY TEACHING POINTS

- Peri-infarction block reflects terminal conduction delay within the infarct zone, in this case the right coronary artery distribution.
- This patient demonstrates electrocardiographic findings consistent with increased intracardiac pressures including left atrial abnormality and left ventricular hypertrophy. Left ventricular hypertrophy strongly supports increased left ventricular mass.

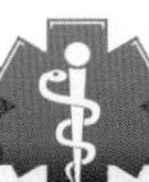

BOARD EXAMINATION ESSENTIALS

Diagnostic codes for the board exam include sinus bradycardia, left ventricular hypertrophy, and ST- and/or T-wave abnormalities secondary to hypertrophy. Equally important, be sure to code; left atrial abnormality/enlargement (a common finding in the presence of ventricular hypertrophy patterns); an inferior myocardial infarction, age indeterminate; a posterior myocardial infarction, age indeterminate; and intraventricular conduction disturbance, nonspecific type.

Electrocardiogram Case Study #90

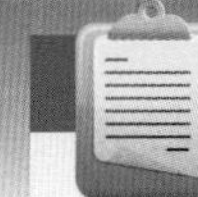

CLINICAL HISTORY

A 36-year-old male with poorly controlled hypertension for the past 10 years. He has recently developed symptoms of exertional shortness of breath and heart irregularity. He is currently seen in the outpatient cardiovascular medicine department.

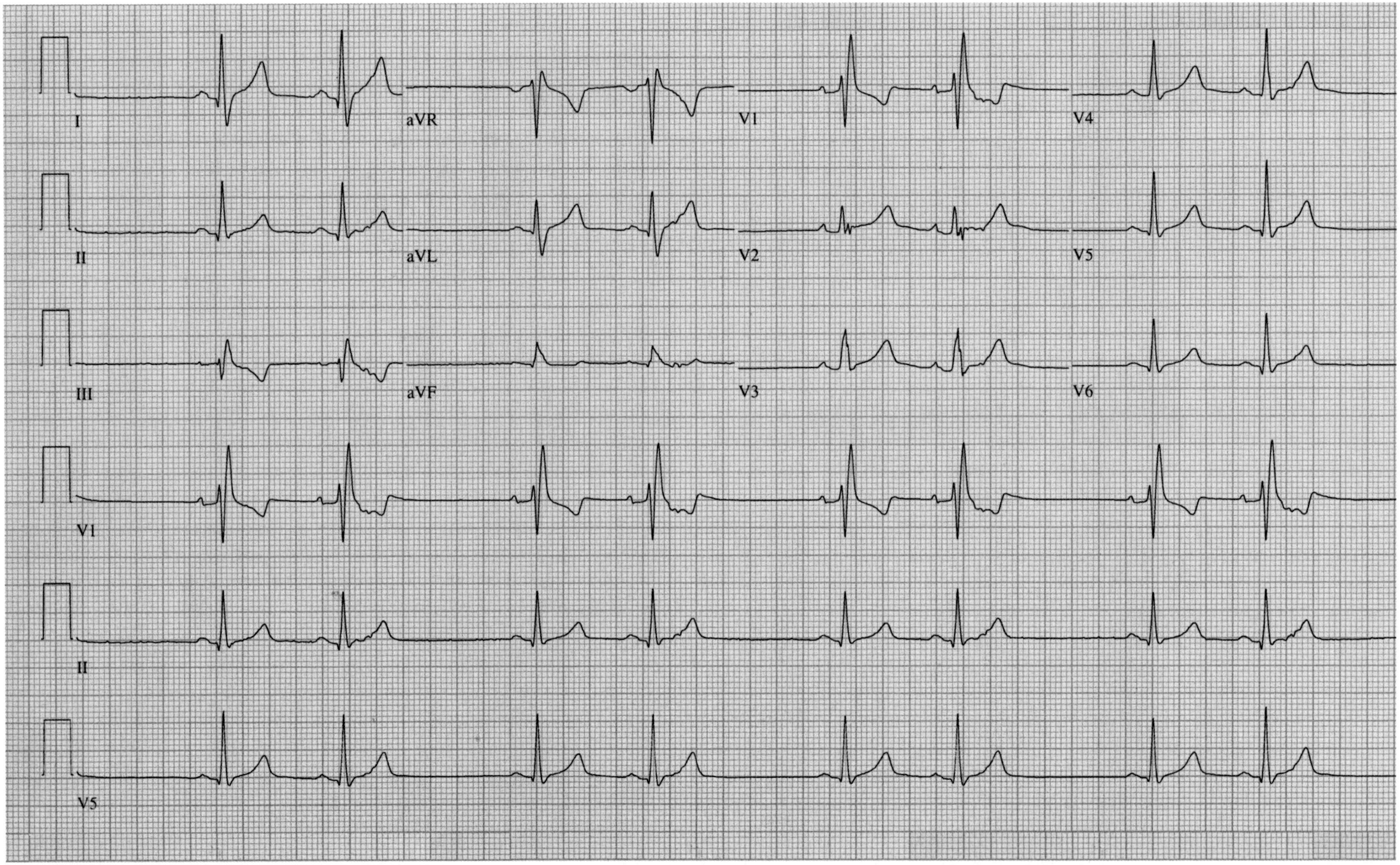

I aVR V1 V4

II aVL V2 V5

III aVF V3 V6

V1

II

V5

Interpretation Notes:

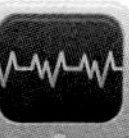

ELECTROCARDIOGRAM INTERPRETATION

This electrocardiogram demonstrates P waves with a normal axis QRS complex at an average rate of approximately 70 per minute supporting normal sinus rhythm. Grouped QRS complexes are seen and this is secondary to nonconducted premature atrial complexes. Within the ST segment of the second QRS complex within each grouping, an additional deflection is evident consistent with a nonconducted premature atrial complex. The QRS complex is widened to >120 milliseconds with an rSR′ QRS complex morphology in lead V1 supporting complete right bundle-branch block. The T waves are upright in leads V2 and V3 indicating the presence of a primary T-wave change.

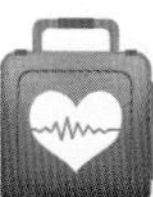

KEY DIAGNOSES

- Normal sinus rhythm
- Nonconducted premature atrial complexes
- Complete right bundle-branch block
- Primary T-wave changes

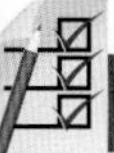

KEY TEACHING POINTS

- Grouped QRS complexes should raise the possibility of either nonconducted premature atrial complexes or Mobitz type I Wenckebach atrioventricular block. For this electrocardiogram, the PR interval remains constant and nonconducted premature atrial complexes are present within the ST segment of the second QRS complex of each grouping, confirming the diagnosis.
- A primary T-wave change is seen in leads V2 and V3 and is of uncertain diagnostic significance. It raises the possibility of underlying coronary artery disease. This patient underwent cardiac stress imaging and no abnormality was found.

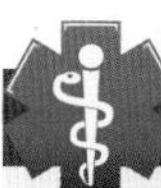

BOARD EXAMINATION ESSENTIALS

This electrocardiogram demonstrates grouped QRS complexes. In this case, board exam diagnostic codes include normal sinus rhythm, atrial premature complexes, and complete right bundle-branch block. Be careful not to code sinus pause or arrest; sinoatrial exit block; or AV block, second degree—Mobitz type I Wenkebach.

Electrocardiogram Case Study **#91**

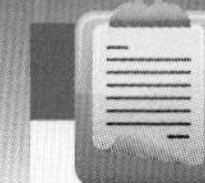

CLINICAL HISTORY

A 74-year-old female admitted acutely to the hospital with severe chest pain, hypotension, and confusion. Serum cardiac enzymes were elevated confirming acute myocardial injury.

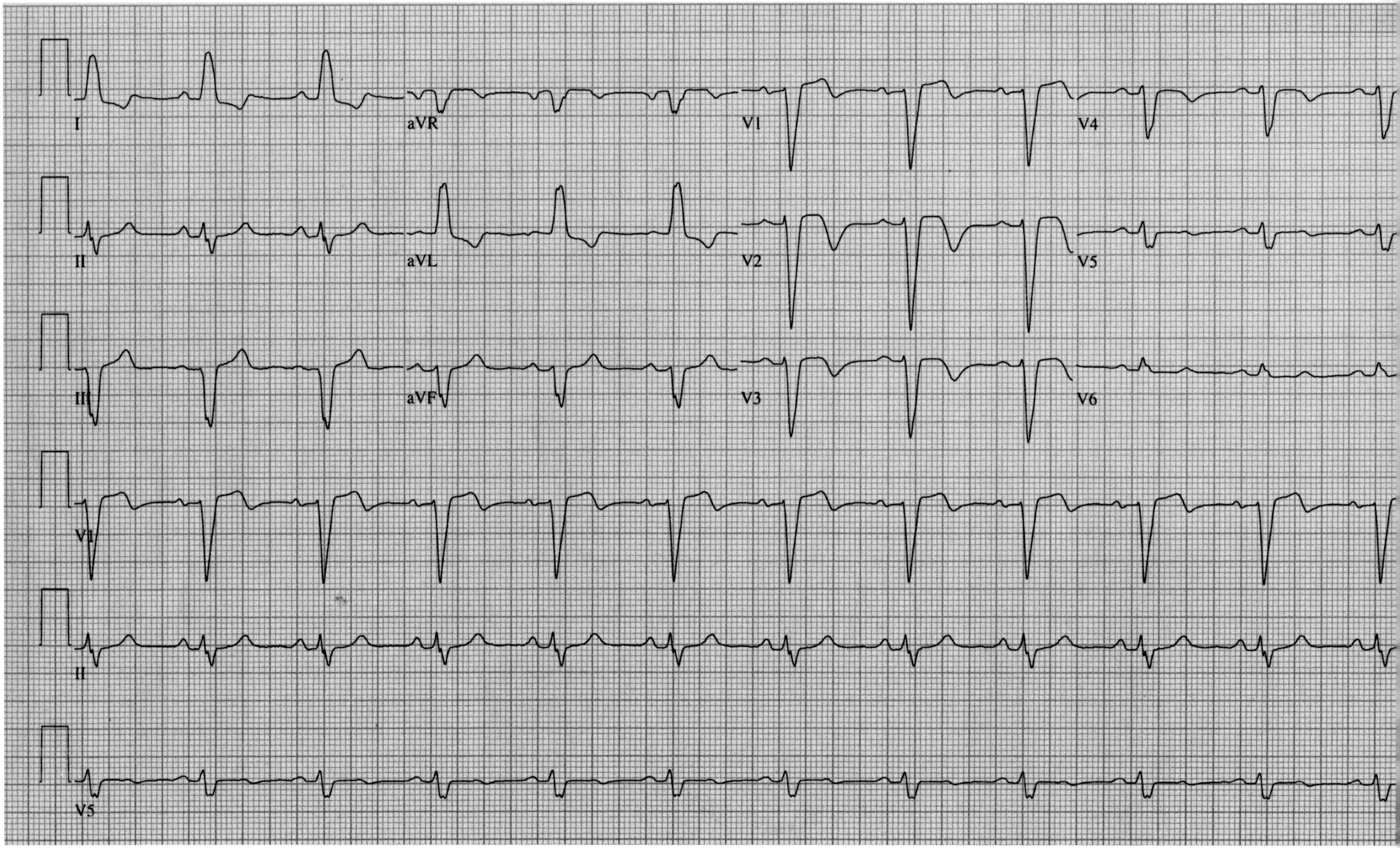

Interpretation Notes:

Electrocardiogram Case Study #91

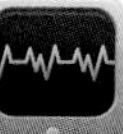

ELECTROCARDIOGRAM INTERPRETATION

This electrocardiogram demonstrates P waves of normal axis at a rate slightly <70 per minute with a constant P to P interval confirming normal sinus rhythm. The QRS complex is prolonged at 120 milliseconds without evidence of septal Q waves supporting complete left bundle-branch block. QRS complex left-axis deviation is also demonstrated as the QRS complex vector is positive in lead I and negative in leads II, III, and aVF. J point and ST-segment elevation is seen in leads V1, V2, V3, and V4. This confirms the presence of acute myocardial injury as supported by the elevated serum cardiac enzymes.

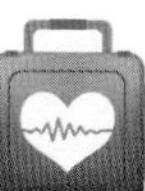

KEY DIAGNOSES

- Normal sinus rhythm
- QRS complex left-axis deviation
- Complete left bundle-branch block
- Acute myocardial injury

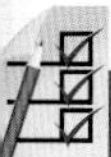

KEY TEACHING POINTS

- In the presence of complete left bundle-branch block, it is possible to accurately arrive at the diagnosis of acute myocardial injury. While the diagnosis of an age-indeterminate myocardial infarction is not possible with certainty in the presence of complete left bundle-branch block, ST-segment deviation including ST-segment elevation is readily identified.
- This patient was taken immediately to the cardiac catheterization laboratory where a proximal complete left anterior descending coronary artery obstruction was identified. This correlates with the electrocardiogram findings given the fact that the ST-segment elevation begins in lead V1, which reflects the proximal left anterior descending coronary artery territory prior to the first septal perforator branch.

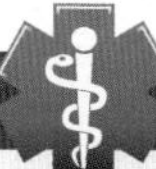

BOARD EXAMINATION ESSENTIALS

On the board examination, anticipate an example of complete left bundle-branch block and acute myocardial injury. For this electrocardiogram, note the absence of Q waves. Importantly, do not code for a myocardial infarction in the presence of complete left bundle-branch block. Appropriate diagnostic codes include normal sinus rhythm, left bundle-branch block, complete, left-axis deviation (greater than –30 degrees) and ST-and/or T-wave abnormalities suggesting myocardial injury. This latter diagnosis is preferred over ST- and/or T-wave abnormalities suggesting myocardial ischemia as both J point and ST-segment elevation are present.

Electrocardiogram Case Study #92

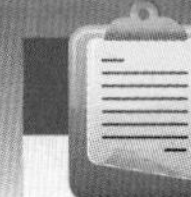

CLINICAL HISTORY

A 58-year-old male admitted via the emergency room with acute chest discomfort who was taken directly to the cardiac catheterization laboratory where a 100% acute occlusion of the left circumflex coronary artery was found. The patient underwent successful intracoronary stent placement with resolution of his symptoms.

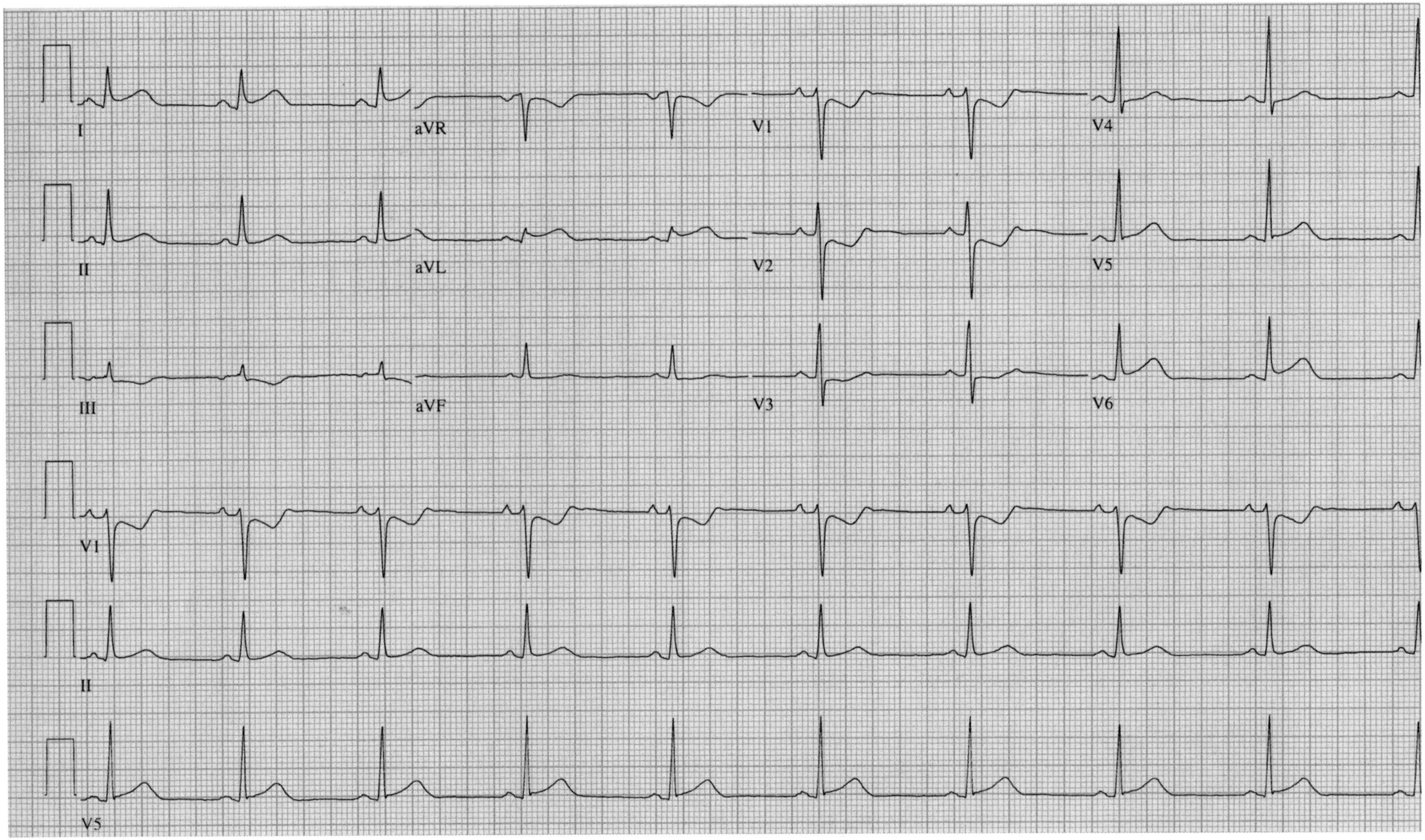

Interpretation Notes:____

____

Electrocardiogram Case Study #92

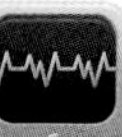

ELECTROCARDIOGRAM INTERPRETATION

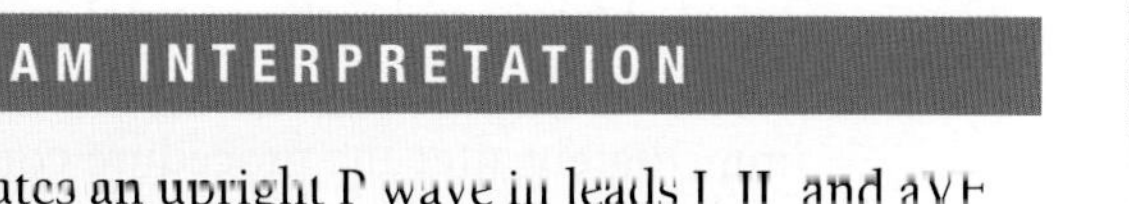

This electrocardiogram demonstrates an upright P wave in leads I, II, and aVF at an atrial rate slightly <60 per minute consistent with sinus bradycardia. J point and ST-segment elevation is noted in leads I, aVL, V5, and V6. No diagnostic Q waves are seen. This is consistent with lateral and high lateral acute myocardial injury. Downsloping ST-segment depression is identified in leads V1 and V2, which could be a reciprocal finding of the lateral and the high lateral ST-segment elevation versus true posterior myocardial injury.

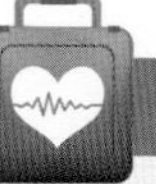

KEY DIAGNOSES

- Sinus bradycardia
- Acute myocardial injury

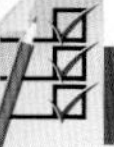

KEY TEACHING POINTS

- To determine if the downsloping ST-segment depression in leads V1 and V2 represents a reciprocal finding to the acute myocardial injury pattern versus true posterior myocardial injury, serial electrocardiograms are necessary. Should R-wave "growth" be identified in leads V1 and V2, this supports the presence of posterior myocardial injury and subsequent infarction. This would be evident under normal circumstances within 24 to 48 hours after the initial myocardial event.
- Acute myocardial injury is the preferred diagnosis for this electrocardiogram given the J point and ST-segment elevation in the absence of Q waves of diagnostic duration.

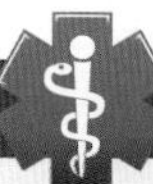

BOARD EXAMINATION ESSENTIALS

This electrocardiogram is another example of acute myocardial injury. Applicable diagnostic codes include sinus bradycardia and ST- and/or T-wave abnormalities suggesting myocardial injury. The lack of Q waves supports not coding a myocardial infarction.

Electrocardiogram Case Study #93

CLINICAL HISTORY

A 75-year-old female with multiple comorbidities and severely symptomatic hypertrophic obstructive cardiomyopathy not deemed to be a cardiothoracic surgical candidate who underwent alcohol septal ablation to her first septal perforator branch of her left anterior descending coronary artery. This electrocardiogram was obtained immediately after the procedure concluded.

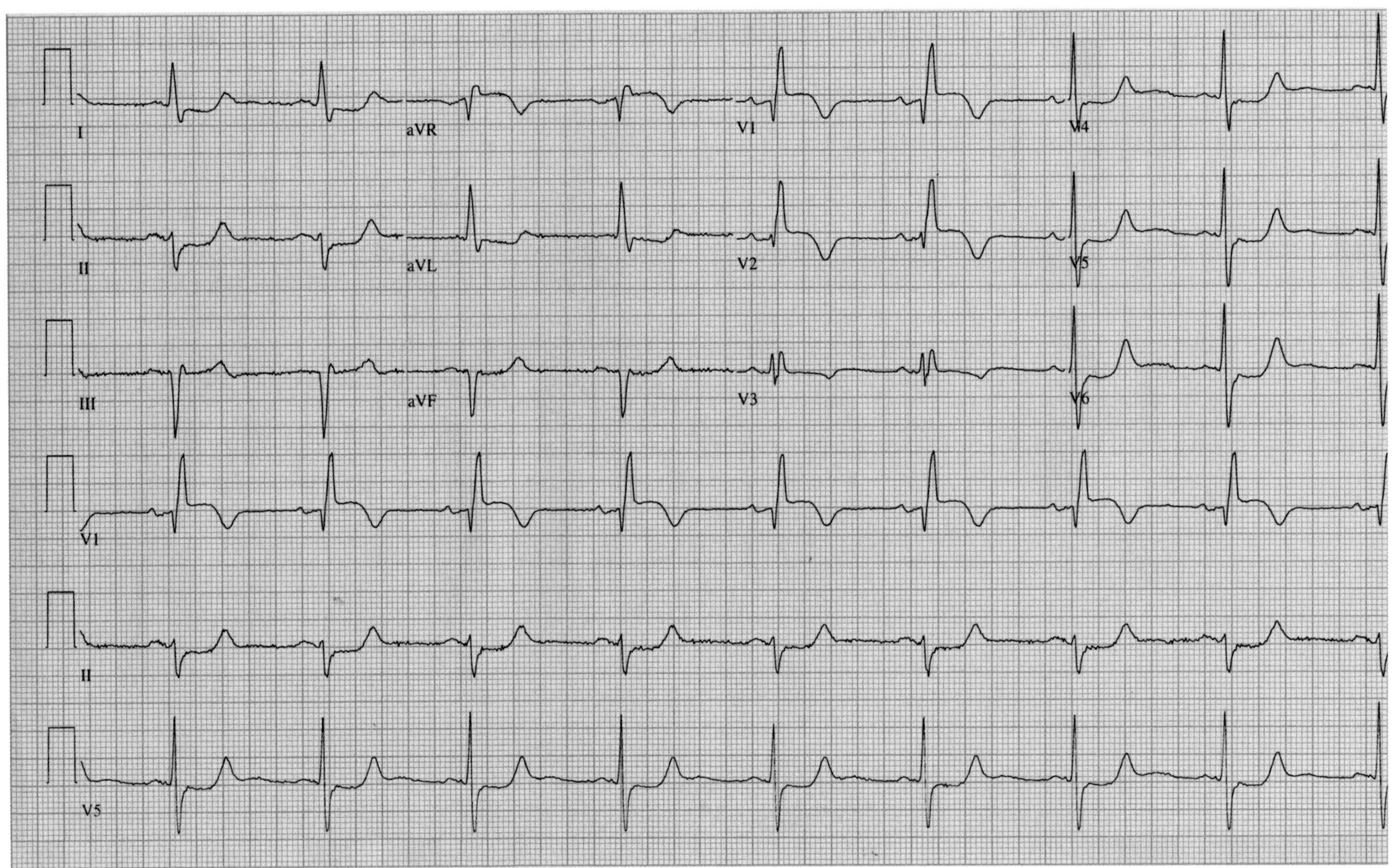

Interpretation Notes:____

____

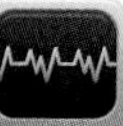

ELECTROCARDIOGRAM INTERPRETATION

This electrocardiogram demonstrates P waves at regular intervals with a normal P-wave axis at an atrial rate approximating 50 per minute supporting sinus bradycardia. Left anterior fascicular block is demonstrated given the positive QRS complex vector in lead I and negative QRS complex vectors in leads II, III, and aVF. Complete right bundle-branch block is also demonstrated as the QRS complex is greater than 120 milliseconds in duration and a QR QRS complex pattern is demonstrated in lead V1. ST-segment elevation is seen in leads V1 and V2 and reciprocal downsloping ST-segment depression in leads I, aVL, V5, and V6. The ST-segment elevation in leads V1 and V2 reflects acute myocardial injury as these leads overlie the proximal interventricular septum and the first septal perforator branch myocardial territory.

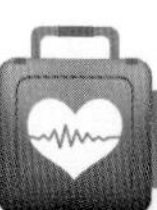

KEY DIAGNOSES

- Sinus bradycardia
- Left anterior fascicular block
- Complete right bundle-branch block
- Acute myocardial injury
- Hypertrophic cardiomyopathy
- Artifact

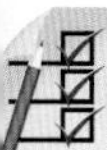

KEY TEACHING POINTS

- The first septal perforator branch alcohol septal ablation procedure characteristically produces an acute myocardial injury pattern in leads V1 and V2 as the myocardial injury pattern is localized to the proximal interventricular septum.
- Conduction abnormalities, most often transient, are also frequently identified including left anterior and posterior fascicular block and varying extents of right ventricular conduction delay.

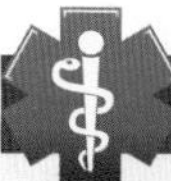

BOARD EXAMINATION ESSENTIALS

This patient has known hypertrophic cardiomyopathy, not classically demonstrated on this electrocardiogram. Diagnostic codes for the board exam include sinus bradycardia, left anterior fascicular block, right bundle-branch block, complete and ST- and/or T-wave abnormalities suggesting myocardial injury. For this electrocardiogram, do not code an inferior myocardial infarction, age indeterminate. While diminutive, a small initially positive QRS complex vector is present in leads II, II, and aVF. Artifact should also be coded.

Electrocardiogram Case Study #94

CLINICAL HISTORY

A 79-year-old male with recurrent episodes of congestive heart failure who was admitted to the hospital for medical optimization. He is presently in acute systolic decompensated congestive heart failure. The patient has known coronary artery disease and suffered a prior myocardial infarction. He is also status post ventricular pacemaker placement.

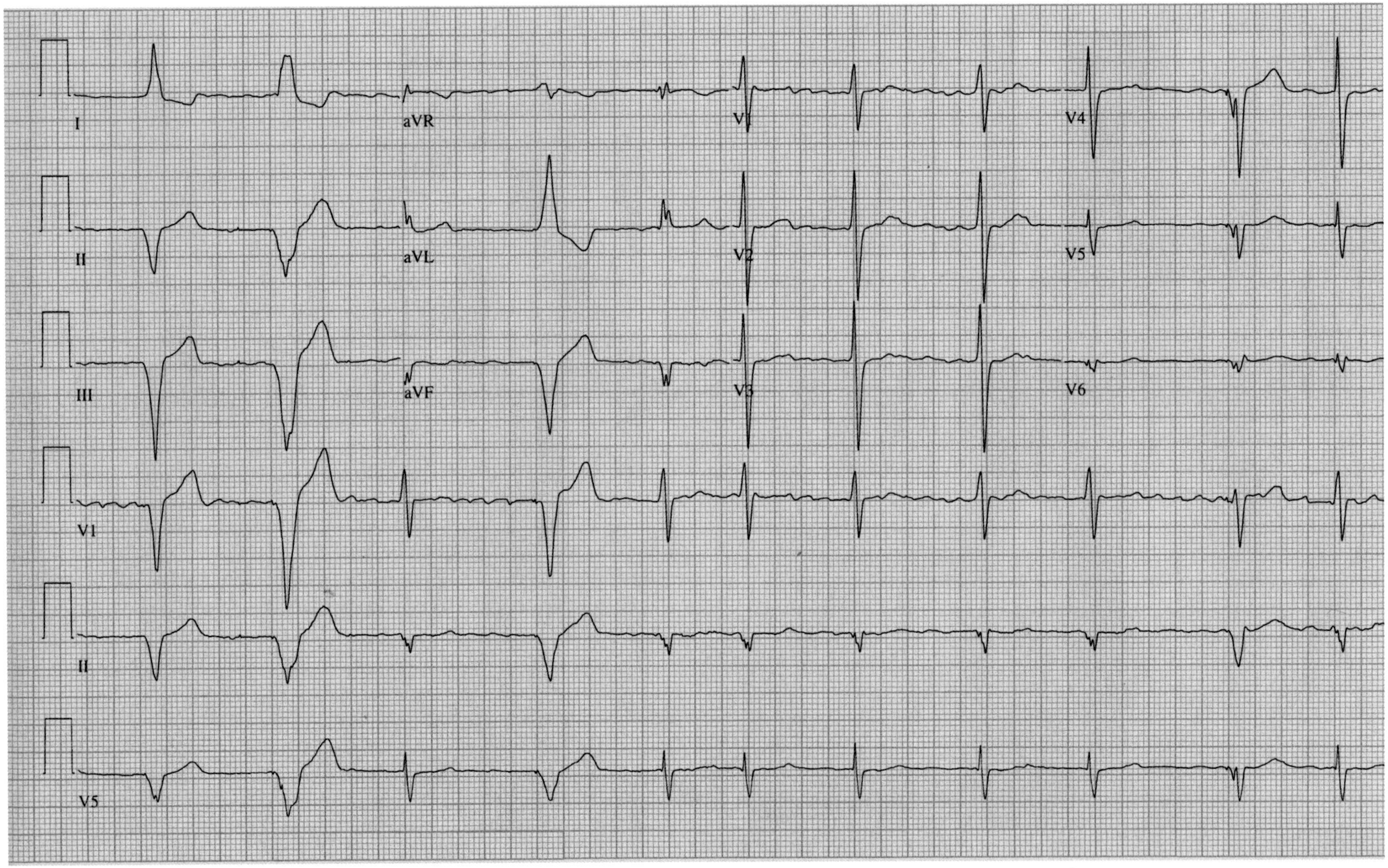

Interpretation Notes:

Electrocardiogram Case Study #94

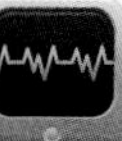

ELECTROCARDIOGRAM INTERPRETATION

This electrocardiogram demonstrates no identifiable P waves, best assessed in the lead V1 rhythm strip. This finding confirms the presence of atrial fibrillation. The ventricular response averages approximately 65 per minute. The second QRS complex is fully ventricularly paced as a discrete ventricular pacemaker deflection is seen best in the lead V5 rhythm strip. The first and the fourth QRS complexes demonstrate an intermediate morphology between the native QRS complex and the ventricular paced complex supporting simultaneous ventricular depolarization best characterized as a pacemaker fusion complex. In lead aVF, the second QRS complex demonstrates a Q wave of approximately 80-millisecond duration. This confirms an age-indeterminate inferior myocardial infarction. The first QRS complex in lead V6 demonstrates a diagnostic Q wave. While an isolated lead, lead V6 is contiguous with the inferior distribution supporting an age-indeterminate lateral myocardial infarction. In lead V1, the R to S wave ratio is <1 precluding the diagnosis of a posterior myocardial infarction.

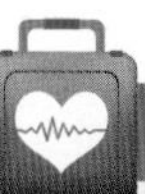

KEY DIAGNOSES

- Atrial fibrillation
- Inferior myocardial infarction, age indeterminate
- Lateral myocardial infarction, age indeterminate
- Ventricular pacemaker
- Pacemaker fusion complexes

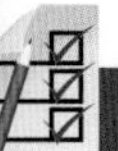

KEY TEACHING POINTS

- Given the presence of a ventricular pacemaker, the ability to interpret the electrocardiogram utilizing the native QRS complex is limited. For instance, in leads I, II, and III, only ventricular paced complexes are identified. Lead aVF provides one native QRS complex and this is important as an inferior myocardial infarction of indeterminate age is identified. Similarly, in lead V6, the native QRS complexes permit the diagnosis of a lateral myocardial infarction of indeterminate age.
- In the presence of a ventricular pacemaker, interpreting the atrial rhythm if possible is important as it may have additional clinical implications.

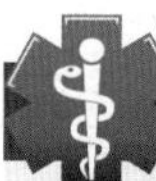

BOARD EXAMINATION ESSENTIALS

This is a challenging electrocardiogram that emphasizes several important board exam diagnostic code concepts. The underlying heart rhythm is atrial fibrillation. An intermittent ventricular demand pacemaker (VVI), normally functioning, is seen. An inferior myocardial infarction, age indeterminate; and a lateral myocardial infarction, age indeterminate, are also present. These two infarction patterns are evident in only single, nonpaced QRS complexes in leads aVF and V6, respectively.

Electrocardiogram Case Study #95

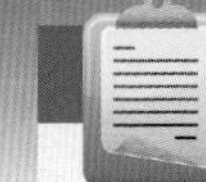

CLINICAL HISTORY

A 35-year-old male status post aortic valve replacement for severe congenital bicuspid aortic stenosis. The patient is postoperative day 2 resting comfortably on a telemetry hospital ward.

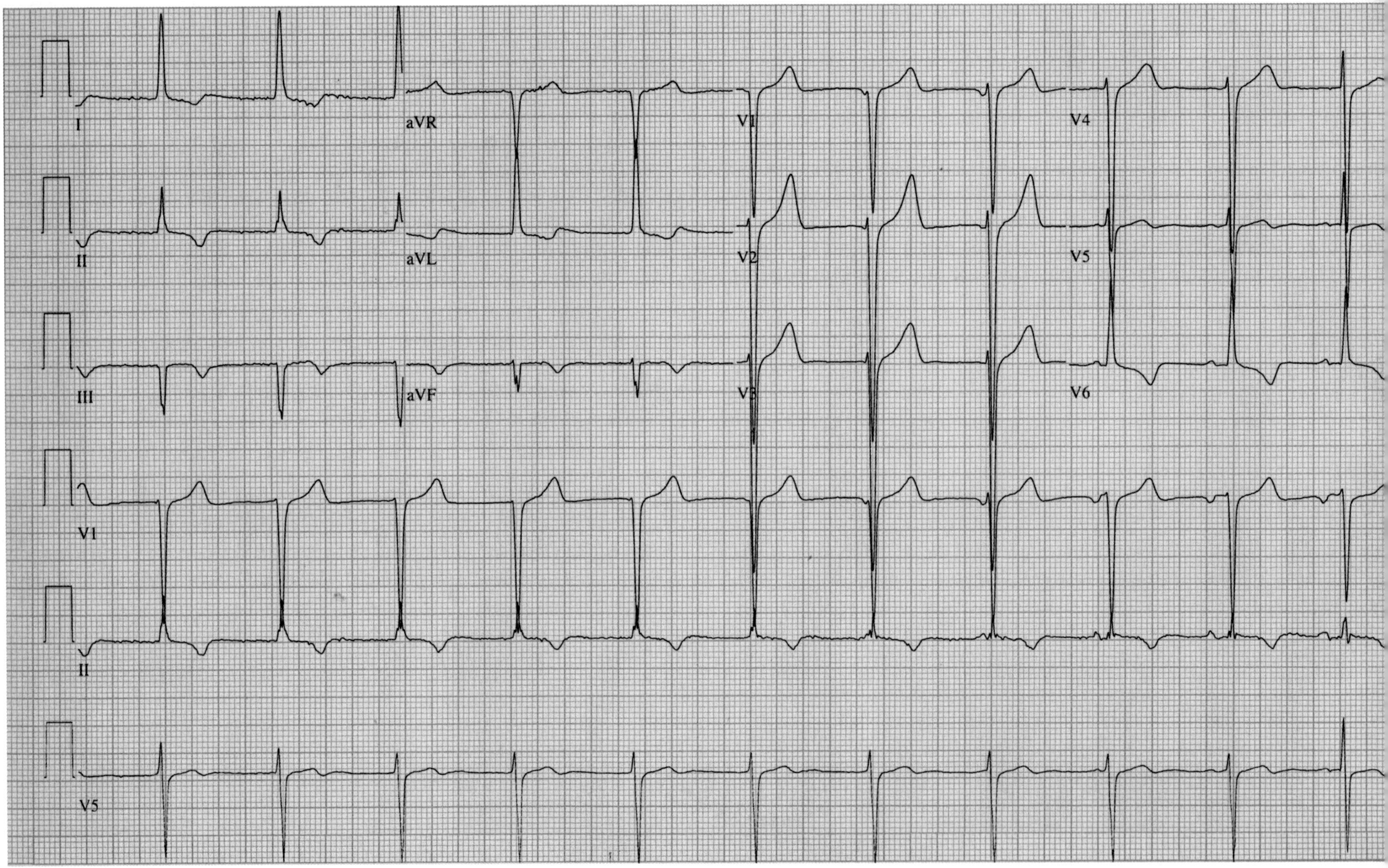

I

aVR

V1

V4

II

aVL

V2

V5

III

aVF

V3

V6

V1

II

V5

Interpretation Notes:

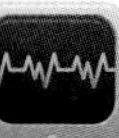

ELECTROCARDIOGRAM INTERPRETATION

This electrocardiogram demonstrates P waves with a normal P-wave axis occurring at a regular interval of 70 per minute consistent with normal sinus rhythm. The P waves are best seen toward the right-hand portion of the electrocardiogram. Narrow QRS complexes also occur at a regular interval at a rate slightly <75 per minute. An inconstant PR interval is identified without clear relationship between the P waves and the QRS complexes. This is an example of atrioventricular dissociation in the presence of normal sinus rhythm and an accelerated junctional rhythm. Voltage criteria for left ventricular hypertrophy with secondary asymmetric T-wave inversion is seen in the precordial and high lateral leads.

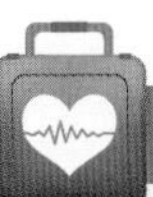

KEY DIAGNOSES

- Normal sinus rhythm
- Accelerated junctional rhythm
- Atrioventricular dissociation
- Left ventricular hypertrophy with secondary ST-T changes

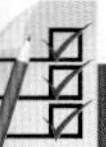

KEY TEACHING POINTS

- An accelerated junctional rhythm is a common dysrhythmia observed soon after open-heart surgery. It typically is a transient arrhythmia during which it usurps pacemaker dominance from the sinus node.
- The presence of left ventricular hypertrophy with secondary ST-T changes is a common finding in the presence of severe aortic stenosis. This reflects increased left ventricular mass secondary to the left ventricular outflow obstruction in the form of a narrowed aortic valve.

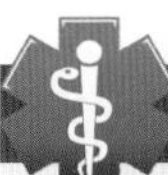

BOARD EXAMINATION ESSENTIALS

This electrocardiogram is of sufficient complexity to appear on the board exam. Diagnostic codes include normal sinus rhythm and AV dissociation. In the presence of AV dissociation, make sure to code two heart rhythms. An AV junctional rhythm is also present. Left ventricular hypertrophy and ST- and/or T-wave abnormalities secondary to hypertrophy should additionally be coded.

Electrocardiogram Case Study #96

CLINICAL HISTORY

A 47-year-old male with severe rheumatic mitral stenosis seen in outpatient cardiovascular medicine preoperative evaluation before anticipated mitral valve replacement. The patient currently is symptomatic with easily inducible shortness of breath with exertion.

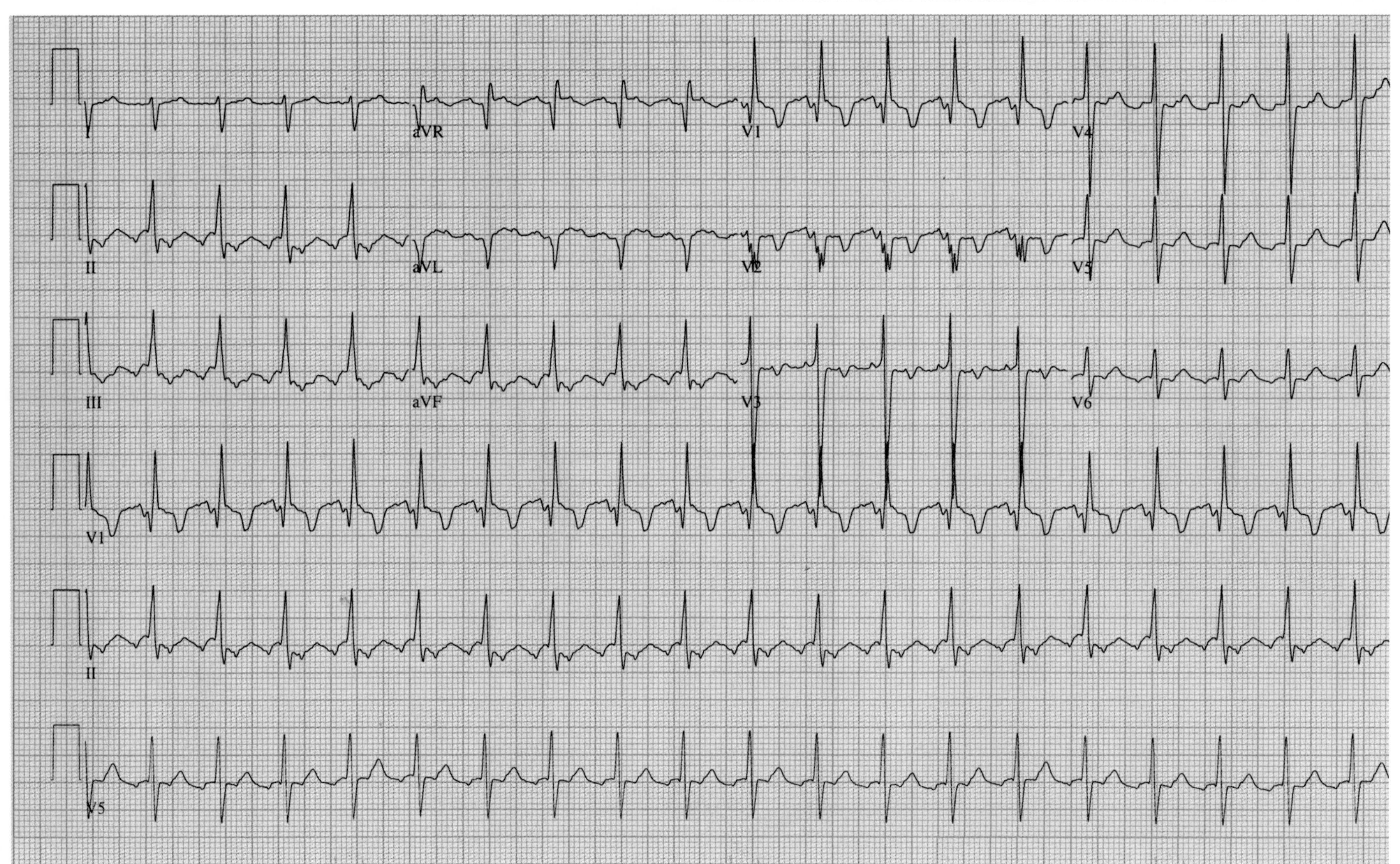

Interpretation Notes:

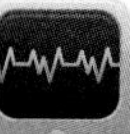

ELECTROCARDIOGRAM INTERPRETATION

This electrocardiogram demonstrates regular occurring narrow QRS complexes at a rate of approximately 125 per minute. Atrial flutter is present best seen in leads II, III, and aVF with the typical sawtooth flutter wave pattern. Two flutter waves are present for each QRS complex. These demonstrate 2:1 atrioventricular conduction. QRS complex right-axis deviation is also seen as the QRS complex vector is negative in lead I and positive in leads II, III, and aVF. A narrow qR QRS complex morphology is seen in lead V1 with associated T-wave inversion. In the presence of QRS complex right-axis deviation, this supports the diagnosis of right ventricular hypertrophy with secondary ST-T changes.

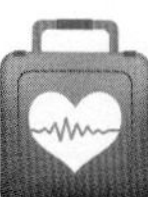

KEY DIAGNOSES

- Atrial flutter
- 2:1 atrioventricular conduction
- QRS complex right-axis deviation
- Right ventricular hypertrophy with secondary ST-T changes

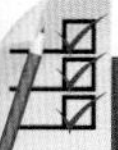

KEY TEACHING POINTS

- This electrocardiogram demonstrates features of longstanding untreated severe mitral stenosis. These include an atrial dysrhythmia such as atrial flutter, right ventricular hypertrophy with secondary ST-T changes, and likely advanced pulmonary hypertension.
- Note the QRS complexes in leads V5 and V6 still demonstrate a prominent S wave. This is due to the anterior prominence of the right ventricle therefore rotating the heart in a clockwise direction with the left ventricle displaced leftward and more posteriorly. If one were to obtain back leads such as leads V7, V8, and V9, left ventricular forces would be more pronounced.

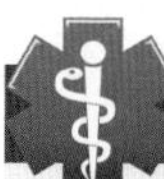

BOARD EXAMINATION ESSENTIALS

This electrocardiogram is another example of mitral valve stenosis. Diagnostic codes for the board exam include atrial flutter, 2:1 AV block, right-axis deviation (greater than +100 degrees), right ventricular hypertrophy, ST- and/or T-wave abnormalities secondary to hypertrophy. While the preferred clinical term is "2:1 AV conduction," within the constraints of the available board exam diagnostic codes, "2:1 AV block" is the next best diagnostic code option.

Electrocardiogram Case Study #97

CLINICAL HISTORY

A 23-year-old male with dialysis-requiring renal disease admitted to the intensive care unit with severe electrolyte disturbances in the setting of dialysis noncompliance.

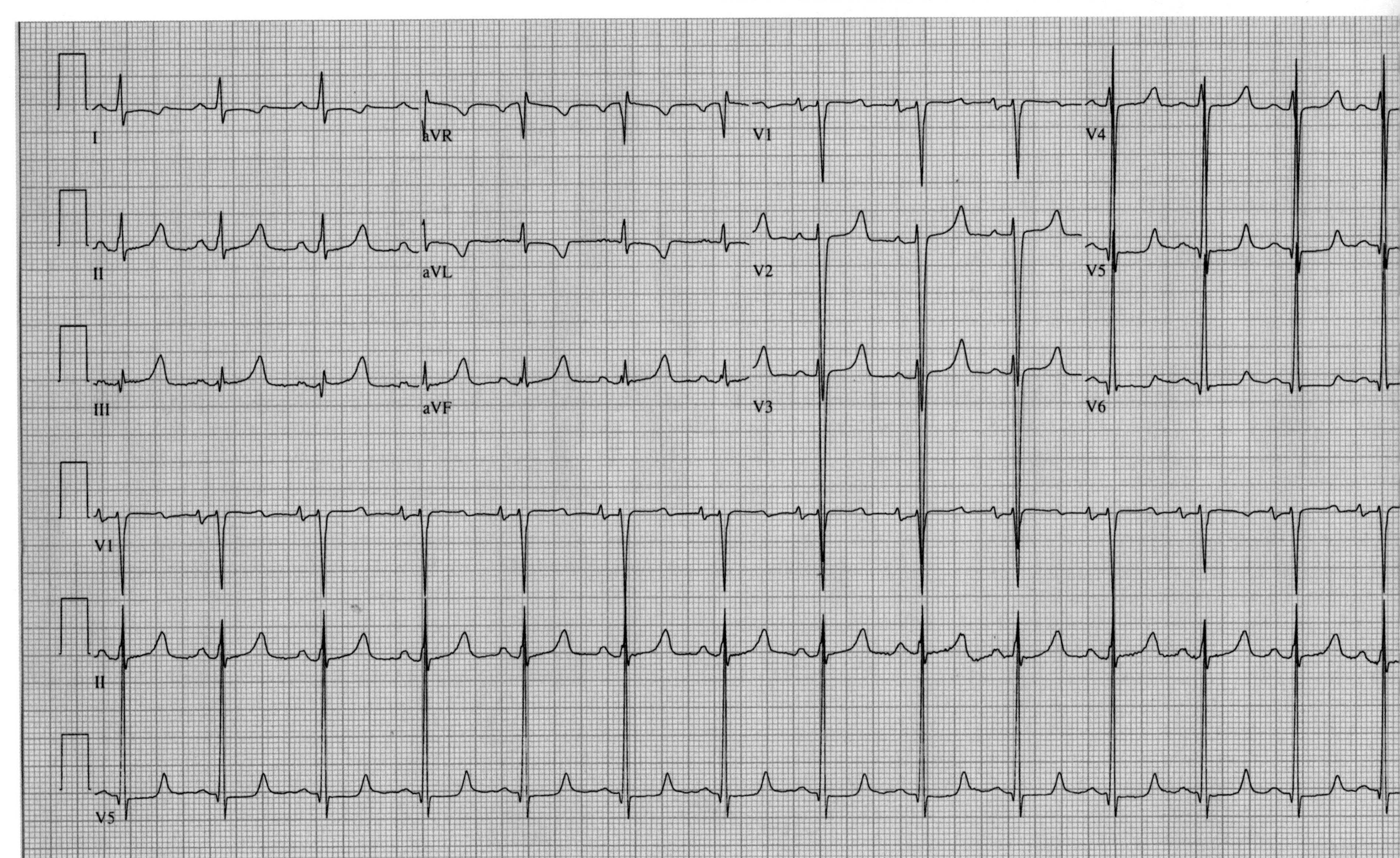

Interpretation Notes:

Electrocardiogram Case Study #97

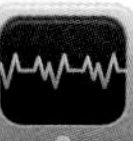

ELECTROCARDIOGRAM INTERPRETATION

This electrocardiogram demonstrates upright P waves in leads I, II, III, and aVF confirming a normal P-wave axis at an atrial rate of approximately 80 per minute consistent with normal sinus rhythm. ST-segment straightening is demonstrated, particularly in leads V5 and V6. The ST segment is prolonged resulting in QT interval prolongation most consistent with hypocalcemia. The T waves are symmetric and narrow based supporting the presence of hyperkalemia. Voltage criteria for left ventricular hypertrophy are also demonstrated with high lateral T-wave inversion. This is consistent with the patient's longstanding history of poorly treated hypertension. Terminal P-wave inversion in lead V1 supports left atrial abnormality.

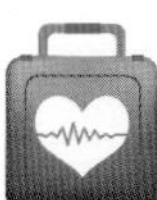

KEY DIAGNOSES

- Normal sinus rhythm
- Hypocalcemia
- Hyperkalemia
- Left ventricular hypertrophy with secondary ST-T changes
- Prolonged QT interval
- Left atrial abnormality

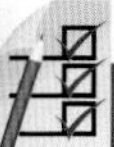

KEY TEACHING POINTS

- Electrocardiogram findings of hypocalcemia and hyperkalemia are commonly seen in end-stage renal disease patients. Note that the calcium disorders impact the ST segment and potassium disorders impact the T wave.
- This patient developed end-stage renal disease at an extremely young age. It is less common to demonstrate severe left ventricular hypertrophy in this age group. The patient has had a repeated history of poor compliance with his medications and dialysis sessions likely accelerating his structural heart disease.

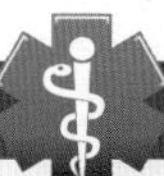

BOARD EXAMINATION ESSENTIALS

The pattern of abnormalities found on this electrocardiogram is likely to be found on the board exam. Diagnostic codes for the board exam include normal sinus rhythm, left ventricular hypertrophy, ST- and/or T-wave abnormalities secondary to hypertrophy, prolonged QT interval, ST- and/or T-wave abnormalities suggesting electrolyte disturbances, and the clinical disorders hyperkalemia and hypocalcemia. Left atrial abnormality/enlargement is also suggested.

Electrocardiogram Case Study #98

CLINICAL HISTORY

A 53-year-old male with recent-onset shortness of breath. The patient has known moderate mitral regurgitation secondary to posterior mitral valve leaflet prolapse.

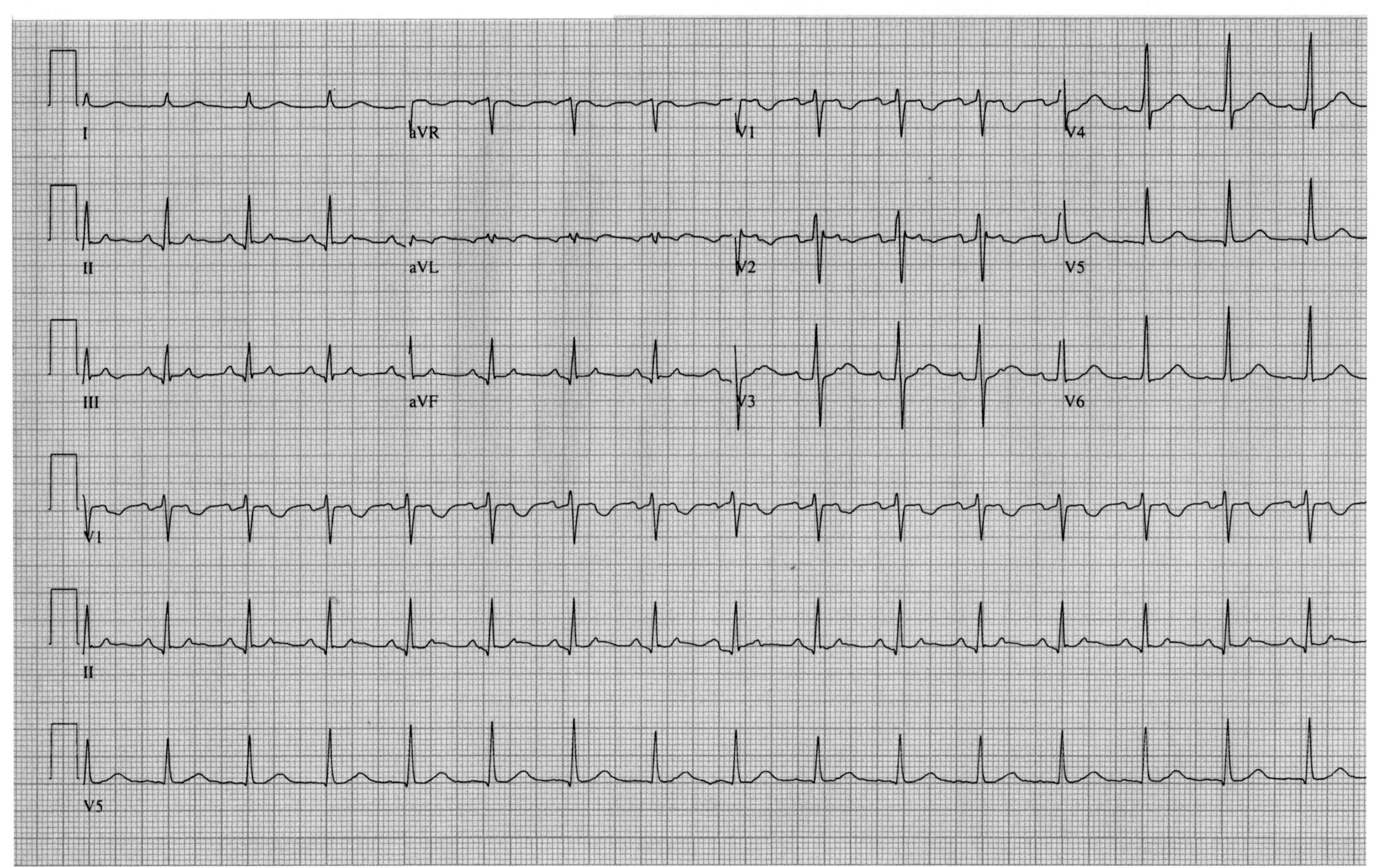

Interpretation Notes:

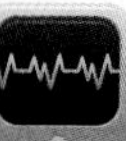

ELECTROCARDIOGRAM INTERPRETATION

This electrocardiogram demonstrates two P waves for each QRS complex occurring at an atrial rate close to 190 per minute supporting ectopic atrial tachycardia with 2:1 atrioventricular conduction. The first P wave is easily seen before each QRS complex. The second P wave is best identified in leads II and III. This transpires within the ST segment superimposed on the proximal portion of the T wave. Using calipers, the second P wave is more readily identified. Otherwise, this might be confused and reported as a normal electrocardiogram.

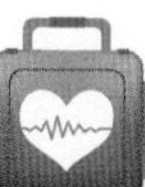

KEY DIAGNOSES

- Ectopic atrial tachycardia
- 2:1 atrioventricular conduction

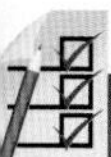

KEY TEACHING POINTS

- In leads V4, V5, and V6, the second P wave occurring after the QRS complex is less easily identified. Upon close inspection, a slightly positive deflection is seen on the ascending portion of the proximal T wave corresponding with the second P wave.
- The best clue to the presence of a second P wave is the altered appearance of the T wave in leads II and III. If this positive deflection were to solely represent a T wave, the T wave would be very diminutive in appearance, short in duration, and more closely resemble a P wave.

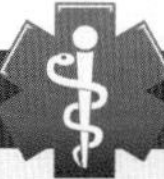

BOARD EXAMINATION ESSENTIALS

This electrocardiogram focuses on the cardiac rhythm. Upon first glance, it appears to reflect normal sinus rhythm. For the board exam, be extra careful when assessing the heart rhythm. In this case, the most applicable diagnostic codes are atrial tachycardia and AV block, 2:1.

Electrocardiogram Case Study #99

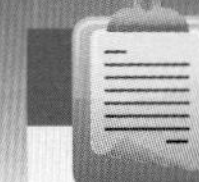

CLINICAL HISTORY

A 44-year-old female with recurrent syncope admitted to the coronary intensive care unit immediately after this electrocardiogram was obtained in the emergency room.

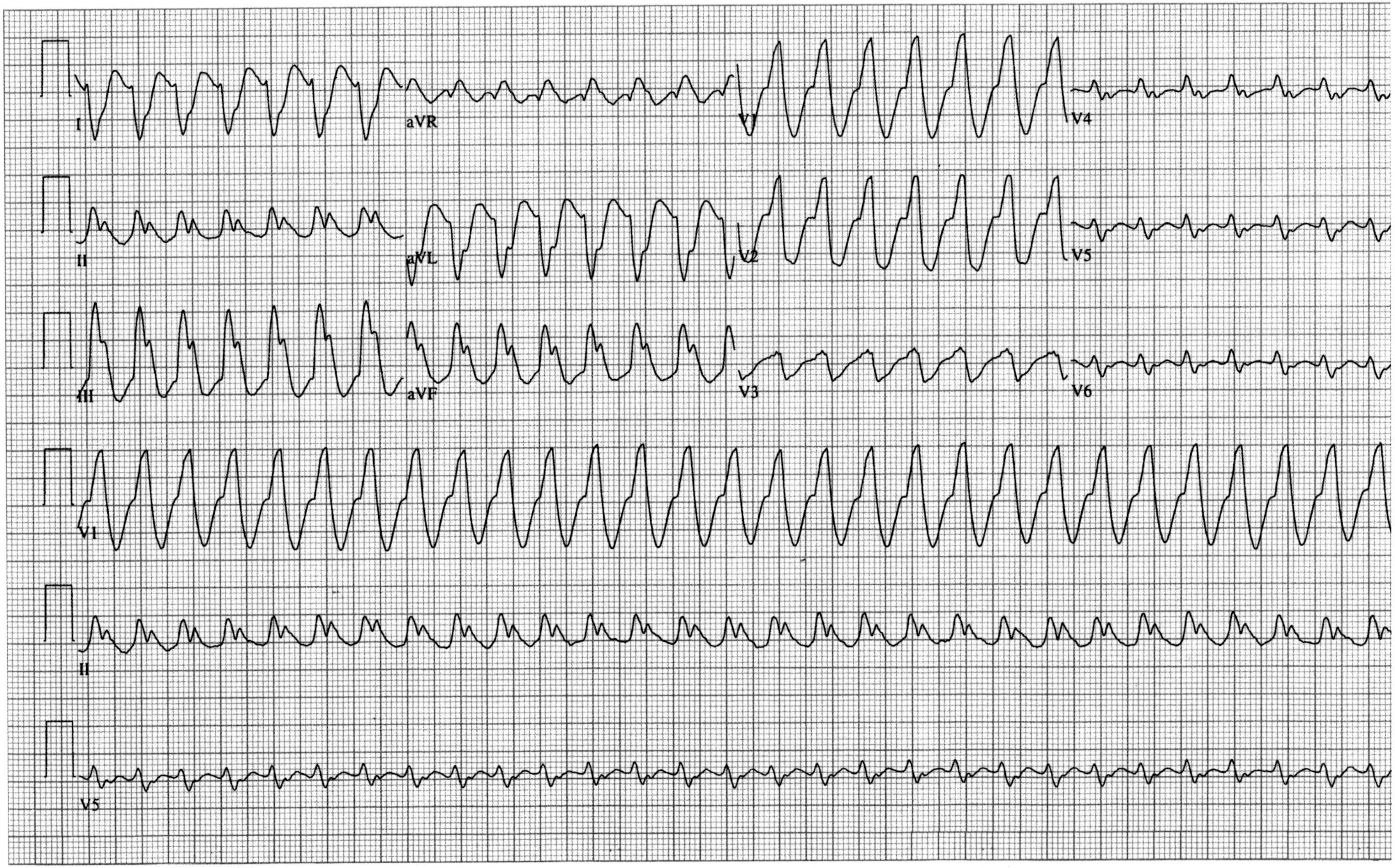

Interpretation Notes:____

____

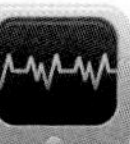

ELECTROCARDIOGRAM INTERPRETATION

This electrocardiogram demonstrates a wide QRS complex tachycardia with a cycle length of 340 milliseconds and a rate of approximately 175 per minute with a right superior axis given the positive QRS complex in lead aVR and a monophasic positive QRS complex vector in lead V1 supporting ventricular tachycardia. Note the positive QRS complexes extending from leads V1 to V6. This is known as "QRS complex concordance" further supporting ventricular tachycardia.

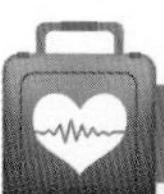

KEY DIAGNOSES

- Ventricular tachycardia

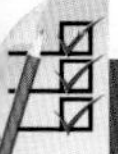

KEY TEACHING POINTS

- Other supporting features of ventricular tachycardia such as fusion complexes and capture complexes are not identified on this electrocardiogram. Atrioventricular dissociation may be present, best seen in the lead II rhythm strip. When carefully inspected, periodic deflections are seen, for instance following the eleventh QRS complex. It is not possible to discern the atrial rhythm with certainty. Despite this, the presence of a monophasic positive QRS complex in lead V1 and a positive concordance of the QRS complexes across the precordium strongly support the presence of ventricular tachycardia.
- Ventricular tachycardia was confirmed in this patient. No evidence of coronary artery disease was found and the patient underwent successful implantable cardiac defibrillator placement.

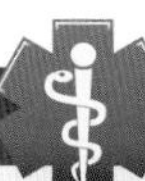

BOARD EXAMINATION ESSENTIALS

Diagnostic codes for this electrocardiogram include ventricular tachycardia (three or more consecutive complexes) and AV dissociation. In the presence of AV dissociation and ventricular tachycardia, an atrial rhythm would also normally be coded. An atrial rhythm is not coded in this circumstance as the P waves, while identifiable, are not able to be assessed completely due to the superimposed ventricular tachycardia.

Electrocardiogram Case Study #100

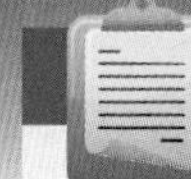

CLINICAL HISTORY

An 87-year-old female with hypertension, intermittent shortness of breath, and frequent episodes of decompensated systolic left ventricular heart failure who is seen in cardiovascular medicine outpatient follow-up.

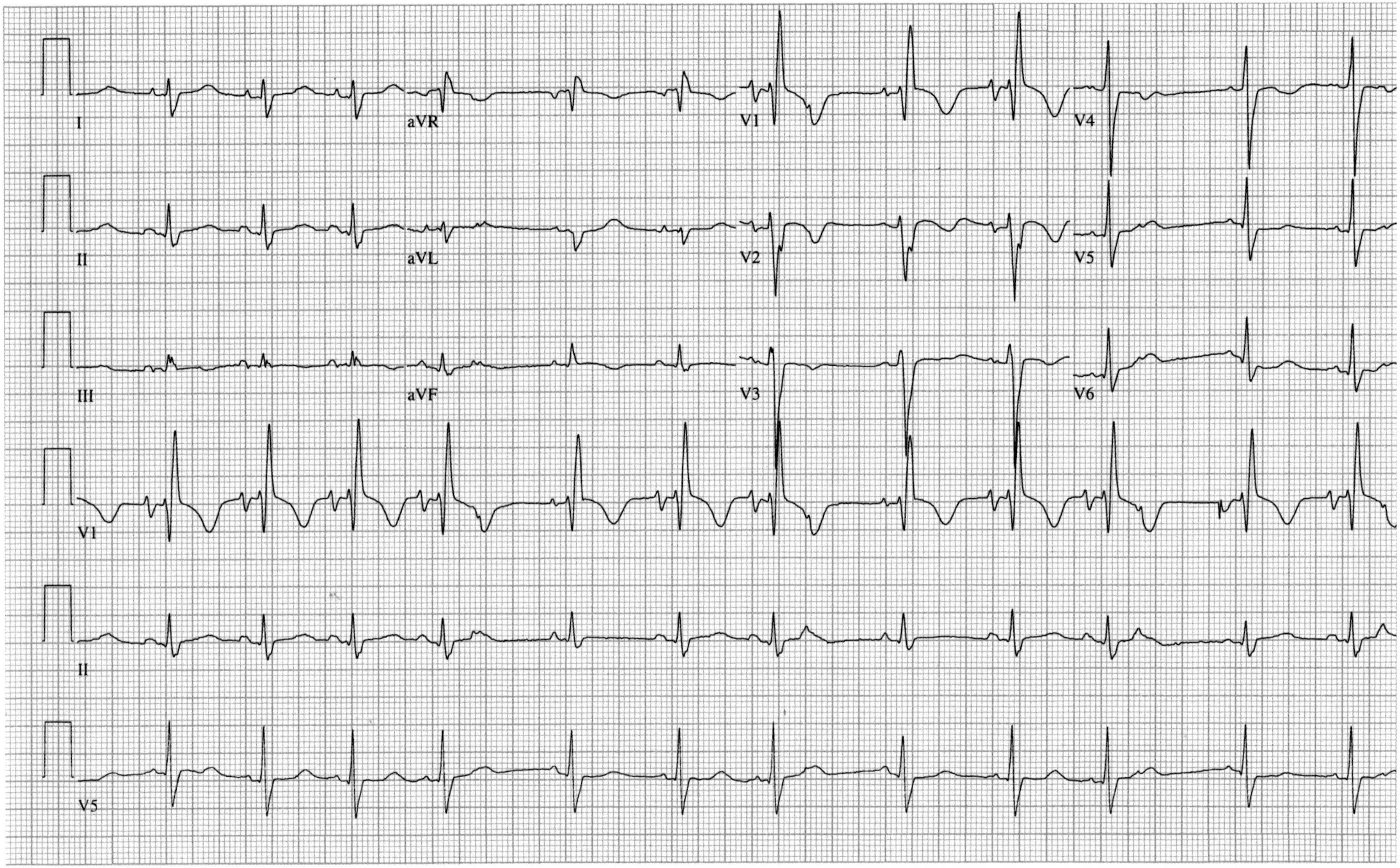

I aVR V1 V4
II aVL V2 V5
III aVF V3 V6
V1
II
V5

Interpretation Notes:

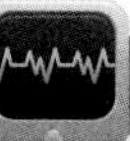

ELECTROCARDIOGRAM INTERPRETATION

This electrocardiogram demonstrates P waves with a normal axis occurring at a regular rate of approximately 75 per minute supporting normal sinus rhythm. The first four P waves appear of similar morphology and precede each QRS complex with a constant and normal PR interval supporting a normal sinus origin. Between the fourth and the fifth QRS complexes, T-wave deformation is seen, best in the lead V1 rhythm strip supporting a nonconducted premature atrial complex. Preceding the fifth QRS complex, a P wave of differing morphology is noted supporting an atrial escape complex. Two more normal sinus complexes are seen followed by a nonconducted premature atrial complex and an atrial escape complex. This cycle occurs a third time toward the right-hand portion of the electrocardiogram but interestingly, a small pacemaker deflection is seen before the second to last P wave indicating an atrial paced complex. The sinus P wave demonstrates terminal negativity supporting left atrial abnormality. Complete right bundle-branch block is also present given the QRS complex duration >120 milliseconds and an rsR′ QRS complex morphology in lead V1. Inferior and anterior nonspecific ST-T changes are seen.

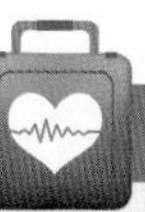

KEY DIAGNOSES

- Normal sinus rhythm
- Nonconducted premature atrial complex
- Atrial escape complex
- Left atrial abnormality
- Complete right bundle-branch block
- Atrial pacemaker
- Nonspecific ST-T changes

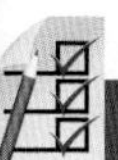

KEY TEACHING POINTS

- The presence of left atrial abnormality suggests altered left atrial conduction and serves as the likely substrate for the nonconducted premature atrial complexes, atrial escape complexes, and the need for an atrial pacemaker.
- Furthermore, conduction system disease extends to the ventricle in the form of complete right bundle-branch block.
- No evidence of a prior myocardial infarction is identified.

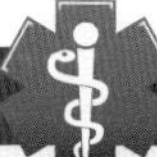

BOARD EXAMINATION ESSENTIALS

This electrocardiogram is complex from a heart rhythm perspective. Diagnostic codes for the board exam include normal sinus rhythm, atrial premature complexes, atrial or coronary sinus pacing, left atrial abnormality and/or enlargement, right bundle-branch block, complete and nonspecific ST- and/or T-wave abnormalities. Right-axis deviation (>100 degrees) is not coded as the QRS complex, while rightward, is not >100 degrees.

Electrocardiogram Case Study #101

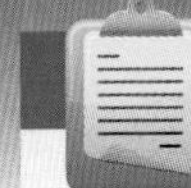

CLINICAL HISTORY

A 62-year-old gentleman who is undergoing preoperative anesthesia clearance prior to planned rotator cuff repair. His past medical history is notable for hypertension but no known cardiac disease. His medications included verapamil.

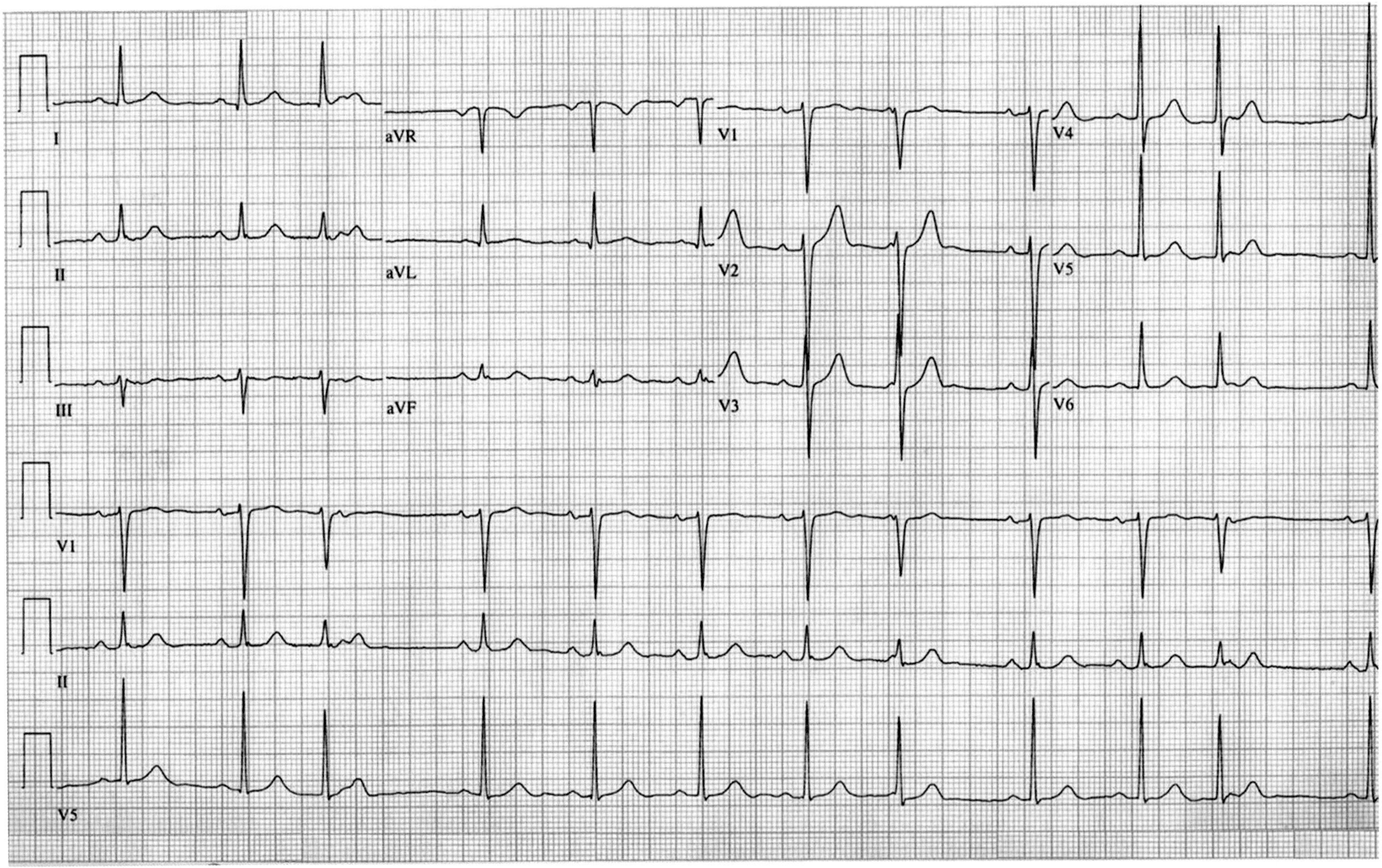

I aVR V1 V4
II aVL V2 V5
III aVF V3 V6
V1
II
V5

Interpretation Notes:

Electrocardiogram Case Study #101

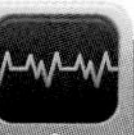

ELECTROCARDIOGRAM INTERPRETATION

Normal sinus rhythm is present. The third, eighth, and eleventh QRS complexes are premature junctional complexes. A P wave does not precede the 3rd or the 11th QRS complex and each demonstrates a similar QRS complex morphology to the native QRS complex. This is otherwise a normal electrocardiogram.

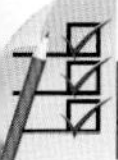

KEY TEACHING POINTS

- Premature junctional complexes are an otherwise normal finding.
- Frequently, retrograde P waves are seen in the presence of premature junctional complexes. An example of retrograde P waves is within the ST segment following the third and the eleventh QRS complexes.

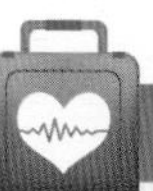

KEY DIAGNOSES

- Normal sinus rhythm
- Premature junctional complexes
- Normal electrocardiogram
- Retrograde P waves

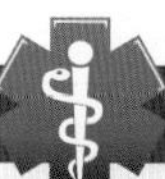

BOARD EXAMINATION ESSENTIALS

For the board exam, diagnostic codes include normal sinus rhythm, AV junctional premature complexes, and normal electrocardiogram. The AV junctional premature complexes are not considered abnormal. The QRS complex demonstrates a short intraventricular conduction delay but does not meet diagnostic criteria and should not be coded for the board exam as it is <100 milliseconds in total duration.

Electrocardiogram Case Study #102

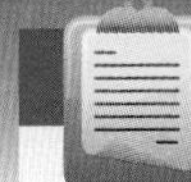

CLINICAL HISTORY

A 59-year-old male with coronary artery disease status a post remote percutaneous transluminal coronary angioplasty to the right coronary artery who re-presents with chest discomfort. A myocardial infarction was excluded by cardiac enzymes and a subsequent stress test was normal. The patient was felt to be suffering from noncardiac musculoskeletal chest discomfort.

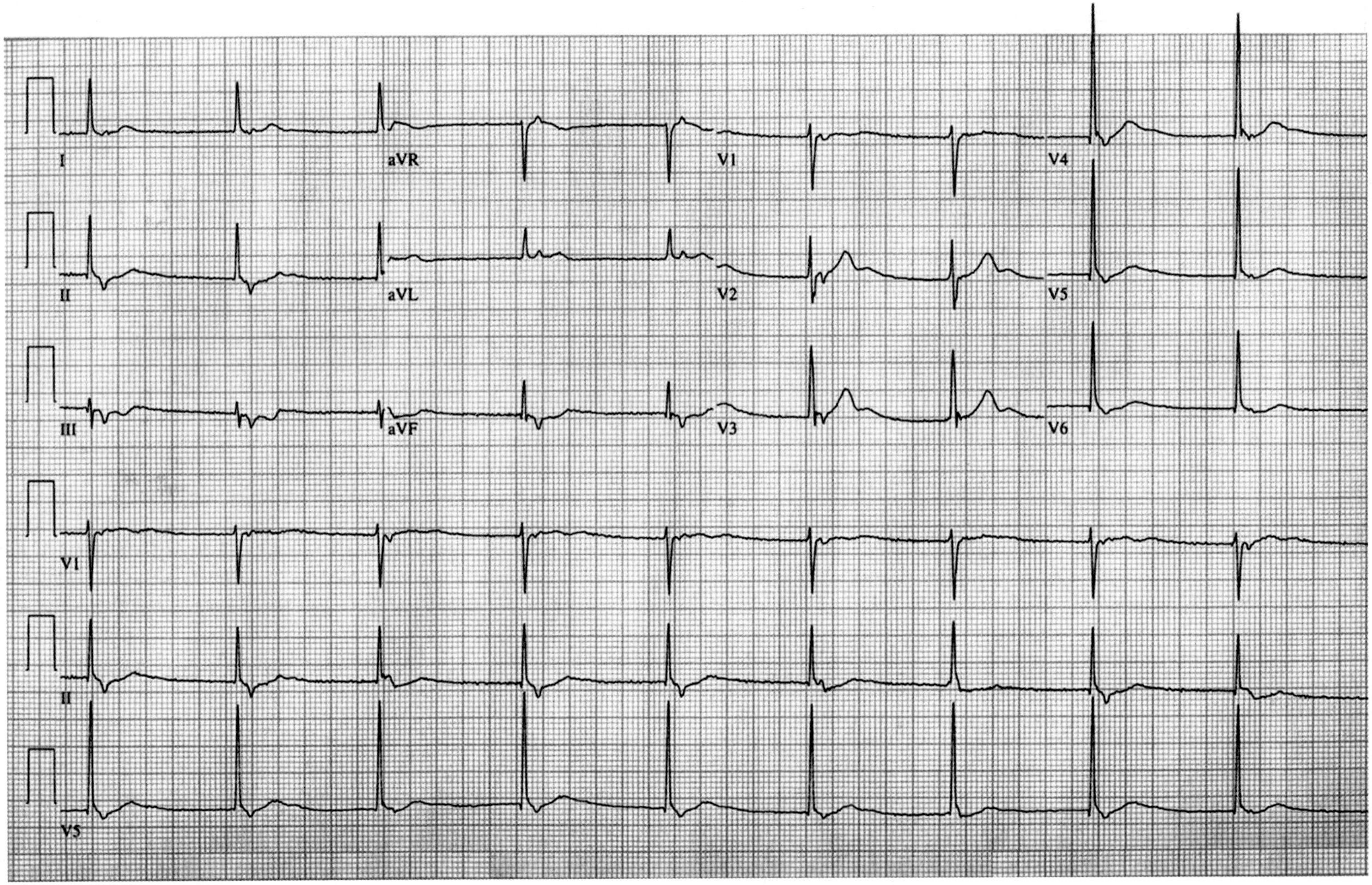

I aVR V1 V4
II aVL V2 V5
III aVF V3 V6
V1
II
V5

Interpretation Notes:____

____

Electrocardiogram Case Study #102

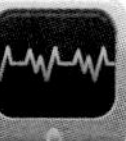

ELECTROCARDIOGRAM INTERPRETATION

The cardiac rhythm demonstrates a regular bradycardia with retrograde P waves after each QRS complex. The P waves are negative in the inferior leads as the atrial wave of depolarization is traveling superiorly, opposite the normal direction of intracardiac conduction. The QRS complex is of normal duration. This represents junctional bradycardia. The causes of this could be many including sinus node disease, medication administration, increased vagal tone, atrial conduction system disease, myocardial ischemia, and valvular heart disease. Prominent positive U waves are present in leads V2 to V4.

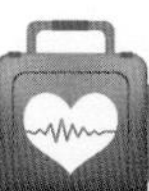

KEY DIAGNOSES

- Junctional bradycardia
- Retrograde P waves
- Positive U waves

KEY TEACHING POINTS

- In this instance, the R:R interval is constant with absent atrial activity prior to each QRS complex. Depending on the relative retrograde versus antegrade conduction rates, the retrograde P wave may occur before, within or after the QRS complex.
- In this example, antegrade conduction from the atrioventricular junction to the ventricle is faster than retrograde conduction from the atrioventricular junction to the atrium and therefore explains the P wave occupying the proximal ST segment after the QRS complex.

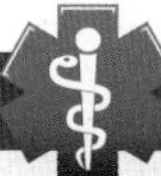

BOARD EXAMINATION ESSENTIALS

Board exam codes include AV junctional rhythm. Prominent U waves should also be coded. No other codes are applicable. When approaching the board exam, be careful not to over code. Some of the electrocardiogram examples may require only one or two diagnostic codes.

Electrocardiogram Case Study #103

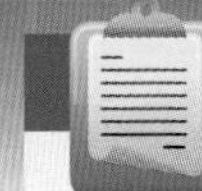

CLINICAL HISTORY

A 66-year-old female who presented to a local urgent care facility with acute-onset chest, arm, neck, and jaw discomfort in the setting of dyspnea.

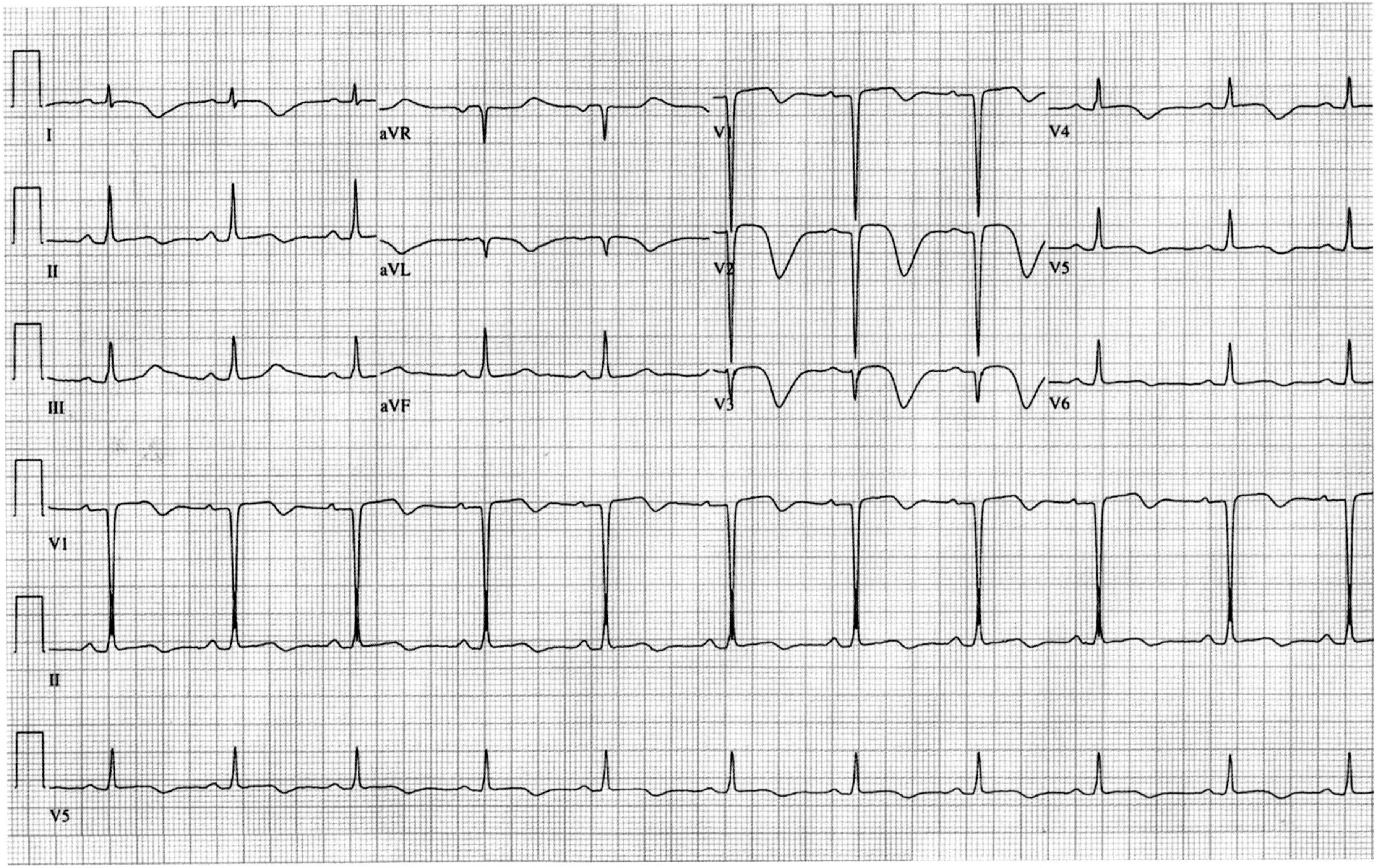

I aVR V1 V4
II aVL V2 V5
III aVF V3 V6
V1
II
V5

Interpretation Notes:____

____

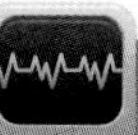

ELECTROCARDIOGRAM INTERPRETATION

Normal sinus rhythm is seen. Most notable is the presence of Q-wave formation in leads V1 to V3. This suggests an anteroseptal myocardial infarction. The upwardly coved ST segments and deep T-wave inversion in the anteroseptal leads, the lateral precordial leads, and the high lateral leads suggests an anteroseptal myocardial infarction recent with lateral ST-T changes. It is probable that this patient has a more extensive wall motion abnormality than suggested by the electrocardiogram Q-wave distribution as this may truly represent an extensive anterolateral myocardial infarction. A prolonged QT interval is present.

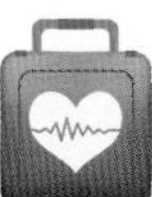

KEY DIAGNOSES

- Normal sinus rhythm
- Anteroseptal myocardial infarction, recent
- Prolonged QT interval
- Acute myocardial injury

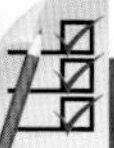

KEY TEACHING POINTS

- The electrocardiogram findings support at least a moderate-sized myocardial infarction.
- The distribution of abnormality supports the left anterior descending coronary artery, likely proximal given the J point and ST-segment elevation in lead V1.

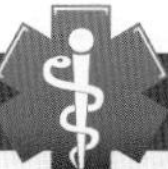

BOARD EXAMINATION ESSENTIALS

For this example, the clinical history is essential supporting ischemic heart disease as the underlying cause of the abnormal electrocardiogram pattern. Diagnostic codes for the board exam include normal sinus rhythm; anteroseptal myocardial infarction, age recent, or probably acute; acute myocardial injury; and prolonged QT interval. Of interest, only one of three QRS complexes in lead V3 possesses a definite Q wave. This still meets the criteria for a myocardial infarction in view of the clinical history coupled with the associated ST-T changes.

Electrocardiogram Case Study #104

CLINICAL HISTORY

A 65-year-old male referred for coronary artery bypass graft surgery in the setting of pulmonary edema and advanced coronary artery disease.

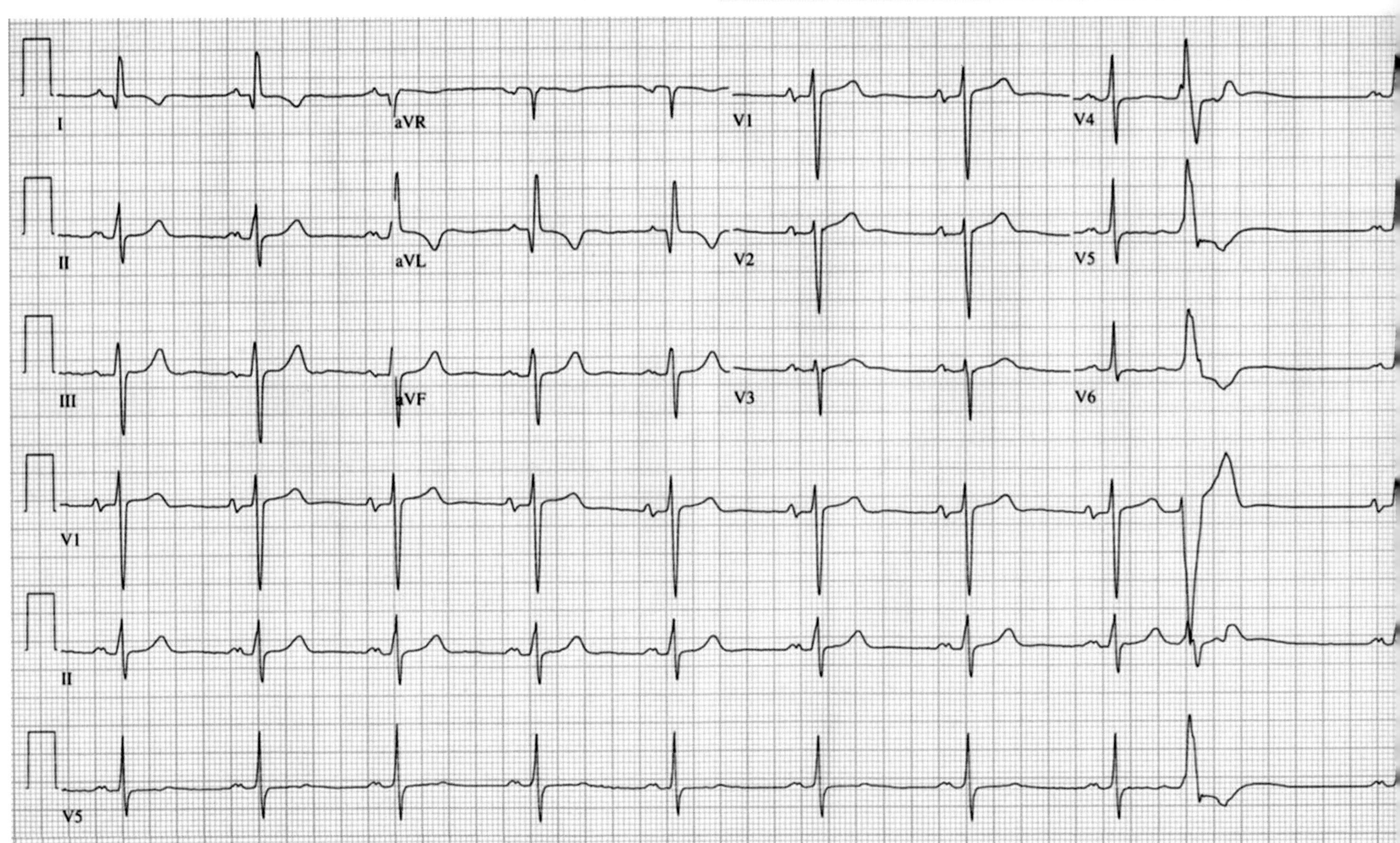

Interpretation Notes:

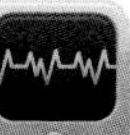

ELECTROCARDIOGRAM INTERPRETATION

Sinus bradycardia is present as the P waves occur at regular intervals at a rate slightly <60 per minute. A prominent bifid P wave in lead II and a terminally negative P wave in lead V1 are consistent with left atrial abnormality. Toward the right-hand portion of the electrocardiogram, a premature ventricular complex is present, widened and different in morphology than the native QRS complex. Most important, Q waves of diagnostic width are present in leads I and aVL reflective of a high lateral myocardial infarction, age indeterminate. There are associated ST-T changes in leads V4 to V6 but no Q waves. This myocardial infarction is limited to the high lateral leads and best termed a "high lateral myocardial infarction, age indeterminate." A nonspecific intraventricular conduction delay is also present.

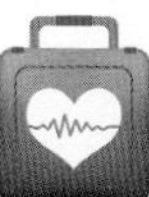

KEY DIAGNOSES

- Sinus bradycardia
- Premature ventricular complex
- High lateral myocardial infarction, age indeterminate
- Left atrial abnormality
- Nonspecific intraventricular conduction delay

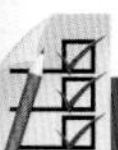

KEY TEACHING POINTS

- This infarction most likely represents the left circumflex coronary artery distribution but may also represent a ramus intermedius branch or a diagonal branch of the left anterior descending coronary artery.
- The high lateral leads demonstrate significant anatomic coronary artery overlap. The exact delineation of the coronary artery representing this electrocardiogram Q-wave abnormality is most confidently concluded at the time of cardiac catheterization

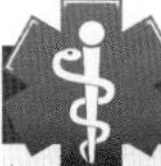

BOARD EXAMINATION ESSENTIALS

Board exam diagnostic codes include sinus bradycardia; left atrial abnormality/enlargement; lateral myocardial infarction, age indeterminate; and a premature ventricular complex. An intraventricular conduction disturbance, nonspecific type, can also be coded as the QRS complex duration is approximately 100 milliseconds, best identified in leads I and aVL in the form of terminal QRS complex widening.

Electrocardiogram Case Study #105

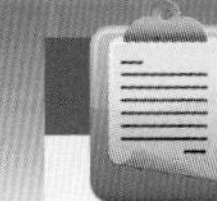

CLINICAL HISTORY

A 76-year-old male with coronary artery disease who is status post a remote myocardial infarction.

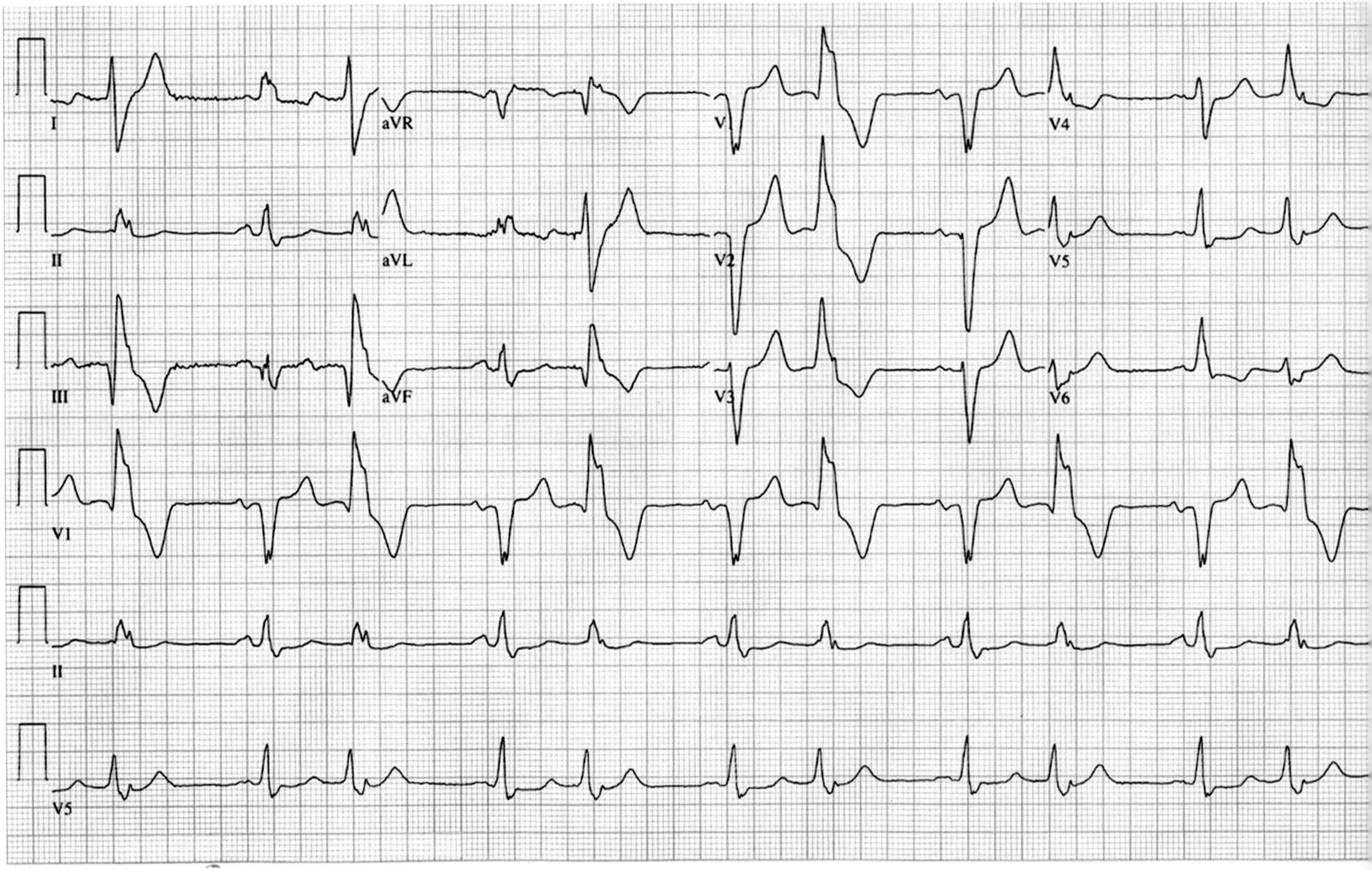

I aVR V1 V4
II aVL V2 V5
III aVF V3 V6
V1
II
V5

Interpretation Notes:____

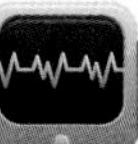

ELECTROCARDIOGRAM INTERPRETATION

The second QRS complex is preceded by a P wave of normal morphology. This indicates normal sinus rhythm. The P wave is terminally negative in lead V1 and prolonged in lead II >110 milliseconds supporting left atrial abnormality. A bigeminal rhythm is present as premature ventricular complexes occur frequently throughout the tracing. This represents ventricular bigeminy. The native QRS complex is broad and demonstrates complete left bundle-branch block morphology. The premature ventricular complexes, best seen in leads III and aVF, demonstrate wide and deep Q waves. While not diagnostic, this suggests an inferior myocardial infarction, age indeterminate, possibly masked by the baseline complete left bundle-branch block.

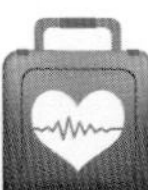

KEY DIAGNOSES

- Normal sinus rhythm
- Premature ventricular complex
- Left atrial abnormality
- Complete left bundle-branch block

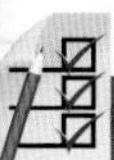

KEY TEACHING POINTS

- The diagnosis of an age-indeterminate myocardial infarction in the setting of complete left bundle-branch block is generally not possible.
- The premature ventricular complexes may unmask this finding if left ventricular in origin given the complete right bundle-branch block morphology demonstrated in rhythm strip lead V1.

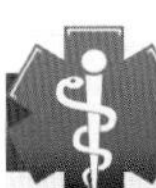

BOARD EXAMINATION ESSENTIALS

Normal sinus rhythm is present as the average heart rate is between 60 and 100 per minute. In addition to normal sinus rhythm, diagnostic codes for the board exam include left atrial abnormality/enlargement; ventricular premature complexes; and left bundle-branch block, complete. While an inferior myocardial infarction, age indeterminate, is suggested by the ventricular premature complexes and a useful clinical tool, do not use this finding for coding an infarction pattern on the board exam.

Electrocardiogram Case Study **#106**

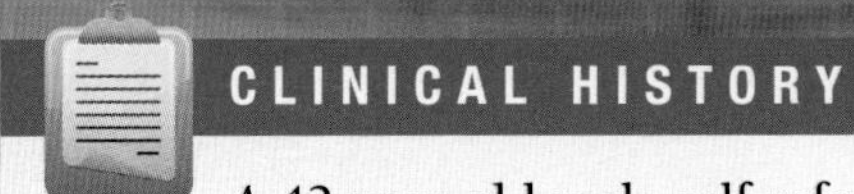

CLINICAL HISTORY

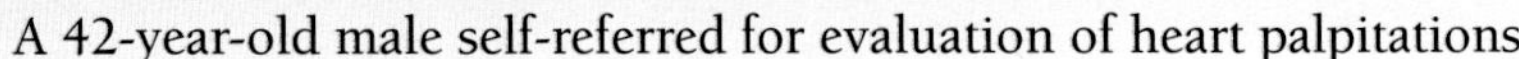

A 42-year-old male self-referred for evaluation of heart palpitations.

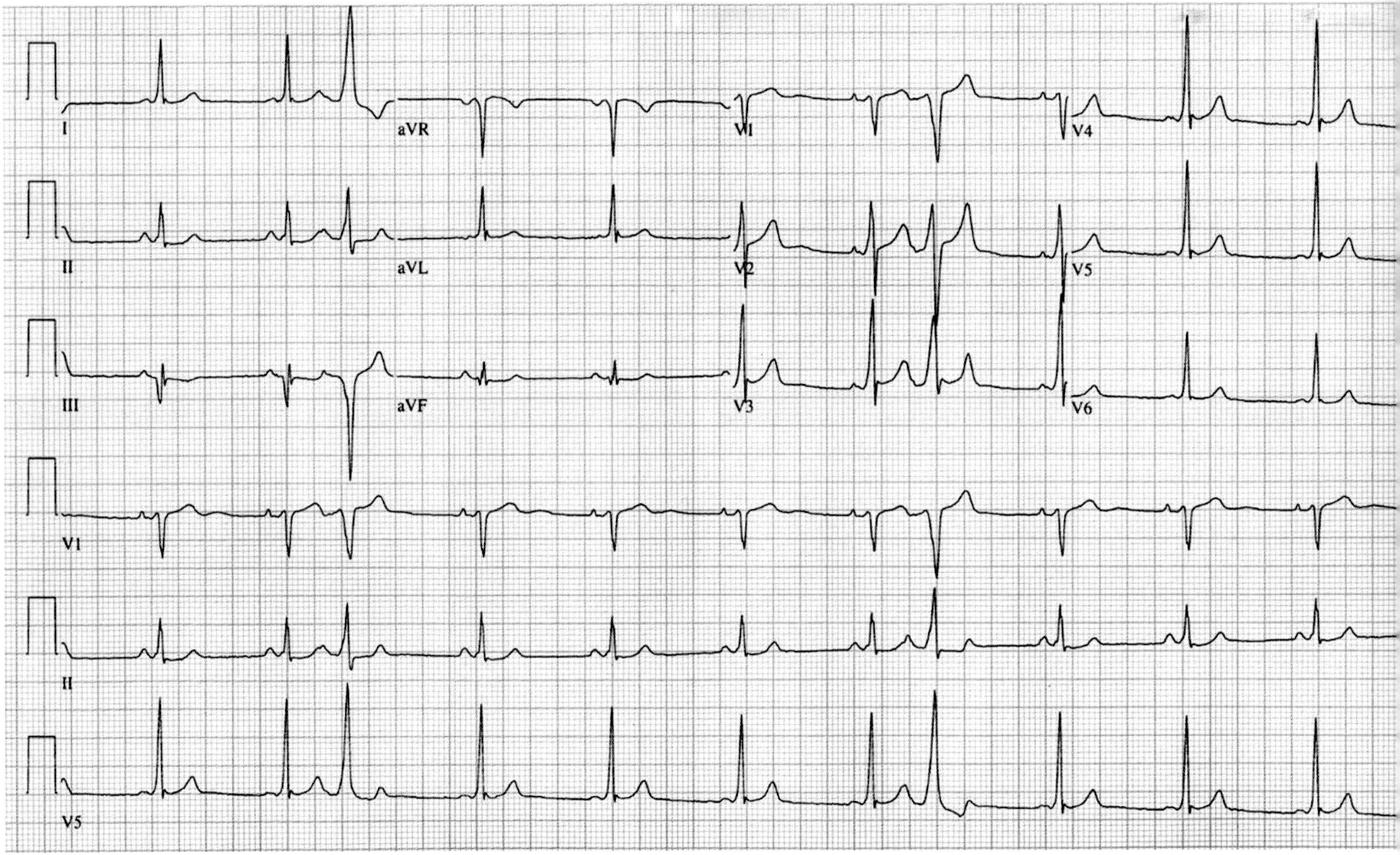

Interpretation Notes:

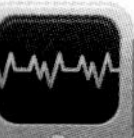

ELECTROCARDIOGRAM INTERPRETATION

This electrocardiogram demonstrates normal sinus rhythm with a shortened PR interval and a slurred QRS complex upstroke indicative of ventricular pre-excitation and the Wolff-Parkinson-White pattern. The third and eighth QRS complexes are preceded by a premature P wave. These are premature atrial complexes.

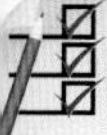

KEY TEACHING POINTS

- Note that the QRS complexes associated with the premature atrial complexes demonstrate a greater degree of ventricular pre-excitation. This is an expected finding as the accessory pathway, unlike the atrioventricular node, demonstrates facile conduction at this shorter cycle length and is able to conduct preferentially without conduction block.
- This electrocardiogram demonstrates the facility of conduction within the accessory pathway and why arrhythmias such as atrial fibrillation are clinically dangerous as the accessory pathway can conduct at very high heart rates and generate hemodynamically unstable cardiac rhythms

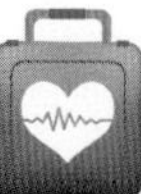

KEY DIAGNOSES

- Normal sinus rhythm
- Wolff-Parkinson-White pattern
- Premature atrial complex

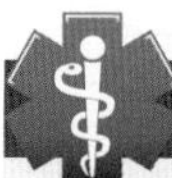

BOARD EXAMINATION ESSENTIALS

On the board exam, anticipate an electrocardiogram example including Wolff-Parkinson-White pattern. Diagnostic codes in addition to Wolfe-Parkinson-White pattern include normal sinus rhythm and atrial premature complexes. Be careful not to code premature ventricular complexes. Instead, these premature complexes are atrial in origin demonstrating enhanced pre-excitation and thus, a greater QRS complex duration. Make sure to inspect the preceding T wave as often a superimposed P wave will deform the T wave and provide the necessary diagnostic insight.

Electrocardiogram Case Study #107

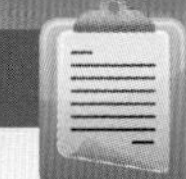

CLINICAL HISTORY

A 64-year-old male who presented to the emergency room with an intermittent 2-week history of bilateral arm discomfort and numbness, worsening on the morning of presentation.

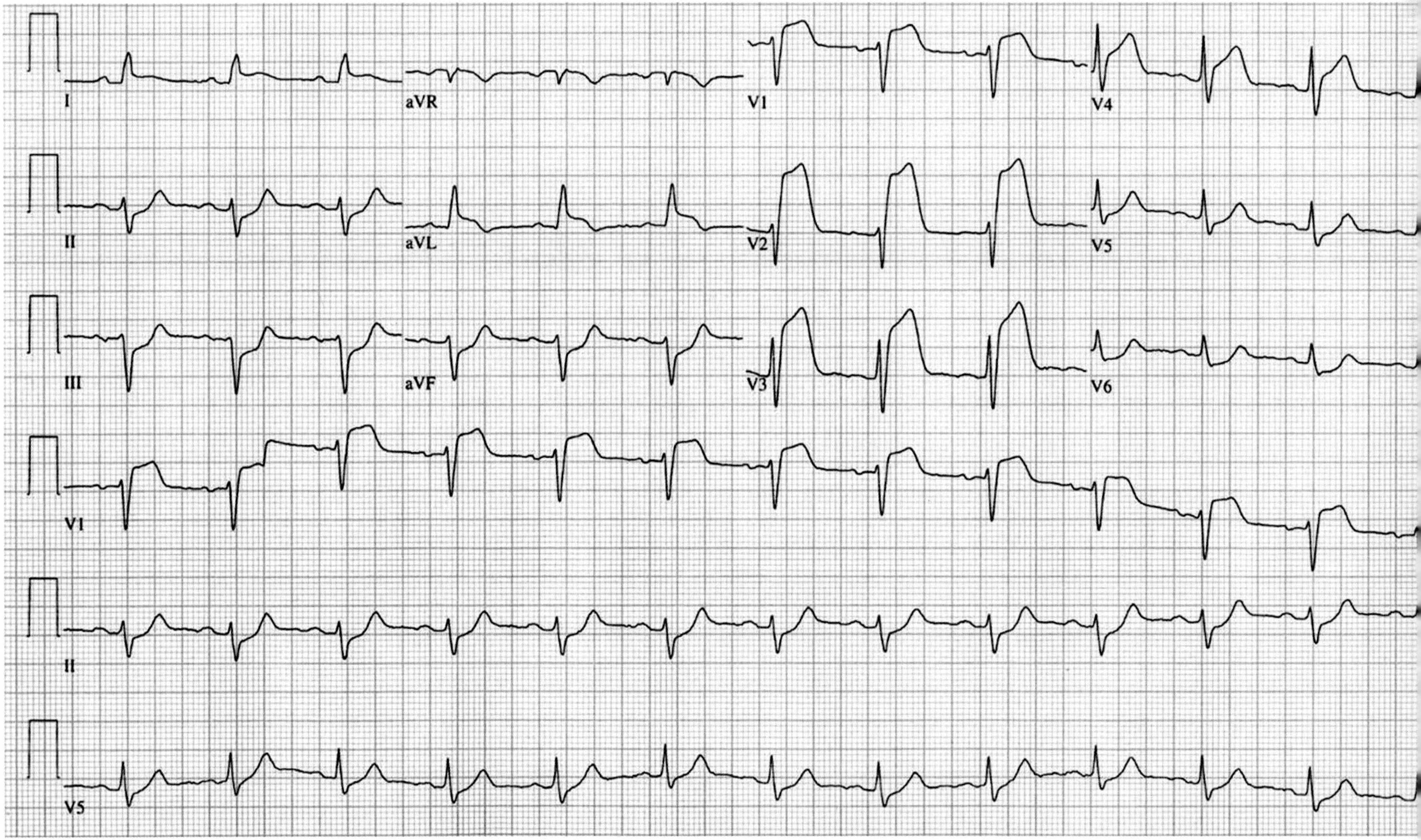

I aVR V1 V4

II aVL V2 V5

III aVF V3 V6

V1

II

V5

Interpretation Notes:

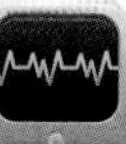

ELECTROCARDIOGRAM INTERPRETATION

Normal sinus rhythm is present. The QRS complex axis is deviated leftward with a positive QRS complex vector in lead I and negative QRS complex vectors in leads II, III, and aVF fulfilling the criteria for left anterior fascicular block. Approximately 9 mm of maximal ST-segment elevation is seen in leads V1 to V4, I, and aVL without Q-wave formation. This is a pattern of acute myocardial injury reflecting extensive anterolateral myocardial involvement. This patient also demonstrates reciprocal inferior and lateral precordial ST-segment depression. Borderline first-degree atrioventricular block is also present.

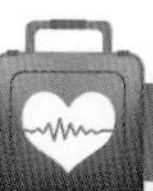

KEY DIAGNOSES

- Normal sinus rhythm
- Left anterior fascicular block
- Acute myocardial injury
- First-degree atrioventricular block

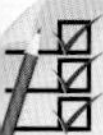

KEY TEACHING POINTS

- If feasible, acute coronary intervention is of utmost importance with the goal of urgent revascularization as this patient stands to suffer a large degree of myocardial necrosis and left ventricular systolic dysfunction.
- The left anterior descending coronary artery occlusion is proximal as the J-point and ST-segment elevation begins in lead V1, which is felt to represent the myocardial territory proximal to the first septal perforator branch of the left anterior descending coronary artery.

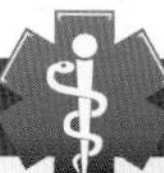

BOARD EXAMINATION ESSENTIALS

This is another electrocardiogram example where just a few diagnostic codes reflect a complete assessment. These codes include normal sinus rhythm; left anterior fascicular block; AV block, first degree; and acute myocardial injury. In the absence of Q waves, do not code a myocardial infarction pattern. Serial electrocardiograms may demonstrate Q-wave development but none are evident on this tracing.

Electrocardiogram Case Study **#108**

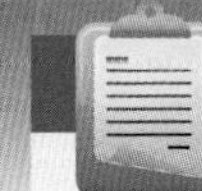

CLINICAL HISTORY

A 55-year-old male who presents to the emergency room with lightheadedness, chest pain of 3-day duration, and a poor appetite in the setting of known hypertension.

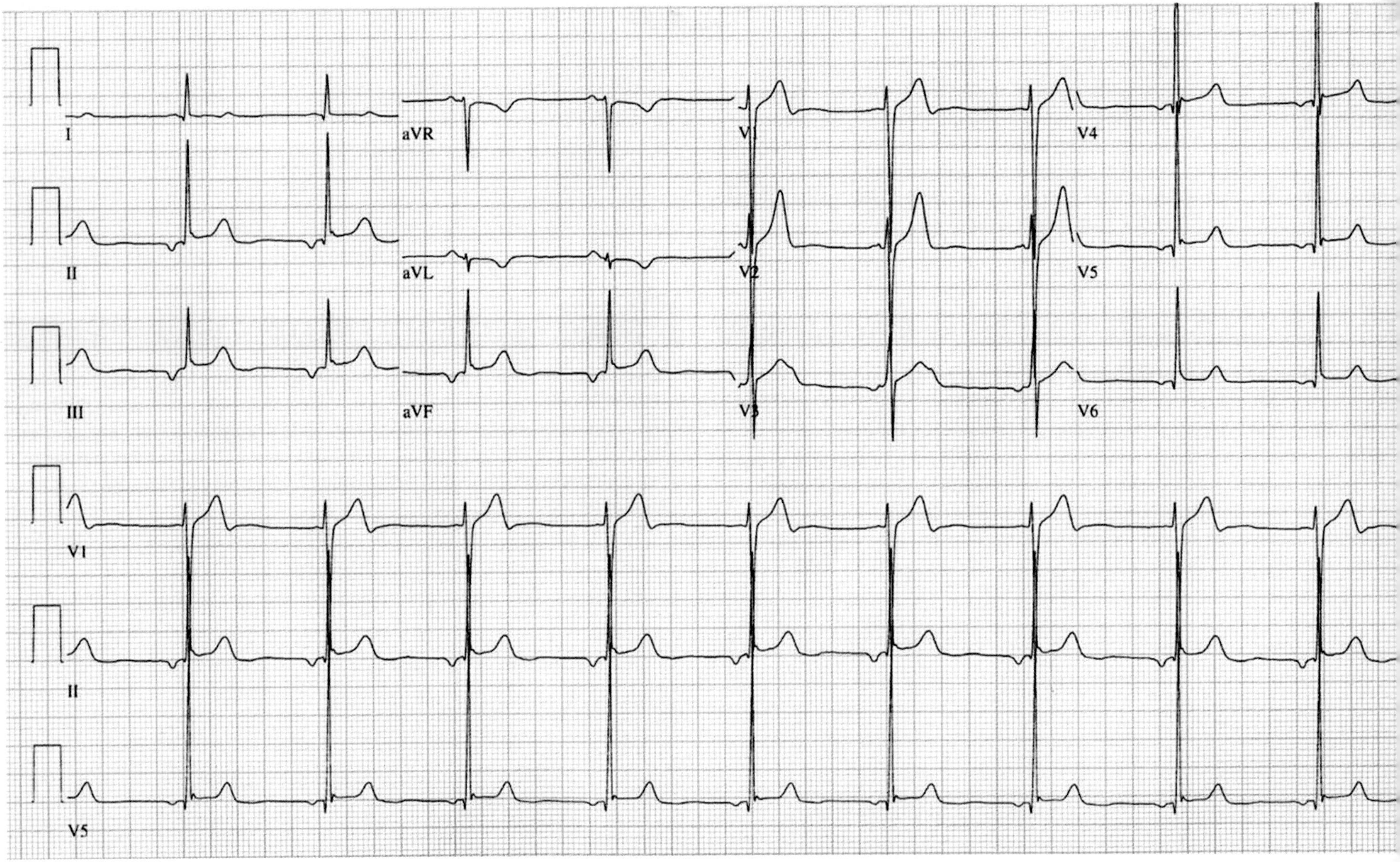

Interpretation Notes:

Electrocardiogram Case Study #108

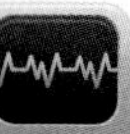

ELECTROCARDIOGRAM INTERPRETATION

P waves with a negative P-wave vector are seen in leads II, III, and aVF. These P waves precede each QRS complex with a constant PR interval. This reflects an ectopic atrial bradycardia as the atrial rate is slightly <60 per minute. Nonspecific ST-T changes are seen in the high lateral leads. Diffuse J-point elevation is present as is PR-segment elevation in lead aVR. These findings support pericarditis.

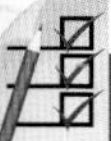

KEY TEACHING POINTS

- Assessment of the P-wave axis is an important consideration for each electrocardiogram. In this instance, this electrocardiogram demonstrates negatively oriented P waves within the inferior leads. This suggests a low atrial origin as seen in the presence of an ectopic atrial bradycardia. This dysrhythmia may be influenced by increased vagal tone and/or medication administration such as those from the beta or calcium blocker pharmaceutical class.

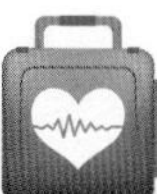

KEY DIAGNOSES

- Ectopic atrial bradycardia
- Nonspecific ST-T changes
- Pericarditis

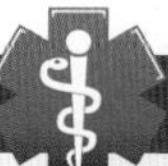

BOARD EXAMINATION ESSENTIALS

For the board exam, the most suitable diagnostic code is an AV junctional rhythm. This is not strictly correct as the supraventricular origin may in fact be extrinsic to but in close proximity to the AV junction, therefore optimally coded an ectopic atrial rhythm. Since this is not a diagnostic code option, AV junctional rhythm is preferred. Nonspecific ST-T changes are also demonstrated in the high lateral leads. The diffuse J-point elevation and PR-segment elevation in lead aVR in the context of chest discomfort favors the clinical diagnosis of pericarditis over early repolarization. In the presence of an atrial rhythm of non-sinus origin, do not code for atrial abnormality/enlargement patterns. Narrow Q waves are seen in leads V4 to V6. These Q waves do not support a myocardial infarction pattern as they are not of diagnostic duration.

Electrocardiogram Case Study #109

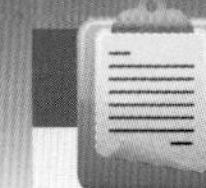

CLINICAL HISTORY

A 42-year-old male with end-stage liver disease secondary to chronic hepatitis C infection who presents to the hospital with an altered mental status and acute renal failure.

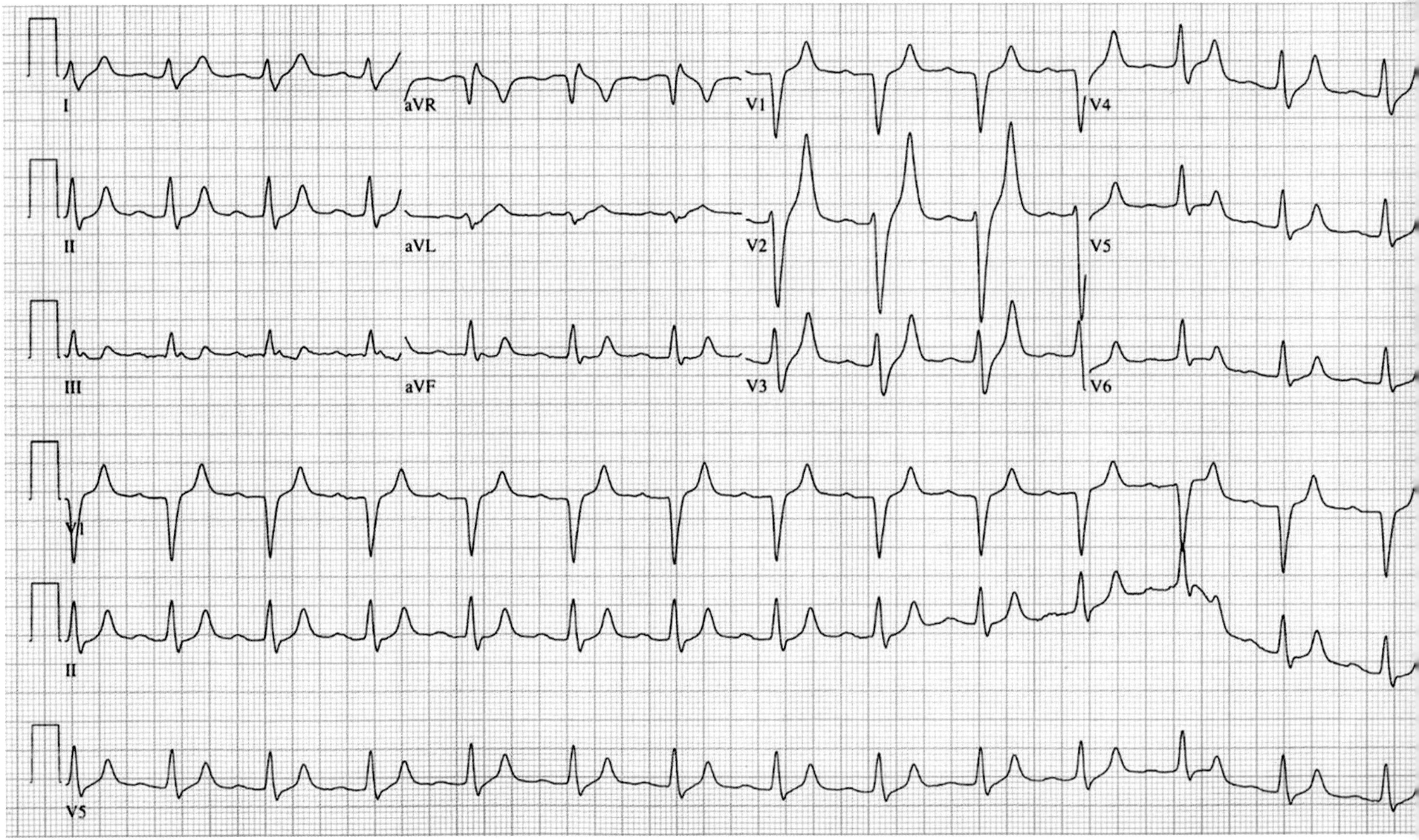

I aVR V1 V4
II aVL V2 V5
III aVF V3 V6
V1
II
V5

Interpretation Notes:

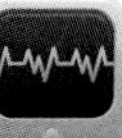

ELECTROCARDIOGRAM INTERPRETATION

Normal sinus rhythm is present as the P waves are upright in the limb leads and precede each QRS complex with a constant PR interval. The PR interval is prolonged at approximately 240 milliseconds supporting first-degree atrioventricular block. The QRS complex is widened to a nonspecific degree and the T waves are narrow based and peaked in all leads. This combination of findings including first-degree atrioventricular block, a nonspecific intraventricular conduction delay, and peaked T waves all suggest advanced hyperkalemia.

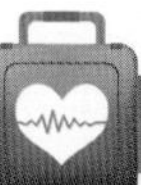

KEY DIAGNOSES

- Normal sinus rhythm
- First-degree atrioventricular block
- Nonspecific intraventricular conduction delay
- Hyperkalemia

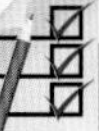

KEY TEACHING POINTS

- It is important to identify abnormalities suggesting hyperkalemia as the electrocardiogram may represent the first clinical clue.
- If the potassium level continues to rise, further QRS complex widening will ensue progressing to eventual asystole.

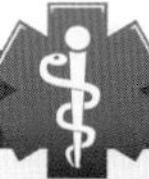

BOARD EXAMINATION ESSENTIALS

Anticipate an electrocardiogram either identical or similar to this on the board exam. Diagnostic codes include normal sinus rhythm; AV block, first degree; intraventricular conduction disturbance, nonspecific type; and hyperkalemia. Additionally, code ST- and/or T-wave abnormalities suggesting electrolyte disturbances, reflected on this electrocardiogram as narrow based, symmetric, and peaked T waves. Make certain not to code complete left bundle-branch block.

Electrocardiogram Case Study #110

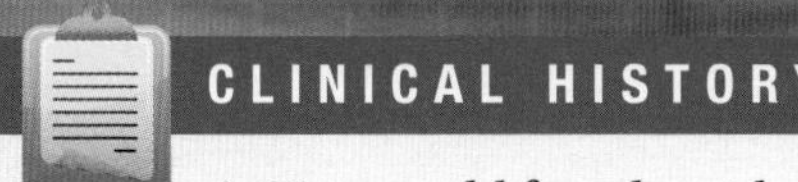

CLINICAL HISTORY

A 66-year-old female with a longstanding history of atrial arrhythmias.

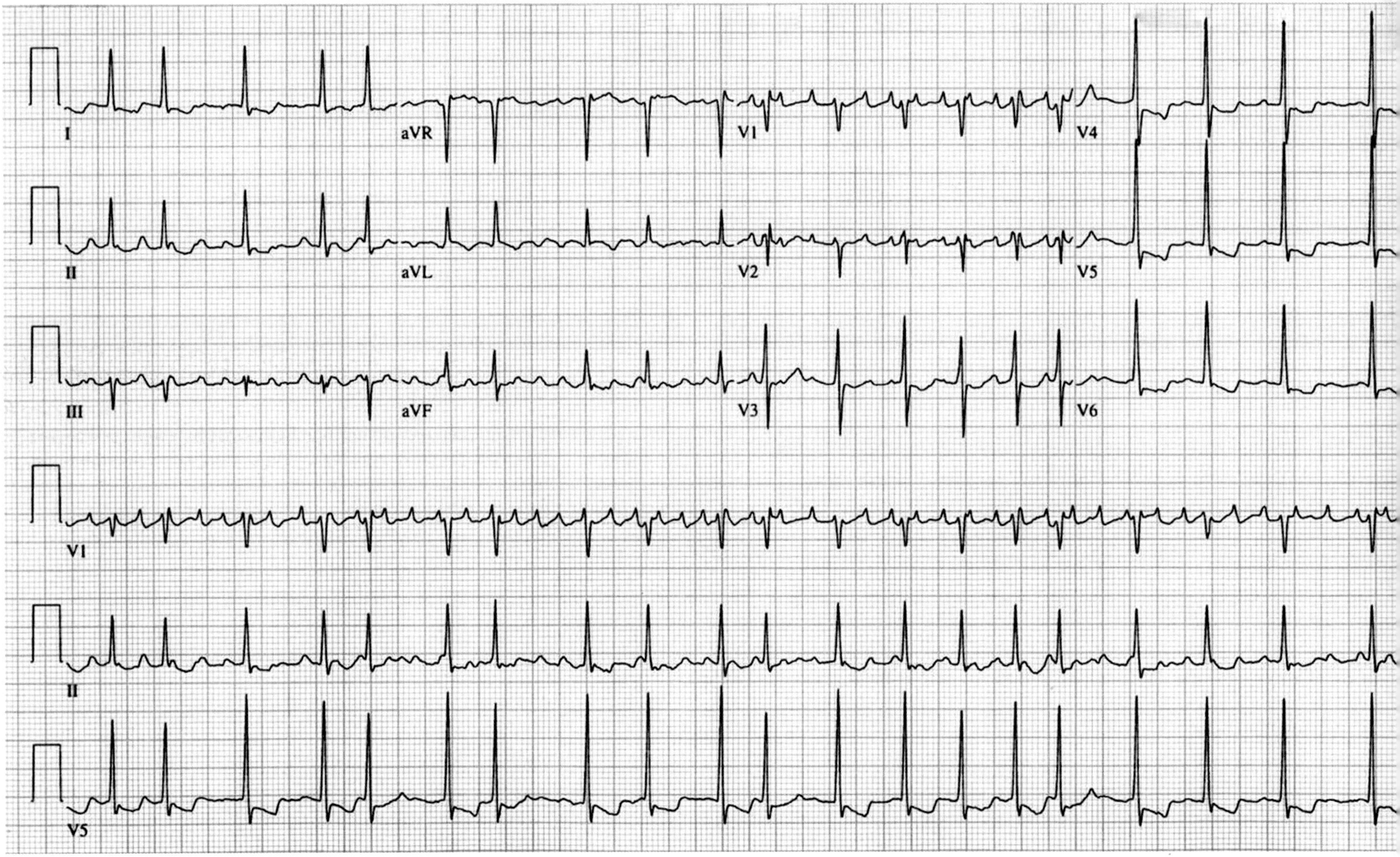

Interpretation Notes:

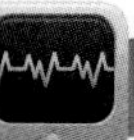

ELECTROCARDIOGRAM INTERPRETATION

The atrial rhythm is best assessed in the lead V1 rhythm strip and demonstrates irregularly irregular atrial activity at a rate >300 per minute. This represents coarse atrial fibrillation. The ventricle depolarizes unpredictably at a rate >100 per minute representing a rapid ventricular response. Diffuse nonspecific ST-T changes are present. There is no evidence of acute myocardial injury or a prior myocardial infarction.

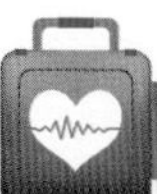

KEY DIAGNOSES

- Atrial fibrillation
- Rapid ventricular response
- Nonspecific ST-T changes

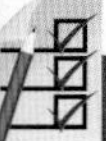

KEY TEACHING POINTS

- This electrocardiogram serves as an example of coarse atrial fibrillation. Atrial fibrillatory activity is readily seen, which occurs at a very high rate in a random and chaotic manner without predictability.
- It is tempting to consider the diagnosis of atrial flutter. Unlike atrial flutter, for this electrocardiogram, the atrial rate is >300 per minute and occurs irregularly without rhythmicity.
- Asymmetric T-wave inversion as seen in leads V4 to V6 suggests left ventricular hypertrophy. This is not supported by the QRS complex voltage.

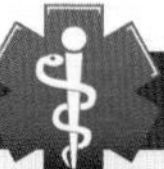

BOARD EXAMINATION ESSENTIALS

For the board exam, it is extremely important to carefully distinguish between atrial fibrillation and atrial flutter. Diagnostic codes on this electrocardiogram include atrial fibrillation and nonspecific ST- and/or T-wave abnormalities. While asymmetric ST-segment depression and T-wave inversion are present suggesting a possible ventricular hypertrophy pattern, supporting QRS complex voltage it is not found. Therefore, do not code a ventricular hypertrophy pattern for this electrocardiogram.

Electrocardiogram Case Study #111

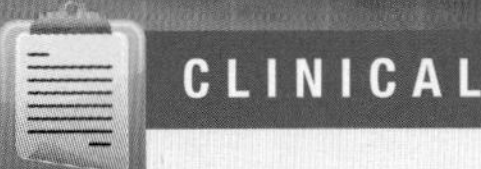

CLINICAL HISTORY

A 33-year-old female seen in the outpatient clinic after a recent hospitalization for an asthma exacerbation. The patient also has a history of palpitations.

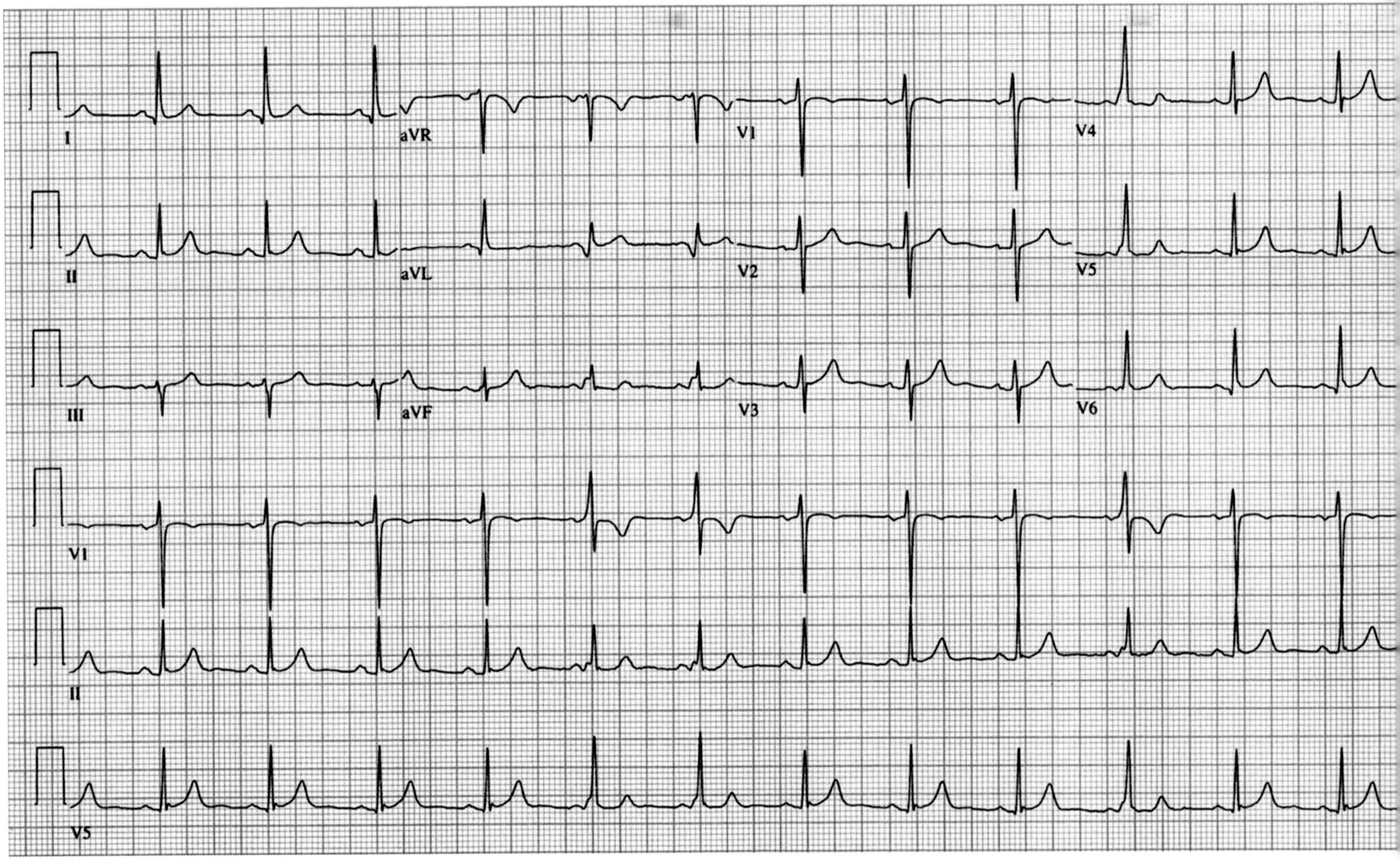

I aVR V1 V4
II aVL V2 V5
III aVF V3 V6
V1
II
V5

Interpretation Notes:

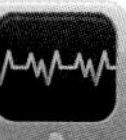

ELECTROCARDIOGRAM INTERPRETATION

This patient demonstrates normal sinus rhythm. The fifth, sixth, and tenth QRS complexes appear different in morphology than the native QRS complexes. There is slurring to the upstroke of the QRS complex with a shortened PR interval denoting intermittent ventricular pre-excitation consistent with the Wolff-Parkinson-White pattern. Note the abnormal effect on ventricular repolarization, particularly evident in the lead V1 rhythm strip.

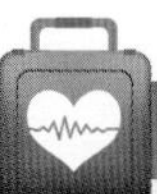

KEY DIAGNOSES

- Normal sinus rhythm
- Wolff-Parkinson-White pattern

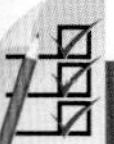

KEY TEACHING POINTS

- The pre-excitation complexes are actually fusion complexes. The QRS complex fusion takes place between normal antegrade conduction and conduction antegrade via the accessory bypass tract with competing ventricular depolarization via the accessory pathway.
- It is common to find differing degrees of ventricular pre-excitation depending on vagal tone, heart rate, and concomitant medications. This electrocardiogram illustrates the transient nature of ventricular pre-excitation.

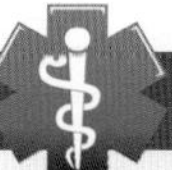

BOARD EXAMINATION ESSENTIALS

This is another example of the Wolff-Parkinson-White pattern and intermittent ventricular pre-excitation. Diagnostic codes include normal sinus rhythm and Wolff-Parkinson-White pattern. Carefully assess the P to P interval. In this example, the P to P interval is constant with the intermittent ventricular pre-excitation likely secondary to changing vagal tone and altered atrioventricular conduction, unrelated to atrial prematurity. Do not code functional (rate-related) aberrancy. Likewise, do not code ventricular pacemaker complexes.

Electrocardiogram Case Study #112

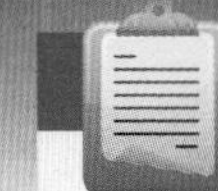

CLINICAL HISTORY

A 40-year-old female with severe shortness of breath, progressive lower-extremity swelling, and abdominal distention who seeks further evaluation.

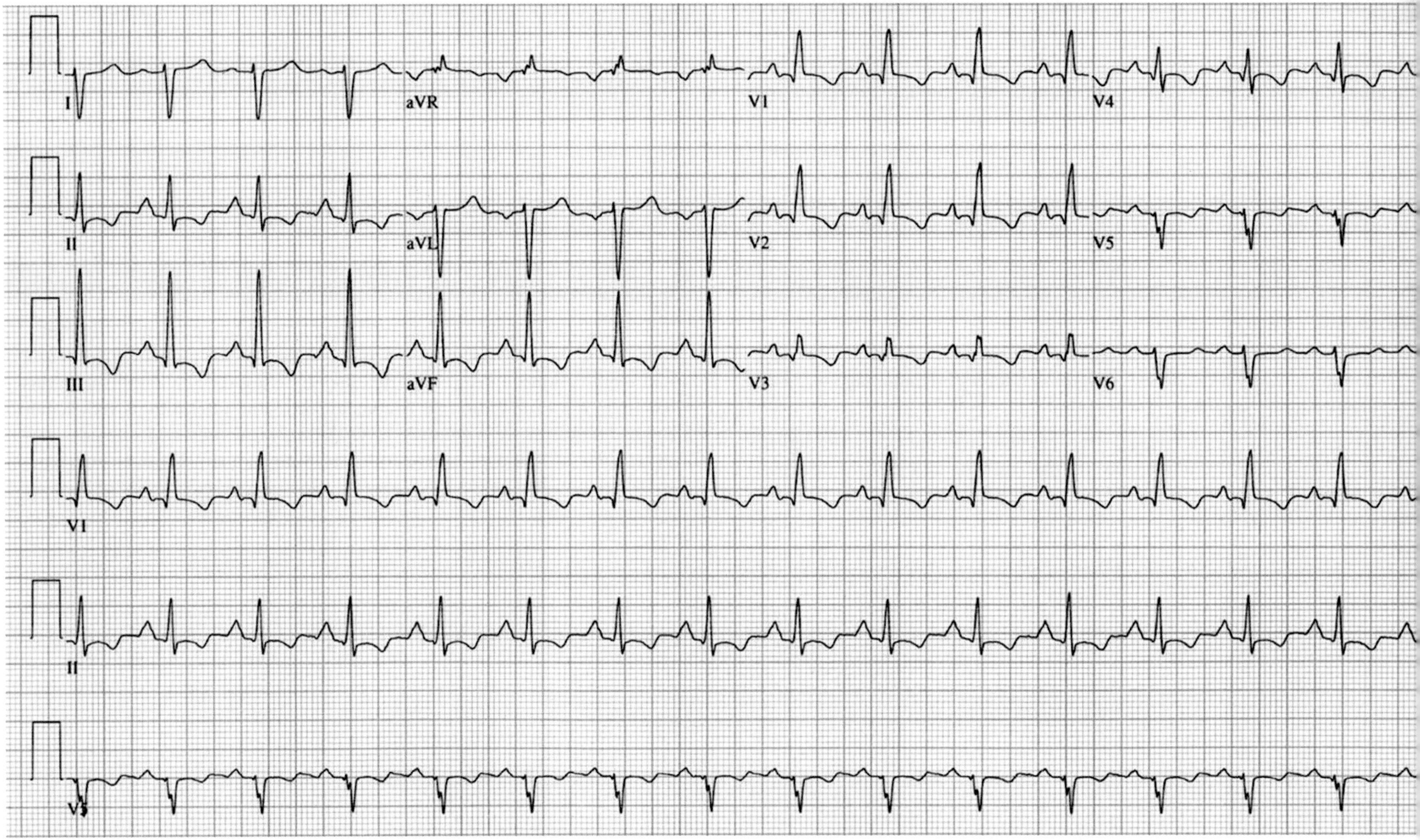

I aVR V1 V4
II aVL V2 V5
III aVF V3 V6
V1
II
V5

Interpretation Notes: ______________________________

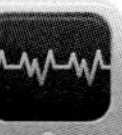

ELECTROCARDIOGRAM INTERPRETATION

The cardiac rhythm is normal sinus rhythm. The P wave in lead II is both broadened and increased in amplitude measuring 0.3 mV. This supports right atrial abnormality. The QRS complex frontal plane axis demonstrates right-axis deviation as the QRS complex vector is negative in lead I and positive in leads II, III, and aVF. A small Q wave and prominent R wave with a normal QRS complex duration is seen in leads V1 to V2 reflecting right ventricular hypertrophy with secondary ST-T changes.

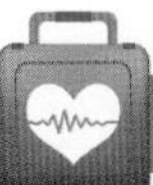

KEY DIAGNOSES

- Normal sinus rhythm
- Right atrial abnormality
- QRS complex right-axis deviation
- Right ventricular hypertrophy with secondary ST-T changes

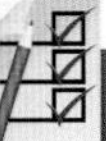

KEY TEACHING POINTS

- This electrocardiogram demonstrates the common features of right ventricular pressure overload. These features include right atrial abnormality, right-axis QRS complex deviation, and right ventricular hypertrophy with secondary ST-T changes.
- Note the poor R-wave progression throughout the precordium given the right ventricular hypertrophy and resultant counterclockwise cardiac rotation. This does not imply the presence of a coexistent myocardial infarction.

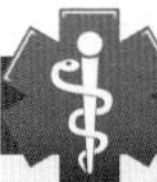

BOARD EXAMINATION ESSENTIALS

This is another likely electrocardiogram board exam example. Diagnostic codes include normal sinus rhythm, right atrial abnormality/enlargement, right-axis deviation (greater than +100 degrees), and right ventricular hypertrophy. Clinical diagnostic coding considerations include chronic lung disease and acute cor pulmonale including pulmonary embolism. A supporting clinical history would be helpful. In this case, the clinical history suggests right-sided congestive heart failure but does not provide enough information to specify a single clinical diagnosis with confidence. The lack of evidence of left atrial abnormality/enlargement supports a primary pulmonary process not invoking left-sided cardiac pathology.

Electrocardiogram Case Study #113

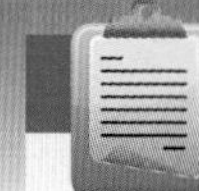

CLINICAL HISTORY

A 64-year-old male who presented to an outside emergency room with acute-onset chest discomfort. This electrocardiogram was performed just prior to an urgent heart catheterization.

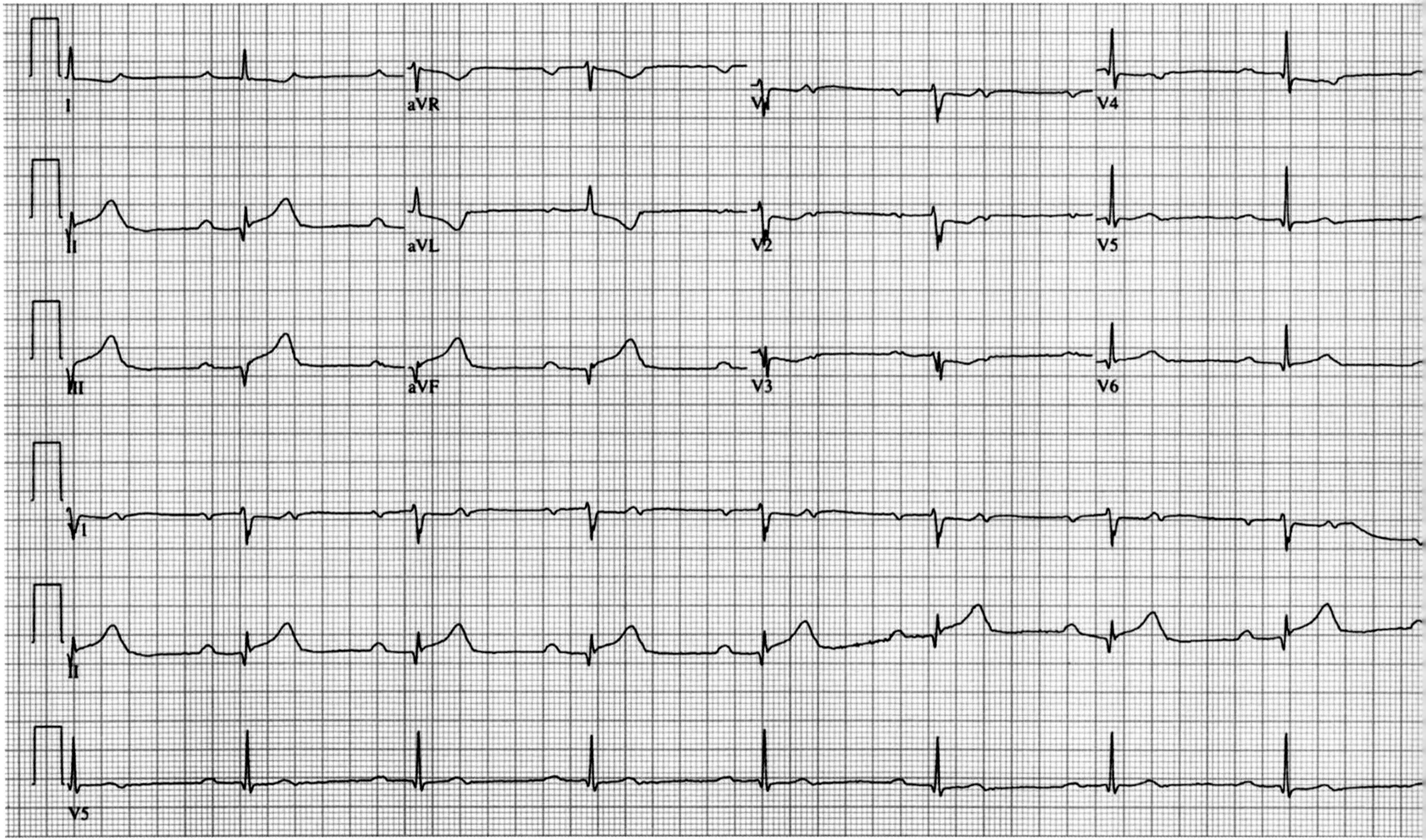

I aVR V1 V4
II aVL V2 V5
III aVF V3 V6
V1
II
V5

Interpretation Notes:

Electrocardiogram Case Study #113

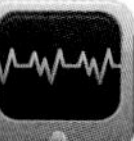

ELECTROCARDIOGRAM INTERPRETATION

On this tracing, the atrial rhythm is best assessed in the lead V1 rhythm strip. Regular P waves occur at a rate of approximately 100 per minute with a P wave preceding each QRS complex and a P wave following each QRS complex within the terminal aspect of the T wave. This represents normal sinus rhythm with 2:1 atrioventricular block. Inferior Q waves are present with J-point elevation, ST-segment elevation, and ST-segment straightening consistent with an inferior myocardial infarction acute and acute myocardial injury. Reciprocal ST-segment depression is seen in leads I, aVL, and V2 to V4. This conduction abnormality is a result of ischemia of the atrioventricular node due to the acute right coronary artery myocardial injury and infarction. Small Q waves approximately 30 milliseconds in duration are seen in leads V4 to V6. Associated ST-T changes are present. The Q wave is not of diagnostic duration to support with certainty an age-indeterminate anterolateral myocardial infarction.

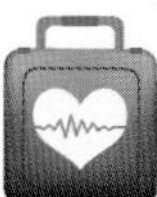

KEY DIAGNOSES

- Normal sinus rhythm
- 2:1 atrioventricular block
- Inferior myocardial infarction, acute
- Acute myocardial injury

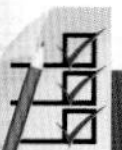

KEY TEACHING POINTS

- It is not clear if the conduction abnormality is second-degree Mobitz type I Wenckebach atrioventricular block or second-degree Mobitz type II atrioventricular block. A longer recording with rhythm strip analysis would be helpful to evaluate for periods of Wenckebach atrioventricular block with varying conduction ratios.
- In the setting of 2:1 atrioventricular block and acute myocardial injury, temporary pacemaker placement should be considered as this patient subgroup can proceed to complete heart block and hemodynamic deterioration, particularly if the atrioventricular block is felt to represent an infra-Hisian location.

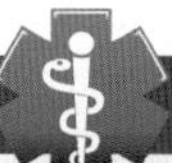

BOARD EXAMINATION ESSENTIALS

For the board exam, anticipate acute myocardial injury/infarction patterns and atrioventricular conduction abnormalities to be found on the same electrocardiogram. Diagnostic codes for this electrocardiogram example include normal sinus rhythm; AV block, 2:1; inferior myocardial infarction; acute and ST- and/or T-wave abnormalities suggesting myocardial injury. Left atrial abnormality/enlargement is also suggested but is not certain. This would be considered an equivocal diagnostic code.

Electrocardiogram Case Study #114

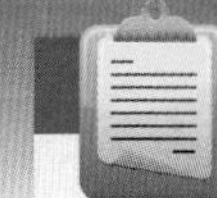

CLINICAL HISTORY

A 57-year-old female hospitalized with advanced congestive heart failure requiring intubation in the setting of severe aortic and mitral regurgitation.

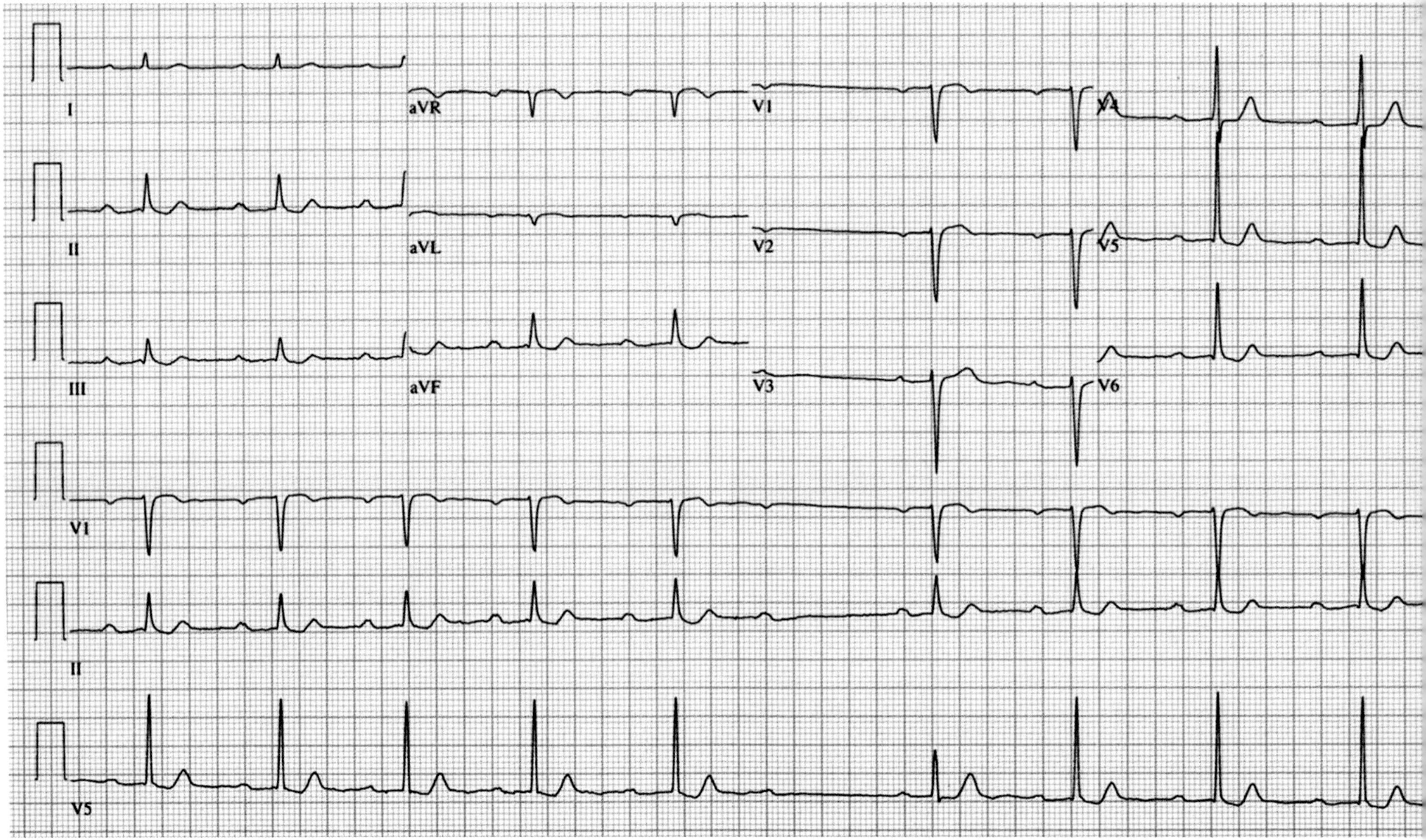

Interpretation Notes:

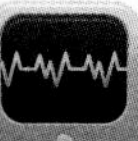

ELECTROCARDIOGRAM INTERPRETATION

The cardiac rhythm is normal sinus rhythm as the limb lead P-wave axis is normal. The PR interval progressively prolongs and eventually results in a nonconducted QRS complex. This represents second-degree Mobitz type I Wenckebach atrioventricular block. The QRS complexes are normal. There is scooping of the ST segments in both the inferior and the lateral precordial leads with a shortened QT interval. These findings are consistent with digitalis administration. Left atrial abnormality is suggested based on the negative terminal P-wave vector in lead V1 and the prolonged P wave in lead II.

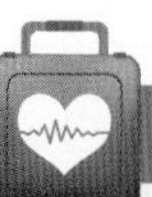

KEY DIAGNOSES

- Normal sinus rhythm
- Second-degree Mobitz type I Wenckebach atrioventricular block
- Digitalis effect
- Short QT interval
- Left atrial abnormality

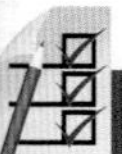

KEY TEACHING POINTS

- This electrocardiogram serves as an example of the effect of digitalis on ventricular repolarization.
- The QT interval is shortened and the ST segments are scooped. This does not imply digitalis toxicity but instead is an expected finding with a therapeutic digitalis level.

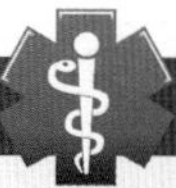

BOARD EXAMINATION ESSENTIALS

Board exam diagnostic codes include normal sinus rhythm; AV block, second degree; Mobitz type I Wenckebach; and left atrial abnormality/enlargement. This does not reflect digitalis toxicity and therefore is not coded. While AV block, first degree, is present, it is generally not coded in the presence of a more advanced form of atrioventricular block.

Electrocardiogram Case Study #115

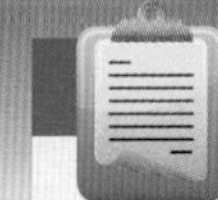

CLINICAL HISTORY

A 51-year-old male with dialysis requiring renal failure and a recent positive stress echocardiogram referred for a cardiac catheterization.

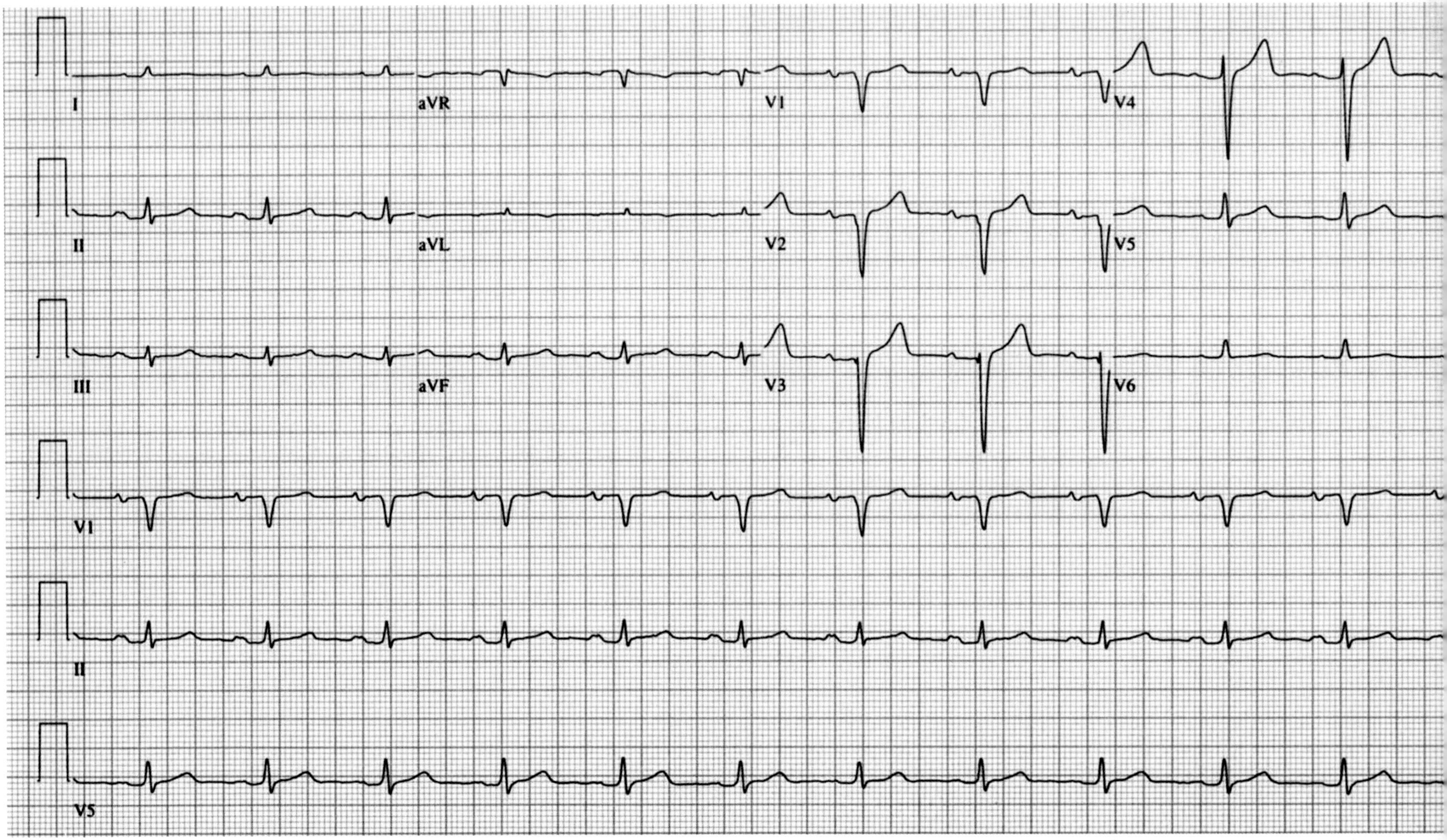

I aVR V1 V4

II aVL V2 V5

III aVF V3 V6

V1

II

V5

Interpretation Notes:

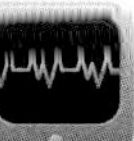

ELECTROCARDIOGRAM INTERPRETATION

This electrocardiogram demonstrates normal sinus rhythm at an atrial rate of approximately 70 per minute. The PR interval is prolonged at 220 milliseconds representing first-degree atrioventricular block. Q waves are seen in both leads V1 to V2. In addition and most importantly, a small Q wave is seen in lead V3. This represents a splinter Q wave and is diagnostic of an anteroseptal myocardial infarction, age indeterminate. The limb lead QRS complexes are <0.5 mV in amplitude satisfying the criteria for low-voltage QRS. A biphasic P wave is seen in lead V1 supporting left atrial abnormality.

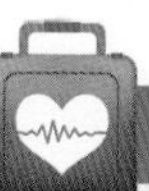

KEY DIAGNOSES

- Normal sinus rhythm
- First-degree atrioventricular block
- Low-voltage QRS
- Anteroseptal myocardial infarction, age indeterminate
- Left atrial abnormality

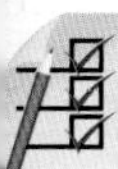

KEY TEACHING POINTS

- Splinter Q waves greatly enhance the specificity for diagnosing a prior anteroseptal myocardial infarction.
- It is important not to overlook splinter Q waves, particularly when the Q waves extend to lead V3 as this can help distinguish a normal electrocardiogram from an electrocardiogram with a high specificity for ischemic heart disease.

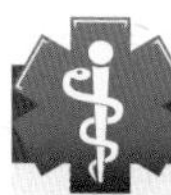

BOARD EXAMINATION ESSENTIALS

Diagnostic codes for the board exam include normal sinus rhythm, AV block, first degree, low voltage, limb leads and anteroseptal myocardial infarction, age indeterminate. Left atrial abnormality/enlargement is also likely present. The QRS complex is slightly prolonged but remains <100 milliseconds.

Electrocardiogram Case Study **#116**

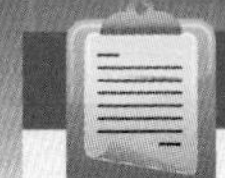

CLINICAL HISTORY

A 56-year-old male with rheumatoid arthritis seen in the outpatient department for a follow-up evaluation. He has no known cardiac history.

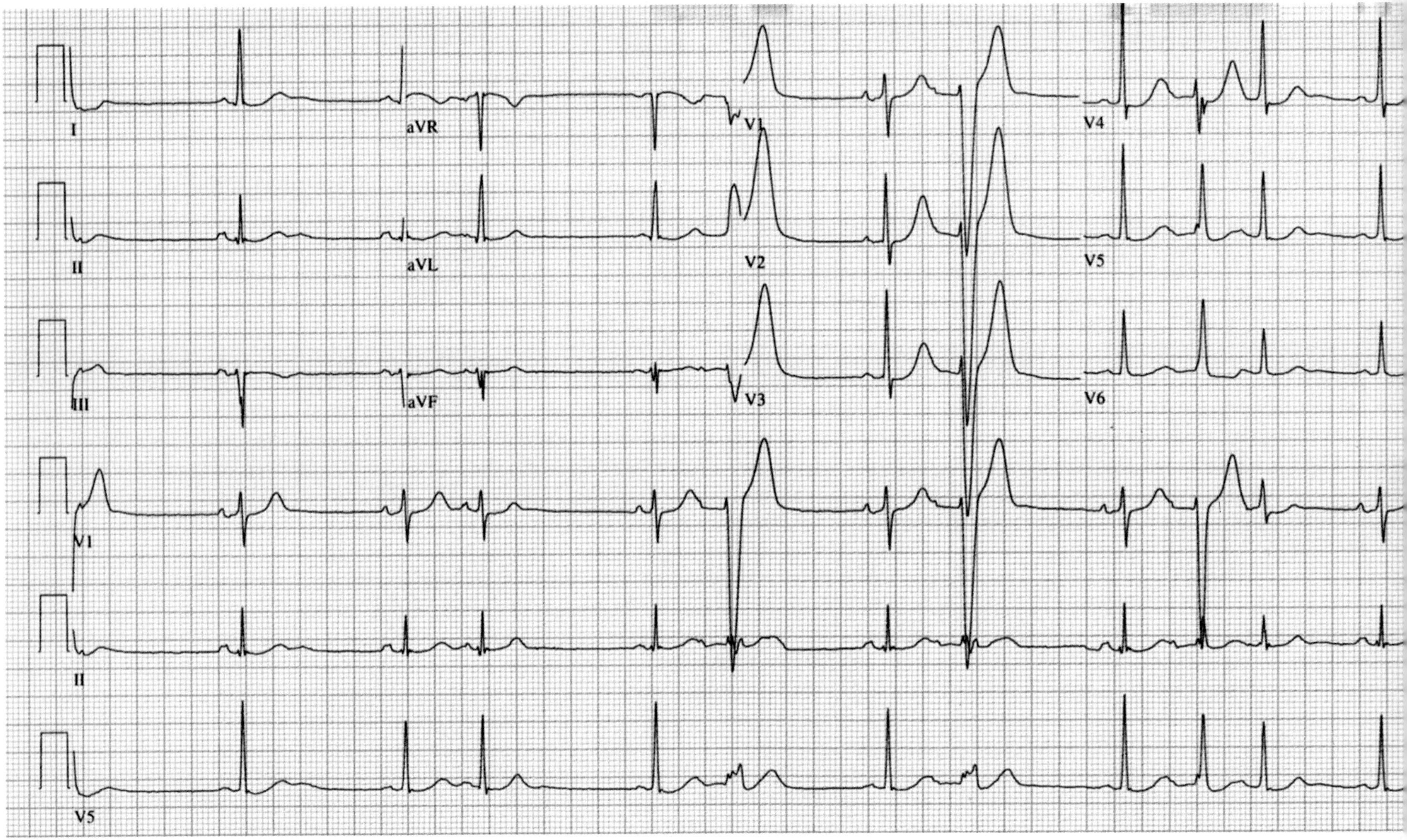

Interpretation Notes:

Electrocardiogram Case Study #116

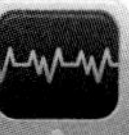

ELECTROCARDIOGRAM INTERPRETATION

This electrocardiogram demonstrates sinus bradycardia as the atrial rate is approximately 50 per minute with a normal P-wave axis. The third P wave is premature with a normally conducted QRS complex representing a premature atrial complex. The fifth P wave is also a premature atrial complex and is followed by a prolonged PR interval and a QRS complex with complete left bundle-branch block aberrancy. In contrast to the prior premature atrial complex, this occurs with a shorter RP interval, greater intra-atrial and atrioventricular nodal conduction delay, and subsequent ventricular aberration. The last premature atrial complex is an interpolated premature atrial complex as it does not reset the sinus node. It also demonstrates aberrant conduction but its shorter QRS complex duration does not satisfy the criteria for complete left bundle-branch block aberration. Diffuse nonspecific ST-T changes are also seen.

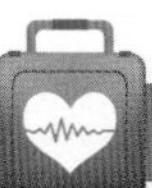

KEY DIAGNOSES

- Sinus bradycardia
- Premature atrial complex, interpolated and noninterpolated
- Complete left bundle-branch block aberrancy
- Aberrant conduction
- Nonspecific ST-T changes
- Concealed conduction

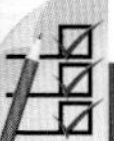

KEY TEACHING POINTS

- Premature atrial complexes with complete left bundle-branch block aberrancy are less common compared to complete right bundle-branch block aberrancy as the refractory period of the left bundle branch is shorter.
- The premature atrial complexes conduct with a prolonged PR interval given the short preceding RP interval and reciprocal relationship between the preceding RP interval and the subsequent PR interval. This is an example of concealed conduction.

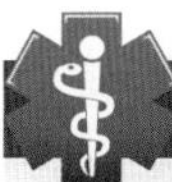

BOARD EXAMINATION ESSENTIALS

Diagnostic codes for the board exam include sinus bradycardia, atrial premature complexes, aberrant conduction, and nonspecific ST- and/or T-wave abnormalities. The key for this electrocardiogram example is to recognize the premature atrial complexes with and without aberrancy and to not inappropriately code them as premature ventricular complexes. Careful inspection of the preceding T wave permits identification of a slight deformation and localization of the premature P wave, securing the diagnosis.

Electrocardiogram Case Study #117

CLINICAL HISTORY

A 44-year-old male with severe peripheral vascular disease admitted for lower-extremity revascularization surgery.

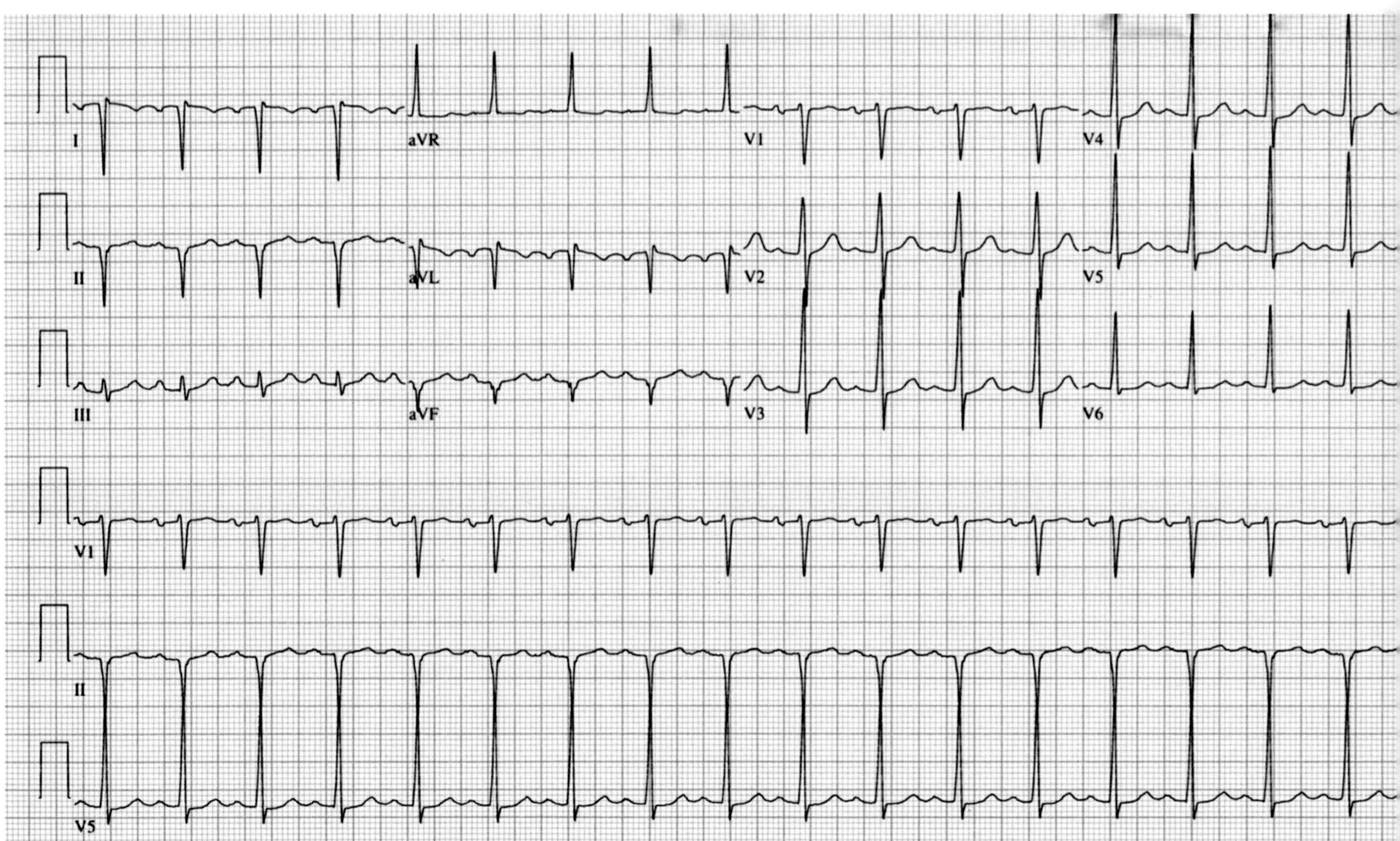

Interpretation Notes:

Electrocardiogram Case Study #117

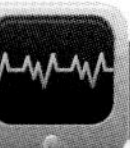

ELECTROCARDIOGRAM INTERPRETATION

This electrocardiogram demonstrates a regular atrial rhythm supporting sinus tachycardia at a rate slightly >100 per minute. The P-wave vector is negative in both leads I and aVL. When the P wave demonstrates a dominant negativity in both leads I and aVL, the differential diagnosis includes misplaced limb leads and dextrocardia. Normal R-wave progression is seen in leads V2 to V6 not supporting a diagnosis of dextrocardia. Therefore, this is an example of switched upper-extremity limb leads.

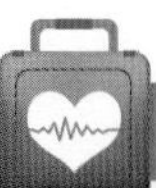

KEY DIAGNOSES

- Sinus tachycardia
- Misplaced limb leads

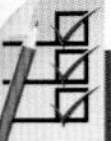

KEY TEACHING POINTS

- It would be appropriate to repeat this tracing checking lead placement more carefully to document this patient's electrocardiogram with normally placed leads.
- Despite this technical error, a dominant Q wave is seen in both leads II and aVF suggesting an inferior myocardial infarction, age indeterminate. In addition, a high lateral myocardial infarction is also suggested given the Q waves. Make sure to repeat electrocardiogram before concluding the presence of a myocardial infarction of indeterminate age.

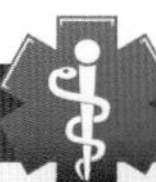

BOARD EXAMINATION ESSENTIALS

Diagnostic codes for the board exam include sinus tachycardia and incorrect electrode placement. Do not code QRS complex axis deviation or myocardial infarction patterns in the presence of a technically substandard electrocardiogram. This is another example where just a few diagnostic codes reflect a complete interpretation for purposes of the board exam.

Electrocardiogram Case Study #118

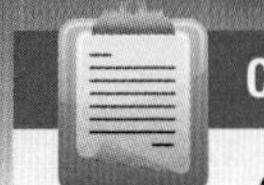

CLINICAL HISTORY

A 22-year-old woman who presents for evaluation of dysplastic nevi. She mentioned to her primary care provider that she has noticed a periodic irregular heart beat.

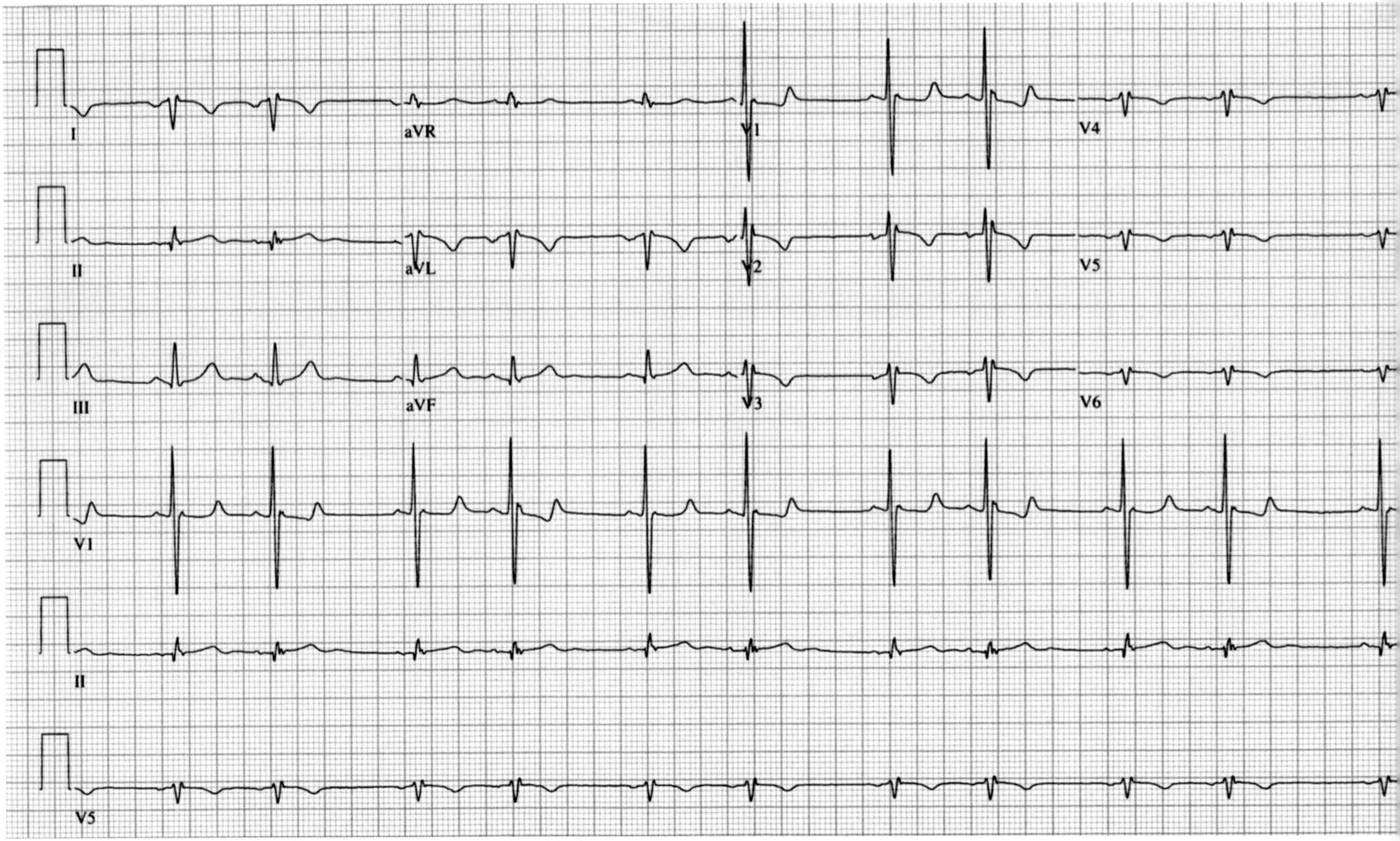

I aVR V1 V4
II aVL V2 V5
III aVF V3 V6
V1
II
V5

Interpretation Notes:

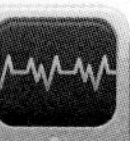

ELECTROCARDIOGRAM INTERPRETATION

This tracing demonstrates an abnormal P-wave axis with a negative P-wave vector in leads I and aVL. The differential diagnosis for this finding includes switched upper-extremity limb leads and dextrocardia. A prominent R wave is seen in lead V1 with R-wave regression as one proceeds from leads V2 to V6. This finding in combination with the negative P-wave vector in the high lateral leads confirms the presence of dextrocardia. This electrocardiogram otherwise demonstrates normal sinus rhythm and premature atrial complexes in a pattern of bigeminy. If one looks closely, the bigeminal P-wave pattern demonstrates a subtle difference in P-wave morphology.

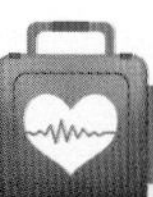

KEY DIAGNOSES

- Normal sinus rhythm
- Premature atrial complex
- Dextrocardia

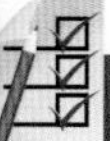

KEY TEACHING POINTS

- Recognizing the presence of dextrocardia is important as otherwise normal electrocardiograms can be interpreted as significantly abnormal, such as inappropriately diagnosing myocardial infarction patterns.
- Upon first glance, the frontal plane QRS complex axis appears deviated extremely rightward possibly even suggesting a lateral myocardial infarction. This finding together with R-wave regression seen in leads V2 to V6 confirms the presence of dextrocardia.

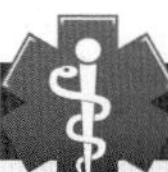

BOARD EXAMINATION ESSENTIALS

This is another likely board exam electrocardiogram example. Diagnostic board exam codes include normal sinus rhythm, dextrocardia, mirror image, and atrial premature complexes. Sinus arrhythmia in this young patient is another diagnostic coding possibility in lieu of atrial premature complexes. Atrial premature complexes are favored given the slight P-wave morphologic difference.

Electrocardiogram Case Study #119

CLINICAL HISTORY

A 16-year-old gentleman admitted acutely to the hospital for further evaluation of profound depression.

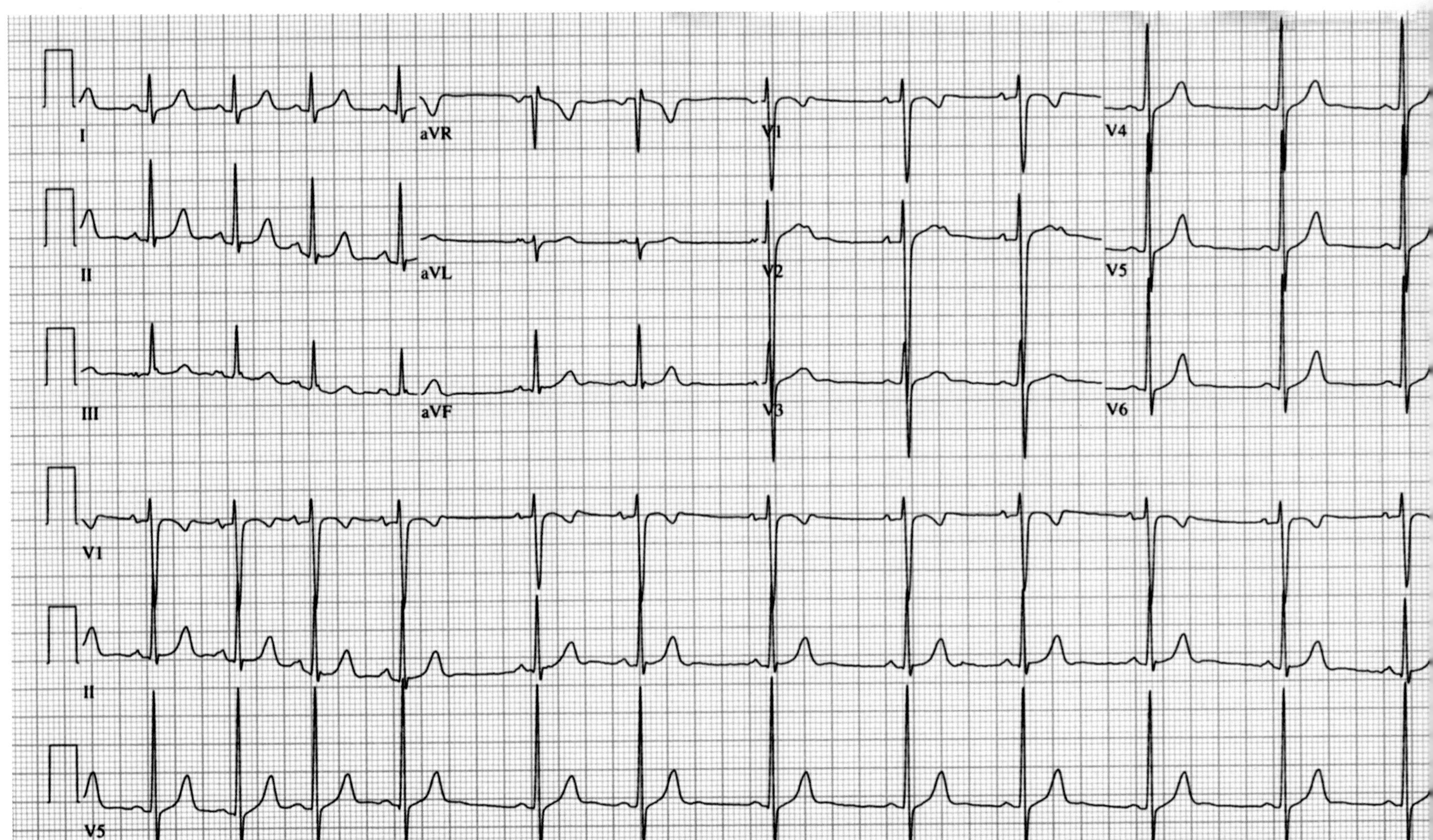

Interpretation Notes:

Electrocardiogram Case Study #119

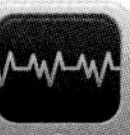

ELECTROCARDIOGRAM INTERPRETATION

The cardiac rhythm is normal sinus rhythm as each QRS complex is preceded by a P wave of similar morphology with a constant PR interval. Toward the left-hand portion of the electrocardiogram, the R:R interval is shorter and slightly irregular. The P-wave morphology remains constant as this represents sinus arrhythmia, seen most commonly in younger age groups. This is a normal electrocardiogram. A wandering baseline artifact is also present.

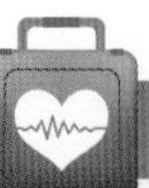

KEY DIAGNOSES

- Normal sinus rhythm
- Sinus arrhythmia
- Baseline artifact
- Normal electrocardiogram

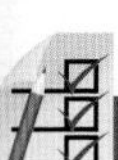

KEY TEACHING POINTS

- Sinus arrhythmia is a common finding and it should not be confused with more pathologic dysrhythmias.
- The sinus node discharge rate typically accelerates during inspiration and decelerates with expiration as demonstrated on this electrocardiogram.

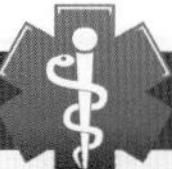

BOARD EXAMINATION ESSENTIALS

This is an example of a normal electrocardiogram. In addition to coding for a normal electrocardiogram, other diagnostic codes for the board exam include normal sinus rhythm, sinus arrhythmia and artifact. T-wave inversion isolated to lead V1 is an otherwise normal finding.

Electrocardiogram Case Study #120

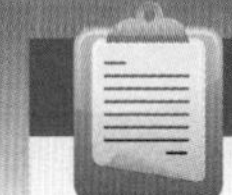

CLINICAL HISTORY

A 22-year-old woman admitted to the hospital for evaluation and treatment of schizophrenia.

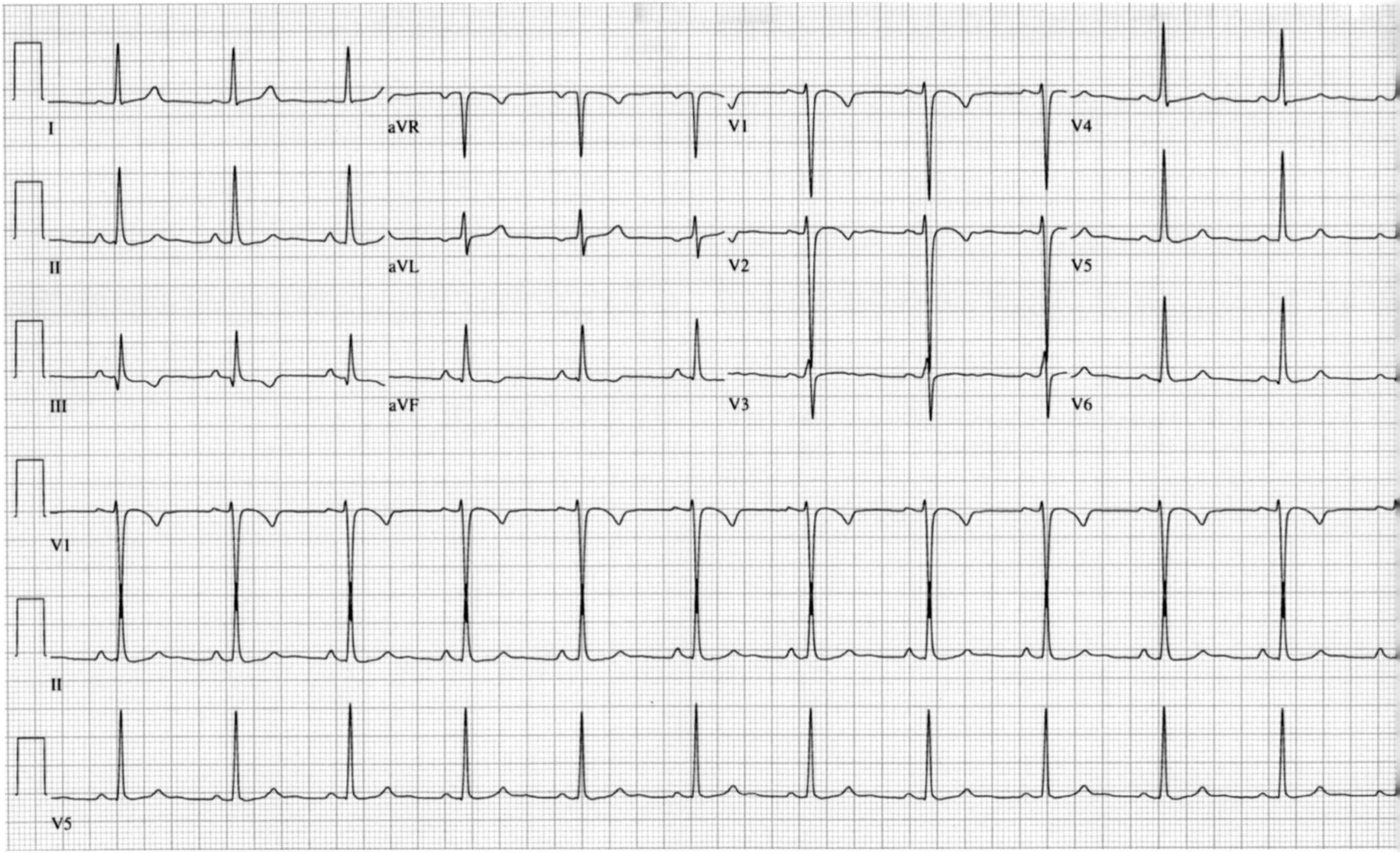

I aVR V1 V4
II aVL V2 V5
III aVF V3 V6
V1
II
V5

Interpretation Notes:

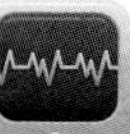

ELECTROCARDIOGRAM INTERPRETATION

This is a normal electrocardiogram. The cardiac rhythm is normal sinus rhythm as the P-wave axis in leads I, II, and III is normal and the atrial rate is approximately 70 per minute. T-wave inversion is present in leads V1 to V2. In a younger age group patient, this is a normal finding and demonstrates a persistent juvenile T-wave pattern.

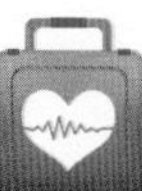

KEY DIAGNOSES

- Normal sinus rhythm
- Juvenile T-wave pattern
- Normal electrocardiogram

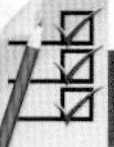

KEY TEACHING POINTS

- Is important to recognize a normal variant when interpreting electrocardiograms.
- The persistent juvenile T-wave pattern is a normal variant and should not be confused with underlying cardiac pathology such as myocardial ischemia or cardiomyopathy.

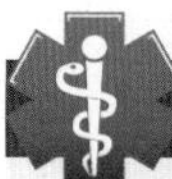

BOARD EXAMINATION ESSENTIALS

This is another normal electrocardiogram example with board exam relevance. Diagnostic codes include normal sinus rhythm; normal electrocardiogram; and normal variant, juvenile T waves. Make sure to reference the clinical history carefully as a juvenile T-wave pattern generally applies to patients 25 years of age or less.

Electrocardiogram Case Study #121

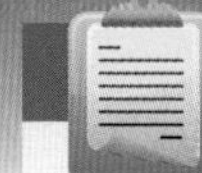

CLINICAL HISTORY

A 73-year-old female with longstanding hypertension who presents for evaluation of recent-onset dyspnea upon exertion. Comorbidities include obesity and insulin requiring diabetes mellitus.

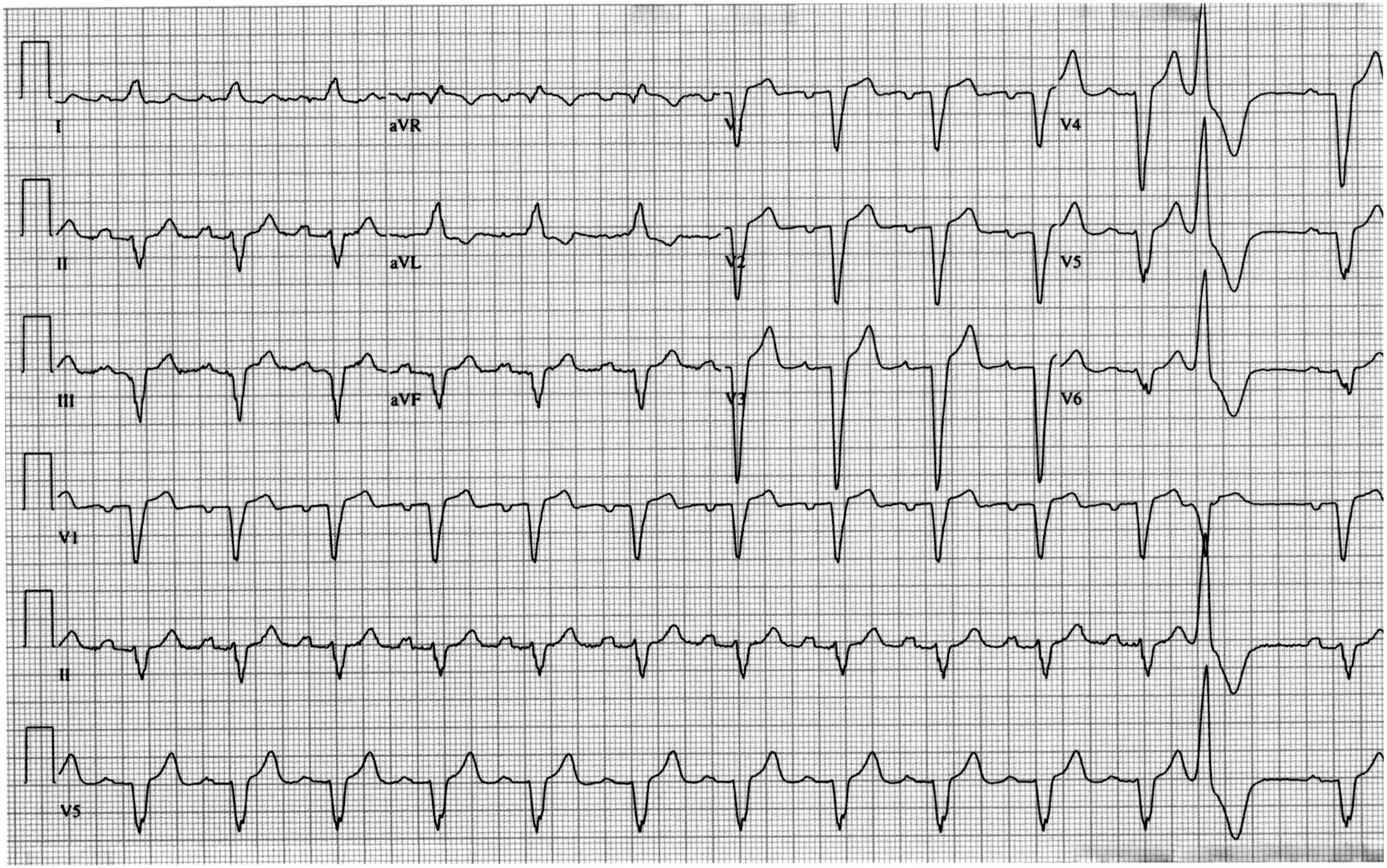

I aVR V1 V4
II aVL V2 V5
III aVF V3 V6
V1
II
V5

Interpretation Notes:

Electrocardiogram Case Study #121

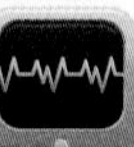

ELECTROCARDIOGRAM INTERPRETATION

Normal sinus rhythm with a prolonged PR interval diagnostic of first-degree atrioventricular block is present. The QRS complex is widened with a complete left bundle-branch block configuration. Despite the presence of Q waves both inferiorly and anterolaterally, it is not possible to diagnose an age-indeterminate myocardial infarction in the presence of complete left bundle-branch block. The second to last QRS complex is a premature ventricular complex. Left atrial abnormality is also present given the broadened P wave in lead II and terminally negative P wave in lead V1. The QRS complex vector is positive in lead I and negative in leads II, III, and aVF supporting QRS complex frontal plane left-axis deviation.

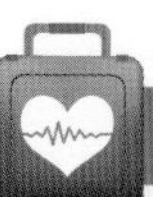

KEY DIAGNOSES

- Normal sinus rhythm
- First-degree atrioventricular block
- Left atrial abnormality
- QRS complex left-axis deviation
- Premature ventricular complex
- Complete left bundle-branch block

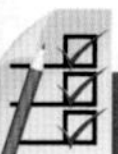

KEY TEACHING POINTS

- The combination of first-degree atrioventricular block, left atrial abnormality, and complete left bundle-branch block suggests possible left ventricular systolic dysfunction.
- In the setting of complete left bundle-branch block, left atrial abnormality is often present.

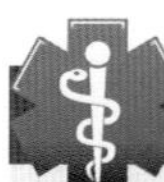

BOARD EXAMINATION ESSENTIALS

Board exam diagnostic codes include normal sinus rhythm; AV block, first degree; left-axis deviation (greater than –30 degrees); left atrial abnormality/enlargement; left bundle-branch block; complete and ventricular premature complex. Do not code for an inferior myocardial infarction pattern of indeterminate age in the presence of complete left bundle-branch block. The lack of septal Q waves supports the presence of complete left bundle-branch block.

Electrocardiogram Case Study #122

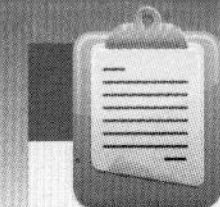

CLINICAL HISTORY

A 19-year-old gentleman with increasing shortness of breath in the setting of a recently diagnosed heart murmur.

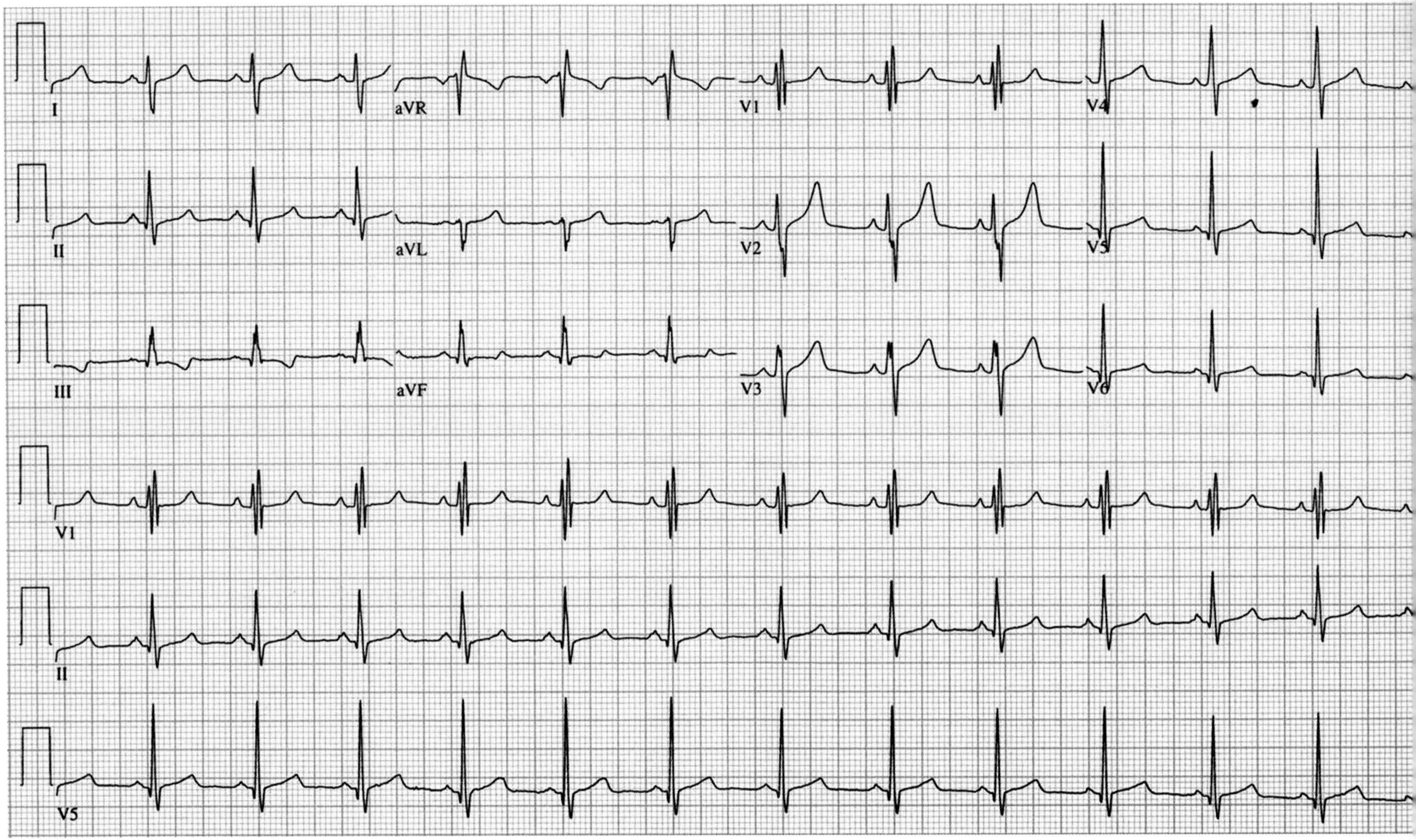

I aVR V1 V4
II aVL V2 V5
III aVF V3 V6
V1
II
V5

Interpretation Notes:

Electrocardiogram Case Study #122

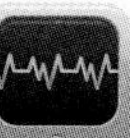

ELECTROCARDIOGRAM INTERPRETATION

The cardiac rhythm is normal sinus rhythm as a P wave of normal axis precedes each QRS complex. The QRS complex frontal plane axis demonstrates right-axis deviation as the QRS complex vector is negative in lead I and positive in leads II, III, and aVF. An rsR′ QRS complex morphology is noted in lead V1. This represents an unusual pattern for right ventricular conduction delay in the setting of QRS complex right-axis deviation and raises the possibility of an atrial septal defect.

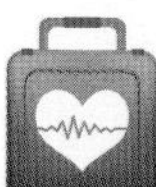

KEY DIAGNOSES

- Normal sinus rhythm
- Right-axis QRS complex deviation
- Ostium secundum atrial septal defect

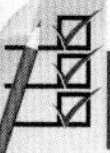

KEY TEACHING POINTS

- The right ventricular conduction delay as seen in lead V1 is characteristic of an atrial septal defect.
- Unlike an ostium primum atrial septal defect where the QRS complex frontal plane axis is deviated leftward, in the setting of an ostium secundum atrial septal defect the QRS complex vector is normal or deviated rightward.
- In this circumstance, the rightward deviation of the QRS complex vector is secondary to the volume overload of the right ventricle given the left to right interatrial shunt.

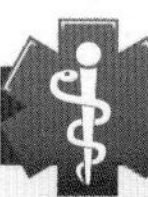

BOARD EXAMINATION ESSENTIALS

Board exam diagnostic codes for this electrocardiogram include normal sinus rhythm; right-axis deviation (greater than +100 degrees); plus intraventricular conduction disturbance, nonspecific type. Familiarize yourself with the characteristic QRS complex delay in lead V1. In conjunction with a consistent clinical history, this QRS complex pattern possesses a reasonable specificity for an atrial septal defect. Once an atrial septal defect is diagnosed, pay special attention to the QRS complex axis to assist in differentiating between a primum and a secundum type. Interestingly, atrial abnormality/enlargement is not identified.

Electrocardiogram Case Study #123

CLINICAL HISTORY

A 63-year-old male with a nonischemic dilated cardiomyopathy status post cardiac transplantation.

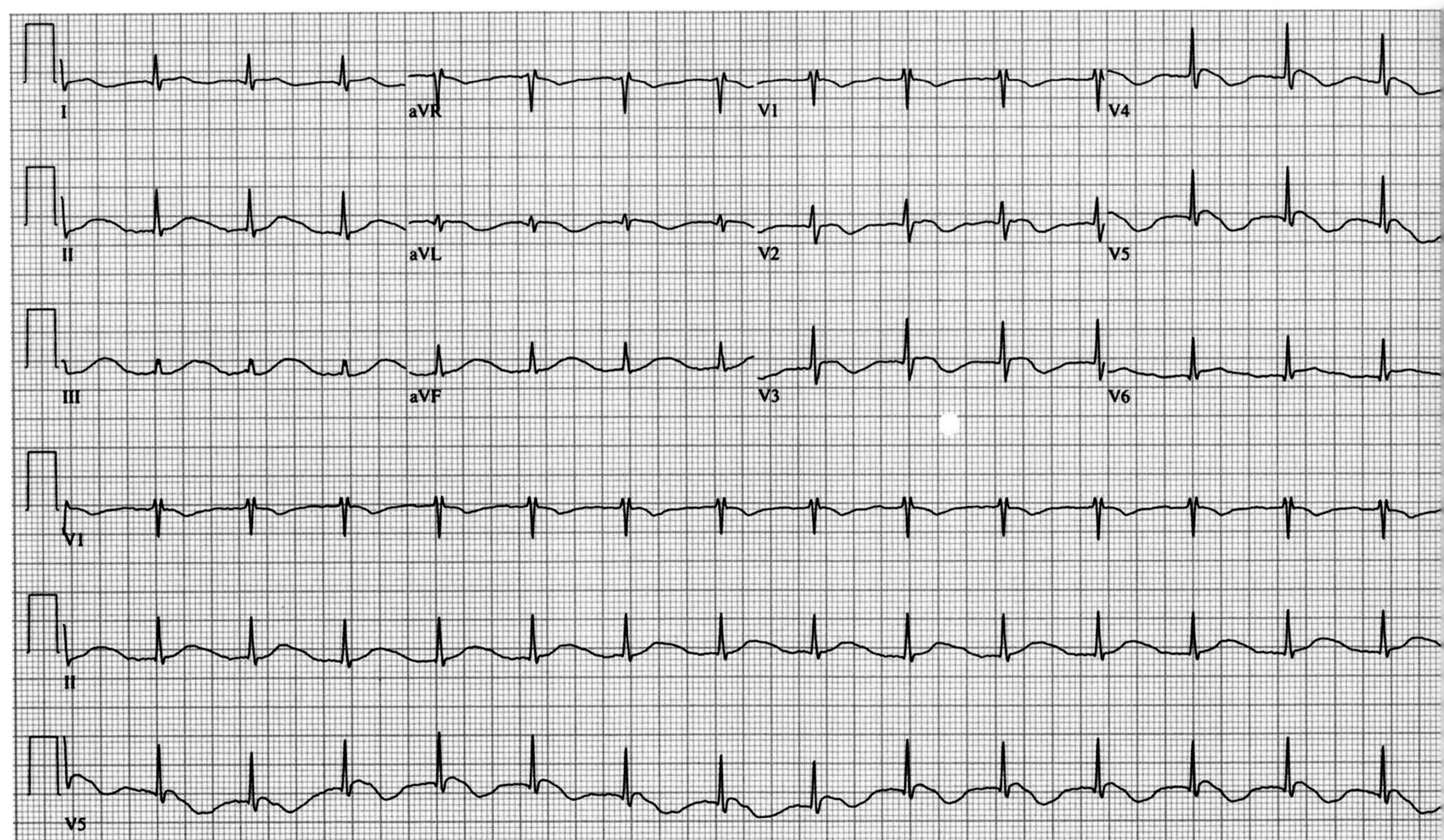

Interpretation Notes:

Electrocardiogram Case Study #123

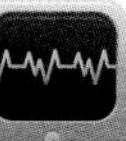

ELECTROCARDIOGRAM INTERPRETATION

This electrocardiogram does not demonstrate obvious atrial activity. The QRS complexes demonstrate a regular R:R interval and are narrow complex in morphology. This collectively suggests an accelerated junctional rhythm. An rSr′ QRS complex morphology is noted in lead V1 but does not satisfy the criteria for incomplete right bundle-branch block as the r′ is <30 milliseconds in duration. Diffuse nonspecific ST-T changes are also noted in the setting of a prolonged QT interval. Widespread ST-segment elevation is also seen most consistent with this patient's recent postoperative state representing postoperative pericarditis.

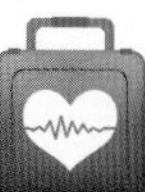

KEY DIAGNOSES

- Accelerated junctional rhythm
- Nonspecific ST-T changes
- Prolonged QT interval
- Pericarditis

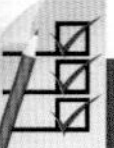

KEY TEACHING POINTS

- It is unclear from this electrocardiogram why the QT interval is so prolonged.
- In the setting of recent heart surgery, electrolyte disturbances, antiarrhythmic medication, or the residual effect of anesthesia and/or cardioplegia are the most likely responsible factors.

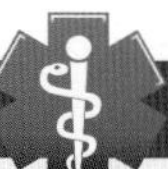

BOARD EXAMINATION ESSENTIALS

Board exam diagnostic codes include AV junctional rhythm, nonspecific ST- and/or T-wave abnormalities, a prolonged QT interval, and acute pericarditis. There is no clear evidence of electrical alternans to suggest a pericardial effusion. Do not code right bundle-branch block incomplete as the r′ is <30 milliseconds in duration.

Electrocardiogram Case Study #124

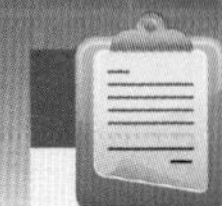

CLINICAL HISTORY

A 77-year-old male with moderate left ventricular systolic dysfunction status post two coronary artery bypass grafting procedures.

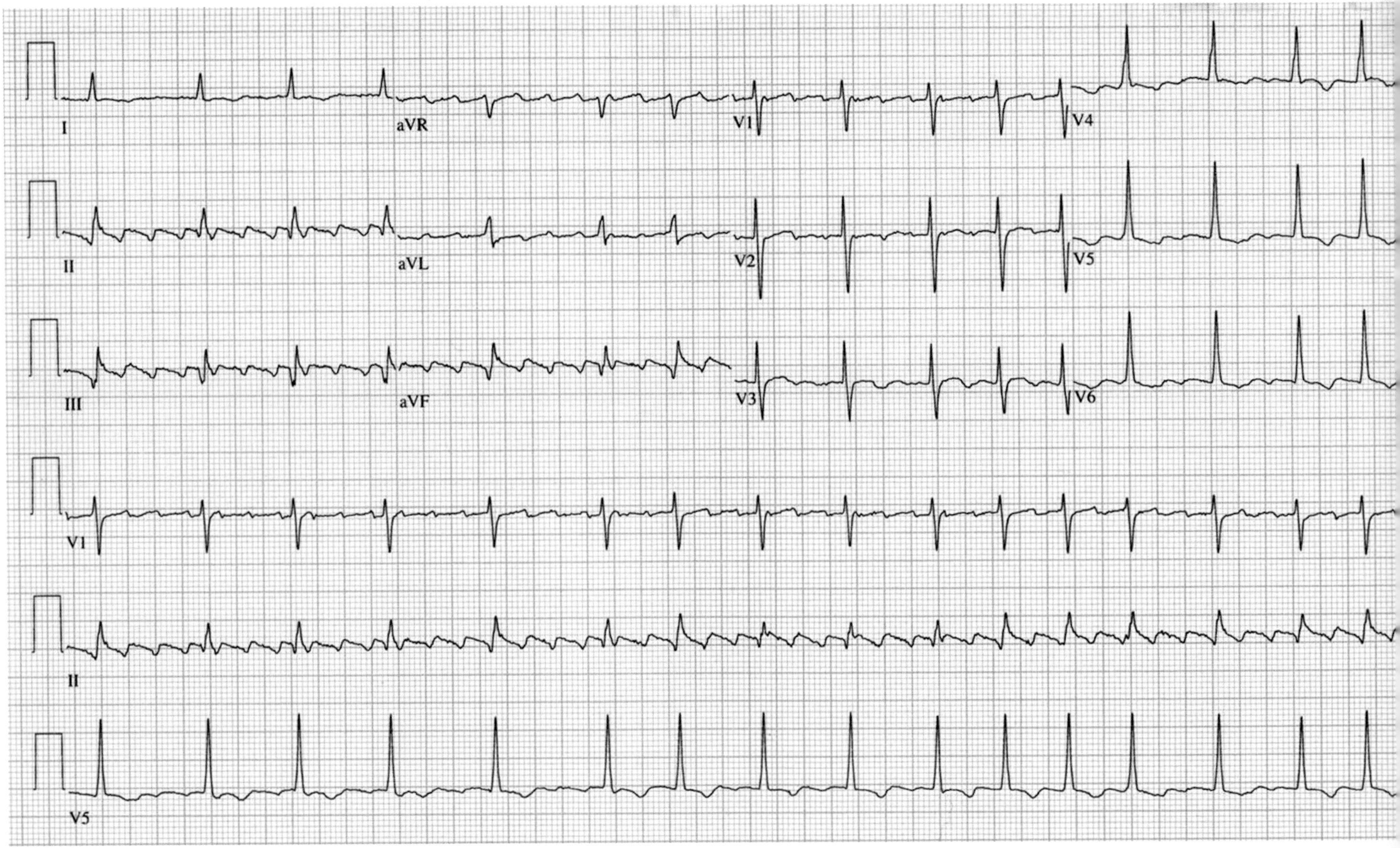

I aVR V1 V4
II aVL V2 V5
III aVF V3 V6
V1
II
V5

Interpretation Notes:

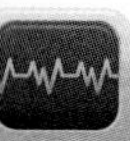

ELECTROCARDIOGRAM INTERPRETATION

Atrial flutter is readily identifiable in leads II, III, aVF, and V1. The ventricular response demonstrates variable atrioventricular conduction ranging from a 2:1 to 4:1 conduction ratio. Q waves are present in leads II, III, and aVF consistent with an inferior myocardial infarction, age indeterminate. Nonspecific anterolateral ST-T changes are demonstrated and are likely related to underlying ischemic heart disease.

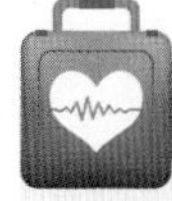

KEY DIAGNOSES

- Atrial flutter
- Inferior myocardial infarction, age indeterminate
- Variable atrioventricular conduction

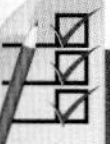

KEY TEACHING POINTS

- Atrial arrhythmias are frequently identified in patients with ischemic heart disease and particularly in those patients who have suffered a myocardial infarction.
- In the setting of reduced left ventricular systolic function, atrial arrhythmias are a common inciting factor for congestive heart failure development

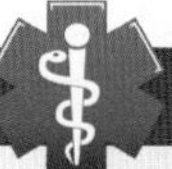

BOARD EXAMINATION ESSENTIALS

For the board exam, applicable diagnostic codes include atrial flutter and an inferior myocardial infarction, age indeterminate. An additional diagnostic code to consider is nonspecific ST- and/or T-wave abnormalities as reflected in the lateral leads. Since the AV conduction is variable, there is no diagnostic code available. It is important to distinguish between an atrial flutter wave with a negative vector and a Q wave. In this case, the flutter wave to QRS complex coupling interval varies plus the Q wave persists, independent of the coupling interval. This supports a myocardial infarction, in this case age indeterminate.

Electrocardiogram Case Study #125

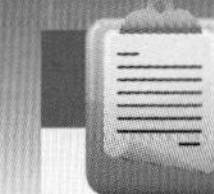

CLINICAL HISTORY

A 24-year-old male professional basketball player who is being evaluated for a preseason physical examination.

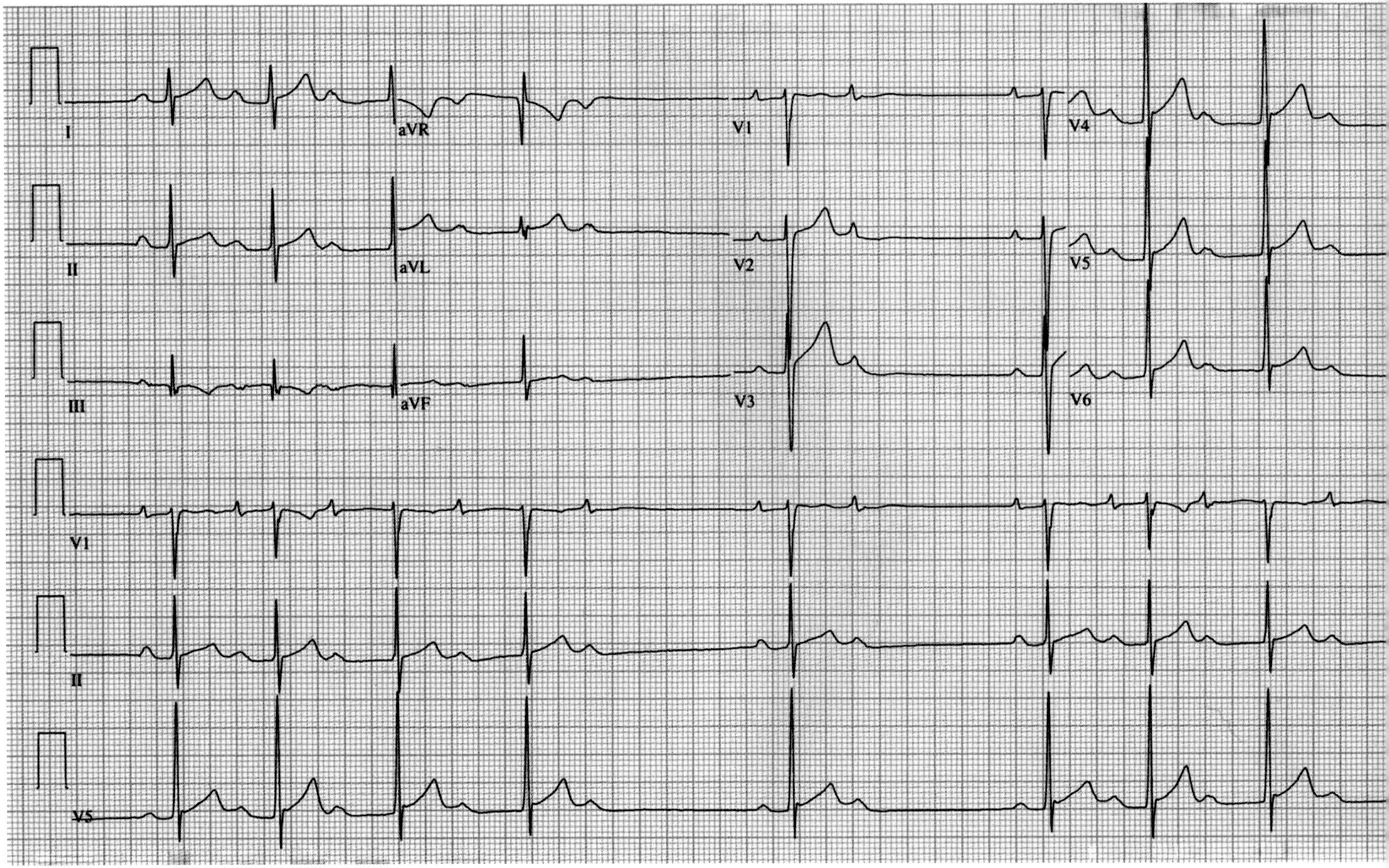

Interpretation Notes:

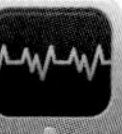

ELECTROCARDIOGRAM INTERPRETATION

Normal sinus rhythm with a normal P-wave axis and sinus arrhythmia is present. There is progressive prolongation of the PR interval with a nonconducted QRS complex following the fifth P wave reflecting second-degree Mobitz type I Wenckebach atrioventricular block. J-point elevation is present best seen in the lateral precordial leads with a normal contour to the ST segment supporting early repolarization.

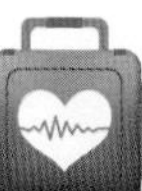

KEY DIAGNOSES

- Normal sinus rhythm
- Sinus arrhythmia
- Second-degree Mobitz type I Wenckebach atrioventricular block
- Early repolarization

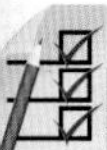

KEY TEACHING POINTS

- The presence of second-degree Mobitz type I Wenckebach atrioventricular block in a highly trained athlete reflects this patient's extreme physical conditioning and heightened vagal tone.
- This tracing is likely normal for this degree of physical conditioning and necessarily does not represent pathologic conduction system disease.

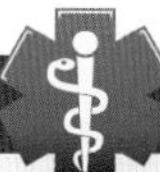

BOARD EXAMINATION ESSENTIALS

In this case, it is important to assess the P to P interval to detect sinus arrhythmia and to differentiate it from AV block second-degree Mobitz type I Wenckebach. Coding a normal electrocardiogram in this circumstance is not recommended. Instead, clinical correlation is required. Appropriate diagnostic board exam codes include normal sinus rhythm, sinus arrhythmia, AV block second-degree Mobitz type I Wenckebach, and early repolarization. While a patient with this clinical history is an unlikely board exam scenario, in the presence of atrioventricular conduction abnormalities sinus arrhythmia can also be present and emphasizes the importance of a careful assessment of the P to P interval across the entirety of the electrocardiogram.

Electrocardiogram Case Study #126

CLINICAL HISTORY

A 70-year-old male with coronary artery disease and moderately severe left ventricular systolic dysfunction who is status post coronary artery bypass graft surgery.

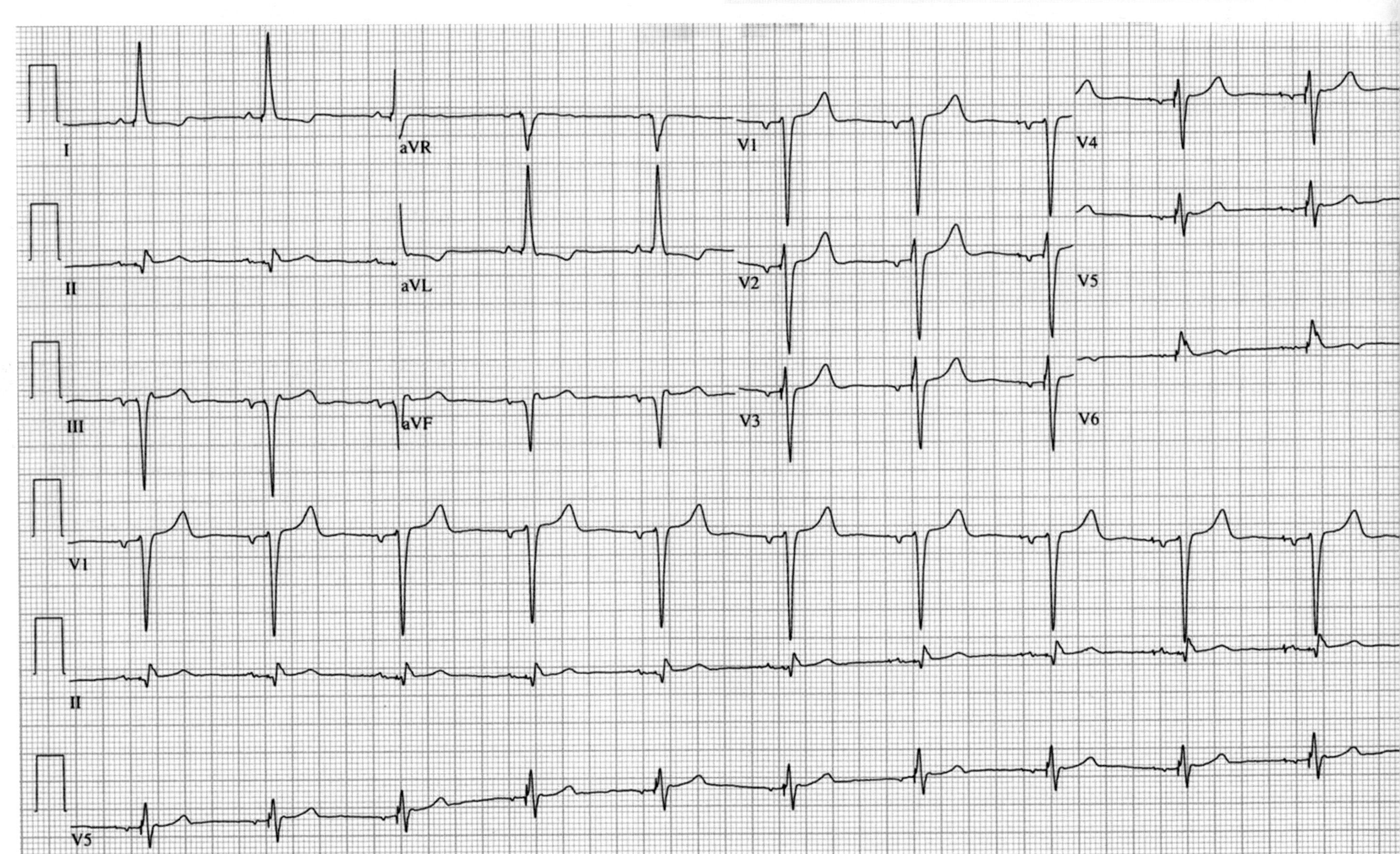

Interpretation Notes:

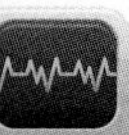

ELECTROCARDIOGRAM INTERPRETATION

This electrocardiogram demonstrates an atrioventricular pacemaker. Lead V4 best demonstrates a small sharp deflection prior to the P wave reflective of atrial pacing. A subsequent ventricular pacemaker spike is noted after a preset atrioventricular delay of approximately 170 milliseconds.

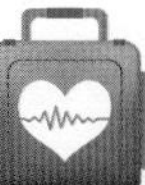

KEY DIAGNOSES

- Atrioventricular pacemaker

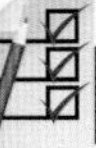

KEY TEACHING POINTS

- This tracing also suggests an inferior myocardial infarction, age indeterminate. It is best not to interpret the QRS complex morphology and specifically myocardial infarction patterns in the setting of ventricular pacing.
- Instead, transiently turning off the pacemaker or setting the pacemaker backup rate lower than the intrinsic heart rate will permit the native QRS complex to become manifest permitting a more confident interpretation.

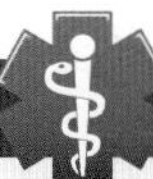

BOARD EXAMINATION ESSENTIALS

Pacemaker deflections can be subtle. For the board exam, should either an atrial or a ventricular pacemaker deflection be identified, make certain to assess each lead for evidence of AV sequential dual chamber pacing. In the presence of ventricular pacing, do not code for QRS complex morphologic findings including axis deviation. The diagnostic code most appropriate for this electrocardiogram includes dual chamber pacemaker, normally functioning. Consideration should be given to a biventricular pacemaker given the somewhat narrow QRS complex. That was not the case in this circumstance as these leads were temporary epicardial leads placed at the time of open heart surgery with the ventricular lead overlying the left ventricle.

Electrocardiogram Case Study #127

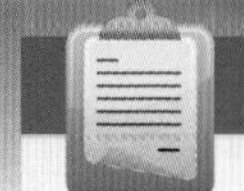

CLINICAL HISTORY

A 75-year-old male status post a remote myocardial infarction and percutaneous coronary intervention who is now experiencing recurrent angina pectoris.

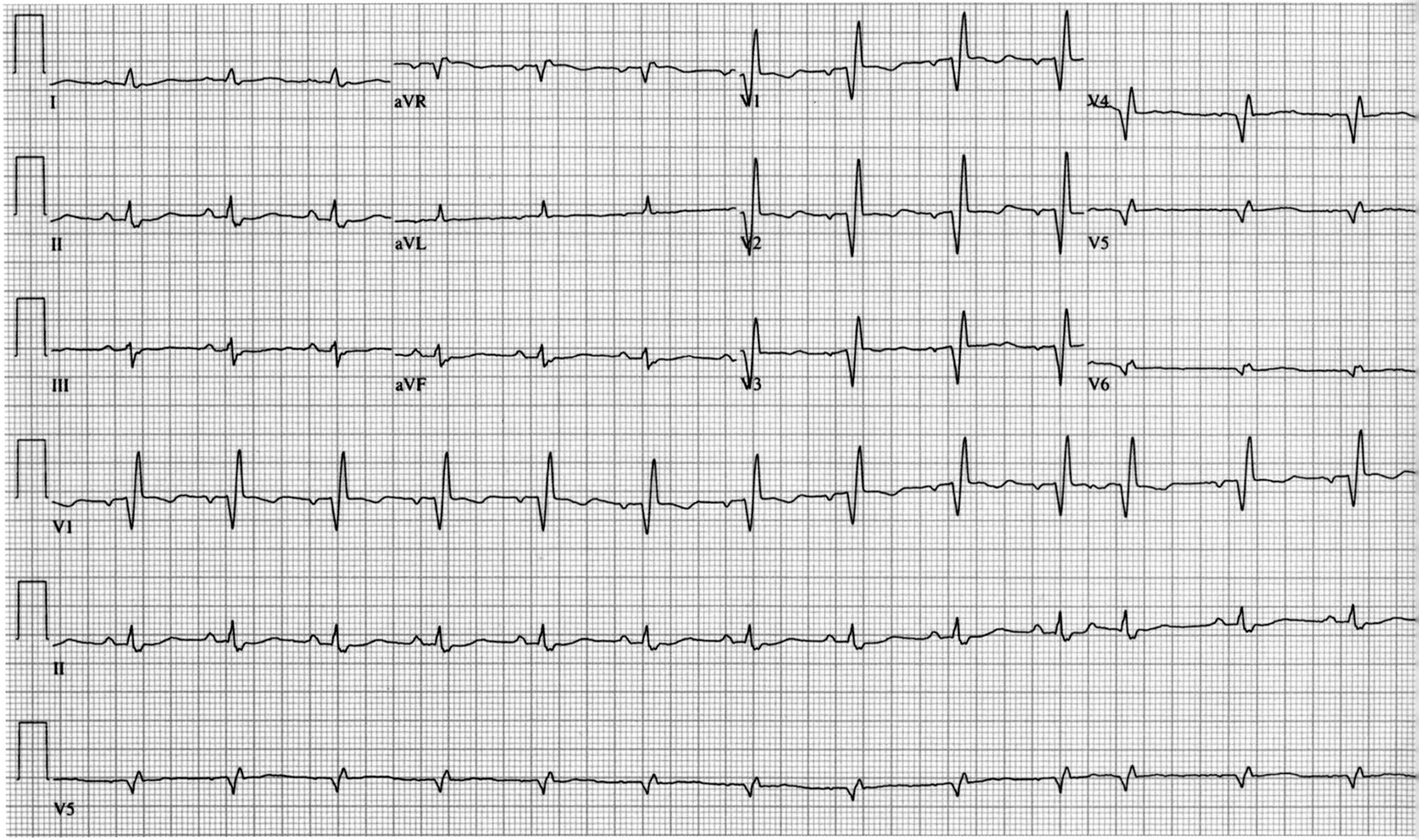

I aVR V1 V4
II aVL V2 V5
III aVF V3 V6
V1
II
V5

Interpretation Notes:

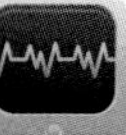

ELECTROCARDIOGRAM INTERPRETATION

Normal sinus rhythm and a normal QRS complex frontal plane axis are present. QRS complex widening >120 milliseconds with QRS complex terminal S-wave prolongation is present in lead I consistent with complete right bundle-branch block. A QR QRS complex pattern is noted in leads V1 to V6 without associated ST-segment elevation denoting an anterolateral myocardial infarction, age indeterminate. This is readily diagnosed in the setting of complete right bundle-branch block as the conduction abnormality resides in the right ventricle not impacting left ventricular depolarization or morphology. The 11th P wave is premature and of different morphology. It also conducts with a relatively prolonged PR interval. This represents a premature atrial complex. If the premature P wave demonstrated greater prematurity, it would result in a nonconducted QRS complex. Low-voltage QRS complexes are present in the limb leads.

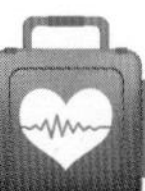

KEY DIAGNOSES

- Normal sinus rhythm
- Premature atrial complex
- Complete right bundle-branch block
- Anterolateral myocardial infarction, age indeterminate
- Low-voltage QRS

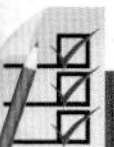

KEY TEACHING POINTS

- In the setting of a right ventricular conduction delay, it is important not to overlook other findings such as an age-indeterminate myocardial infarction.
- For this electrocardiogram, the myocardial infarction extends over the entire precordium, is electrocardiographically extensive, and reflects advanced resting left ventricular systolic dysfunction.

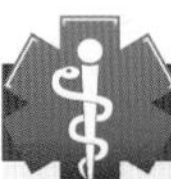

BOARD EXAMINATION ESSENTIALS

This electrocardiogram highlights the ability to assess left ventricular electrical events in the presence of a right ventricular conduction delay. This example will likely appear on the board exam. Diagnostic codes include normal sinus rhythm; atrial premature complex; right bundle-branch block, complete; anterolateral myocardial infarction, age indeterminate; and low-voltage, limb leads. While complete left bundle-branch block obscures age-indeterminate myocardial patterns, complete right bundle-branch block can actually enhance myocardial infarction localization as left ventricular depolarization events are initially solely reflected within the proximal QRS complex.

Electrocardiogram Case Study #128

CLINICAL HISTORY

A 63-year-old male with an approximate 25-year history of hypertension who presents to his primary care physician for routine follow-up.

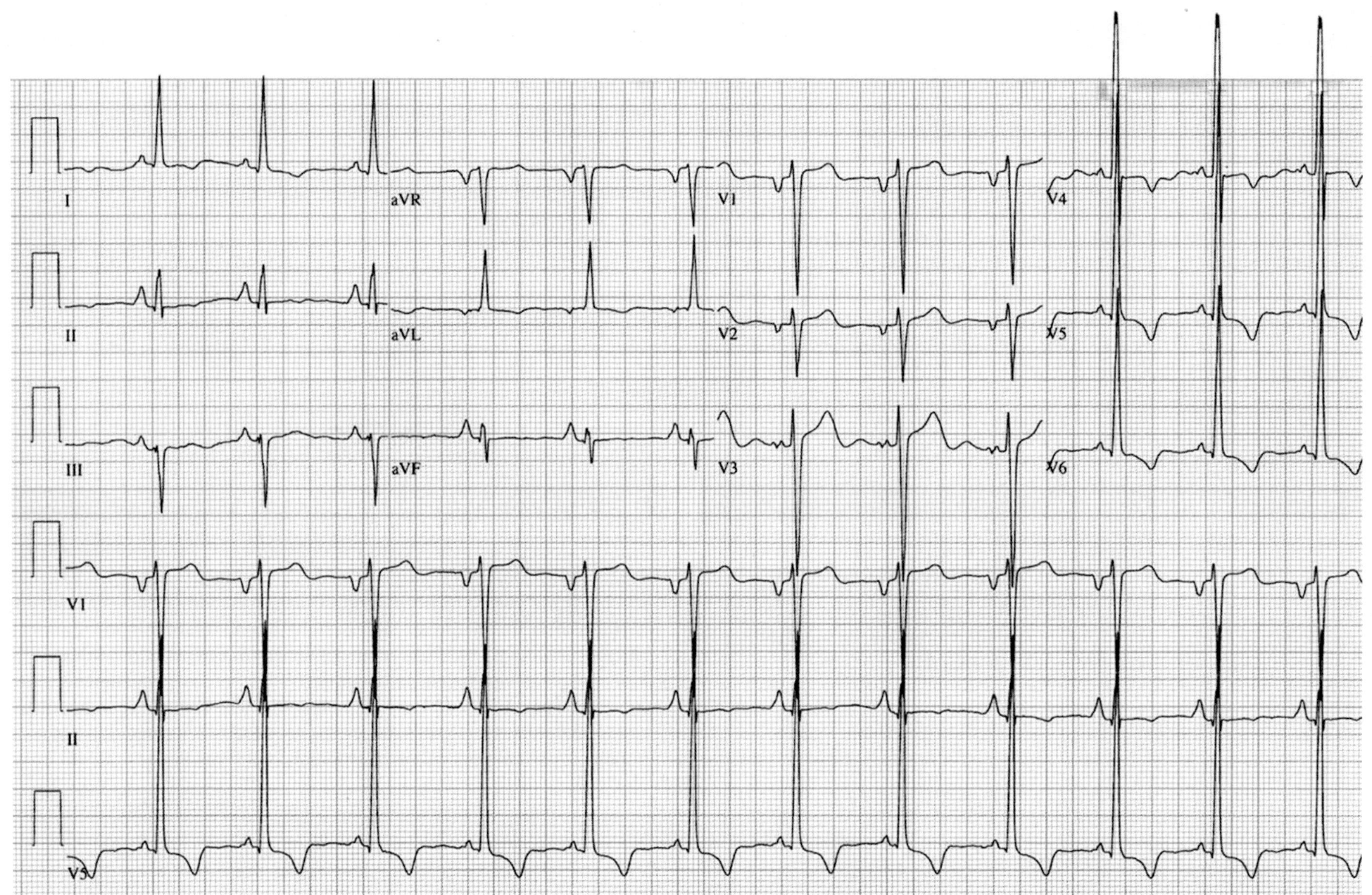

Interpretation Notes:

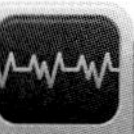

ELECTROCARDIOGRAM INTERPRETATION

Normal sinus rhythm is present as each QRS complex is preceded by a P wave of normal axis. The P-wave morphology is abnormal with a terminal negativity in lead V1 consistent with left atrial abnormality. In lead II, the P-wave amplitude is >0.3 mV consistent with right atrial abnormality. Prominent precordial QRS complex voltage is present with asymmetric ST-T changes indicative of left ventricular hypertrophy with secondary ST-T changes. Negative U waves are seen in the lateral precordial leads supporting the presence of left ventricular hypertrophy.

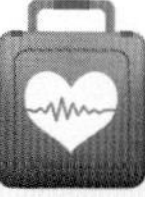

KEY DIAGNOSES

- Normal sinus rhythm
- Left atrial abnormality
- Right atrial abnormality
- Left ventricular hypertrophy with secondary ST-T changes
- Negative U waves

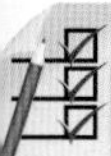

KEY TEACHING POINTS

- This electrocardiogram satisfies many criteria for left ventricular hypertrophy. In addition to the prominent QRS complex voltage and asymmetric T-wave inversion indicative of a strain pattern, a slightly prolonged QRS complex and prominent left atrial abnormality are also present.
- Negative U waves are readily seen. The differential diagnosis of negative U waves includes coronary artery disease and left ventricular hypertrophy.
- With the associated electrocardiogram findings, the negative U waves are most likely secondary to left ventricular hypertrophy.

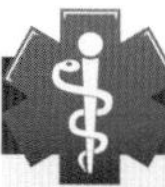

BOARD EXAMINATION ESSENTIALS

This is another electrocardiogram likely to be included on the board exam. Diagnostic codes include normal sinus rhythm, left atrial abnormality/enlargement, right atrial abnormality/enlargement, left ventricular hypertrophy, and ST- and/or T-wave abnormalities secondary to hypertrophy. This electrocardiogram is performed at full or normal standardization (10 mm/mV). For the board exam, an example of one half standardization (5 mm/mV) may be included and if so, it would still be appropriate to code for left ventricular hypertrophy if voltage criteria are satisfied. Make sure not to overlook the standardization setting for each board exam electrocardiogram example.

Electrocardiogram Case Study #129

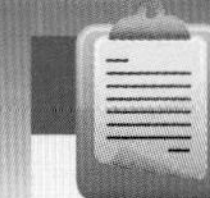

CLINICAL HISTORY

A 55-year-old male who presents for cardiology clinic follow-up in the setting of a nonischemic dilated cardiomyopathy.

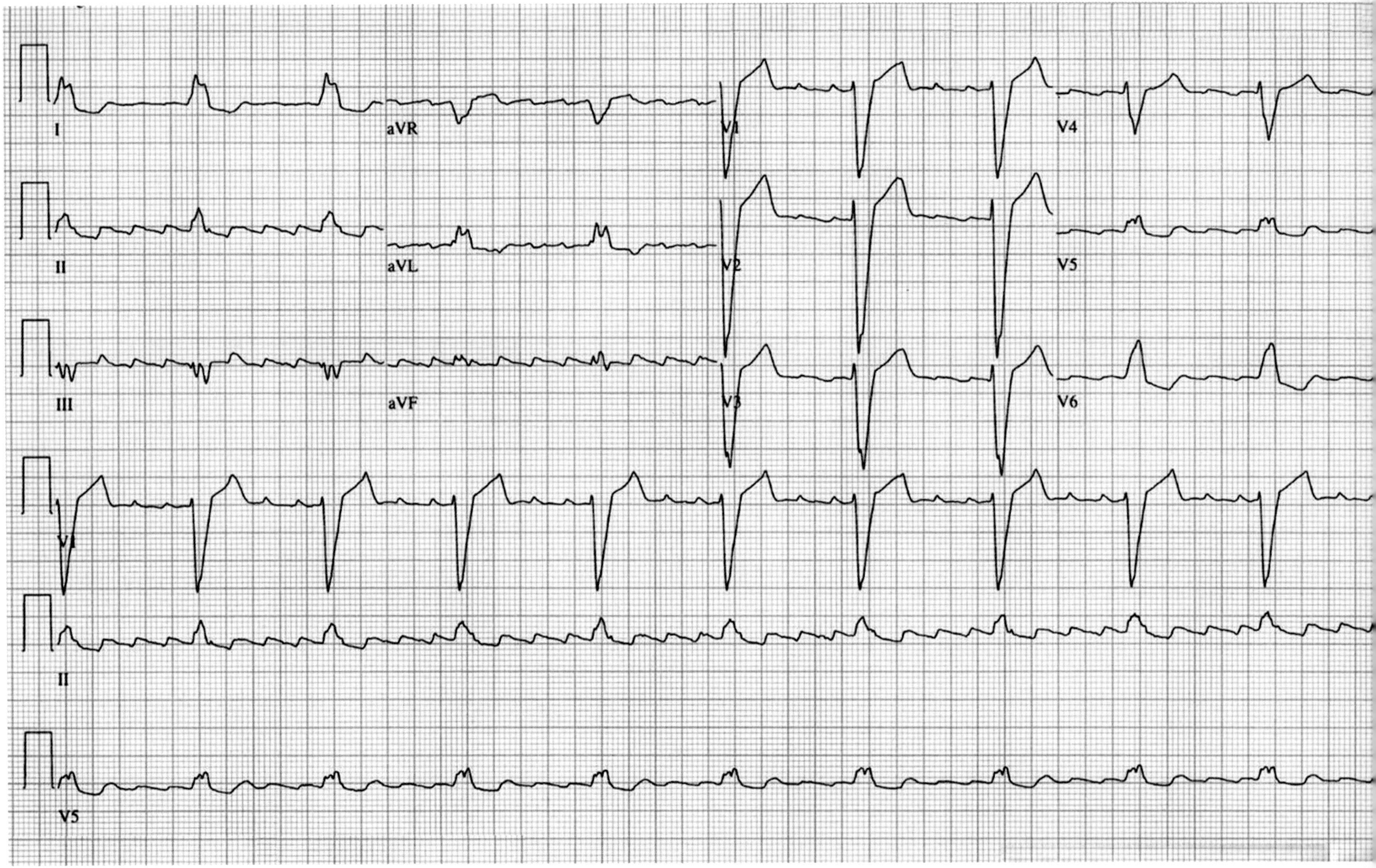

I aVR V1 V4
II aVL V2 V5
III aVF V3 V6
V1
II
V5

Interpretation Notes:

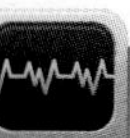

ELECTROCARDIOGRAM INTERPRETATION

Best seen in the inferior leads, a regular "sawtoothed" pattern of atrial activity supports atrial flutter. Four atrial flutter waves are noted for each QRS complex representing 4:1 atrioventricular conduction. The QRS complex is widened with complete left bundle-branch block morphology.

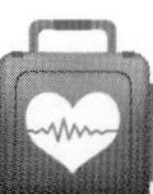

KEY DIAGNOSES

- Atrial flutter
- 4:1 atrioventricular conduction
- Complete left bundle-branch block

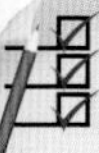

KEY TEACHING POINTS

- The finding of complete left bundle-branch block is abnormal and suggests underlying structural heart disease oftentimes associated with significant left ventricular systolic dysfunction.
- This is further supported by the presence of an atrial dysrhythmia, in this case atrial flutter.

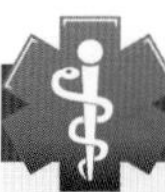

BOARD EXAMINATION ESSENTIALS

Board exam diagnostic codes include atrial flutter and LBBB complete. While AV conduction, 4:1 is present, no board exam diagnostic code exists for this abnormality. Note the constant flutter wave to QRS complex coupling interval supporting AV association and 4:1 AV conduction. If this coupling interval varied, complete heart block would merit consideration. Additionally, note the absence of septal Q waves therefore satisfying the criteria for complete left bundle-branch block.

Electrocardiogram Case Study #130

CLINICAL HISTORY

An 81-year-old male with a history of tachycardia/bradycardia syndrome requiring permanent pacemaker implantation.

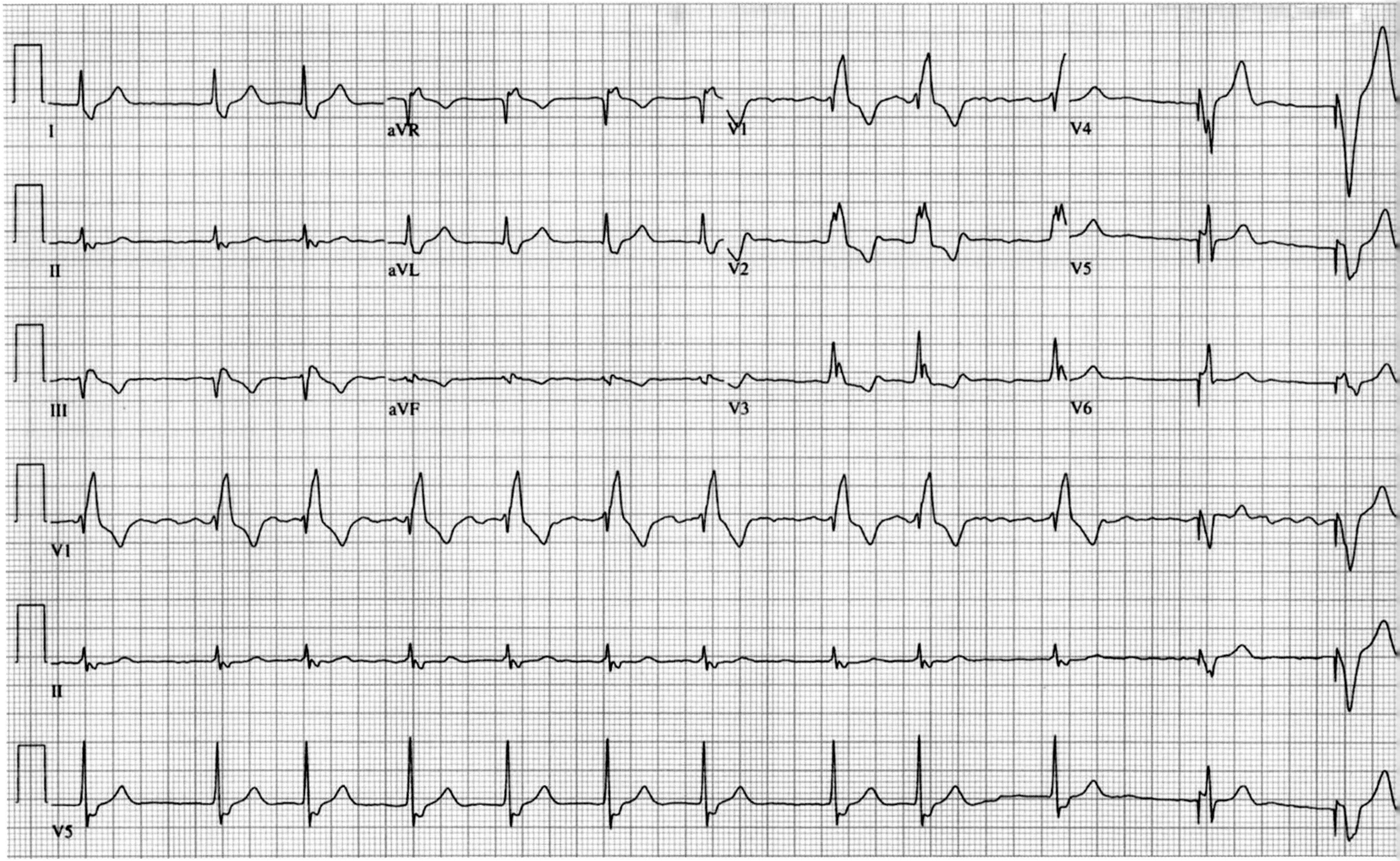

I aVR V1 V4

II aVL V2 V5

III aVF V3 V6

V1

II

V5

Interpretation Notes:____

____

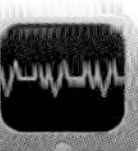

ELECTROCARDIOGRAM INTERPRETATION

The cardiac rhythm is irregularly irregular without identifiable atrial activity. This is consistent with atrial fibrillation. The QRS complex is >120 milliseconds in duration with terminal S-wave QRS complex slowing in lead I and an rsR′ QRS complex pattern in lead V1 suggesting complete right bundle-branch block. The last two QRS complexes on this electrocardiogram represent a ventricular pacemaker. The very last complex is fully paced and the second to last complex is intermediate between the native QRS complex and the ventricular paced complex. This is best classified as a pacemaker fusion complex.

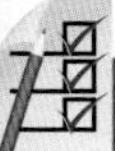

KEY TEACHING POINTS

- A diminutive R wave is seen in leads III and aVF. Following the R wave is a deep S wave with terminal T-wave inversion. Despite the presence of this diminutive R wave, this electrocardiogram suggests at least the possibility of a prior inferior myocardial infarction, age indeterminate.

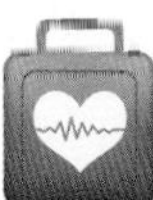

KEY DIAGNOSES

- Atrial fibrillation
- Complete right bundle-branch block
- Ventricular pacemaker

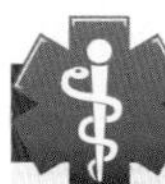

BOARD EXAMINATION ESSENTIALS

For purposes of the board exam, do not code a myocardial infarction unless there is clear evidence of a Q wave of diagnostic duration in two contiguous electrocardiogram leads. In this particular circumstance, those criteria are not met. Diagnostic board exam codes include atrial fibrillation; right bundle-branch block, complete; and ventricular demand pacemaker, normally functioning. Note that the ventricular pacing is intermittent and in the presence of atrial fibrillation, there is no evidence of atrial pacing.

Electrocardiogram Case Study #131

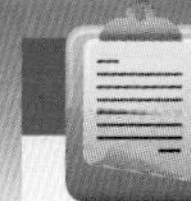

CLINICAL HISTORY

A 77-year-old male with a recurrent history of congestive heart failure who is referred for coronary artery bypass grafting and mitral valve repair secondary to mitral insufficiency.

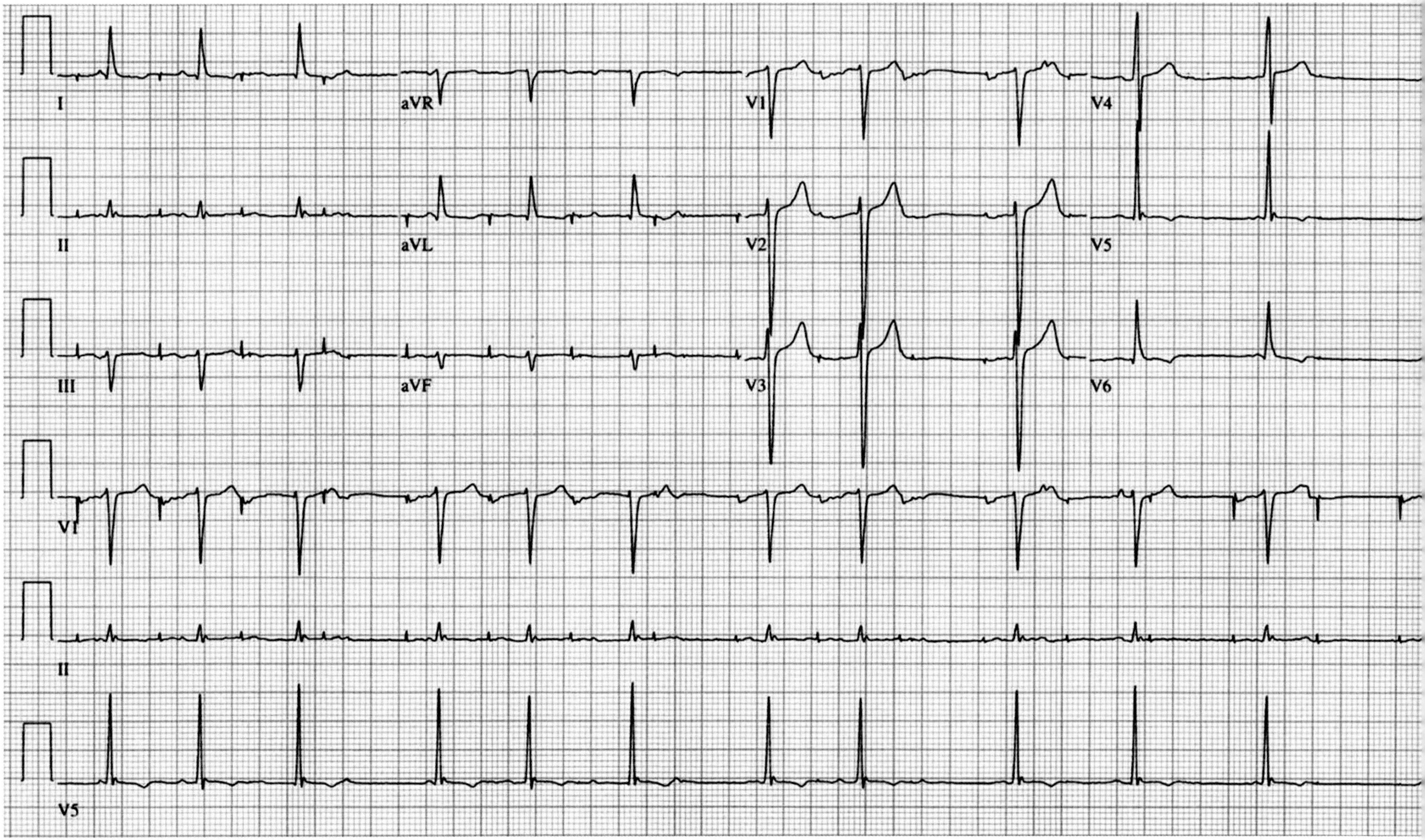

I aVR V1 V4
II aVL V2 V5
III aVF V3 V6
V1
II
V5

Interpretation Notes:

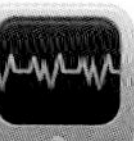

ELECTROCARDIOGRAM INTERPRETATION

A narrow negative deflection is seen preceding each P wave indicating atrial paced complexes. Grouped QRS complexes are present with progressive prolongation of the pacing to QRS complex interval. This supports second-degree Mobitz type I Wenckebach atrioventricular block. The atrial pacing spike to QRS complex conduction ratio spans 3:2, 2:1, and 4:3. Nonspecific ST-T changes are present. Also noted is subtle ST-segment elevation throughout the electrocardiogram with associated elevation of the atrial repolarization segment in lead aVR. These findings support pericarditis in this recently postoperative cardiac surgical patient.

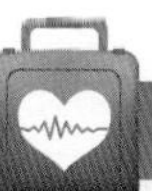

KEY DIAGNOSES

- Atrial pacemaker
- Second-degree Mobitz type I Wenckebach atrioventricular block
- Nonspecific ST-T changes
- Pericarditis

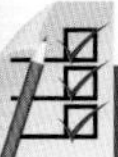

KEY TEACHING POINTS

- This electrocardiogram is an example of second-degree Mobitz type I Wenckebach atrioventricular block. Grouped QRS complexes should raise consideration for second-degree Mobitz type I Wenckebach atrioventricular block and nonconducted premature atrial complexes.
- Atrioventricular conduction abnormalities are not confined to normal cardiac rhythms and can be found in the setting of atrial dysrhythmias and also in the presence of an atrial pacemaker.

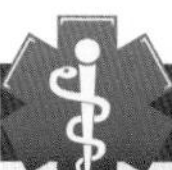

BOARD EXAMINATION ESSENTIALS

This electrocardiogram example highlights the importance of assessing AV conduction in the presence of an atrial pacemaker. Board exam diagnostic codes include atrial or coronary sinus pacing, AV block, second-degree Mobitz type I (Wenckebach), and nonspecific ST- and/or T-wave abnormalities. While pericarditis was thought to be present clinically, anticipate a more obvious example for the board exam. Do not code atrial abnormality/enlargement in the presence of an atrial pacemaker.

Electrocardiogram Case Study #132

CLINICAL HISTORY

A 55-year-old male with coronary artery disease and a remote history of coronary artery bypass grafting surgery who is acutely admitted to the hospital in the setting of palpitations and a wide complex tachycardia.

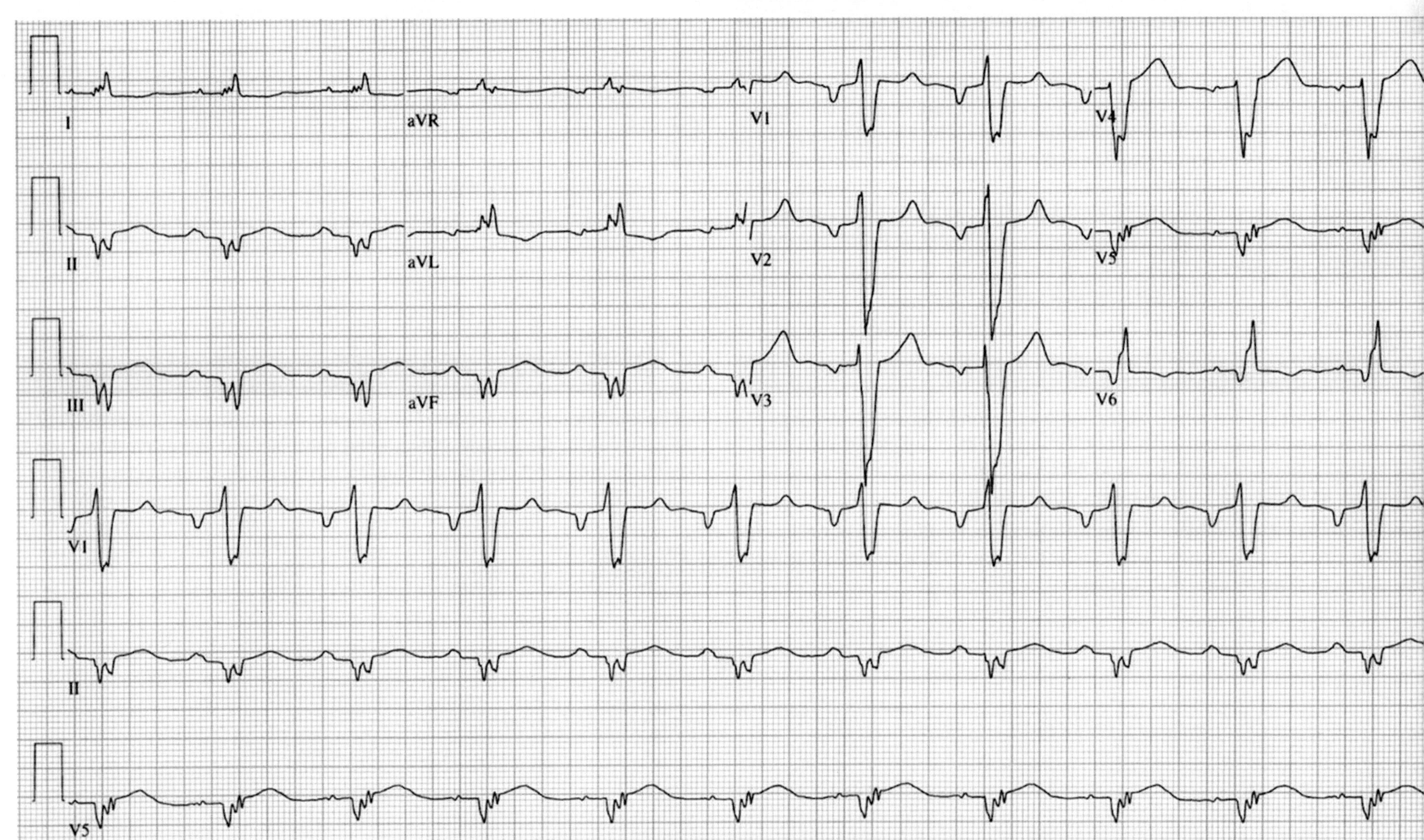

Interpretation Notes:

Electrocardiogram Case Study #132

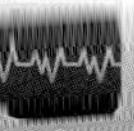

ELECTROCARDIOGRAM INTERPRETATION

The cardiac rhythm is normal sinus rhythm with a normal P-wave axis and an atrial rate of approximate 65 per minute. Left atrial abnormality is present with a deeply negative P wave in lead V1 and a broadened P wave in lead II. The PR interval is prolonged representing first-degree atrioventricular block. Prominent Q waves are seen both inferiorly and laterally. This represents an inferolateral myocardial infarction, age indeterminate. The R wave in leads V1-2 is of normal amplitude and does not reflect a posterior myocardial infarction. The QRS complex is terminally broadened as seen in lead V6. This represents peri-infarction block with delayed conduction through the infarct zone with a positive terminal QRS complex vector directed toward lead V6.

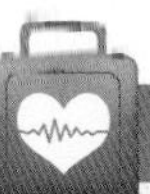

KEY DIAGNOSES

- Normal sinus rhythm
- Left atrial abnormality
- Inferior myocardial infarction, age indeterminate
- Lateral myocardial infarction, age indeterminate
- Nonspecific intraventricular conduction delay
- First-degree atrioventricular block

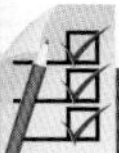

KEY TEACHING POINTS

- The presence of peri-infarction block represents delayed depolarization within the infarct zone and is a form of a nonspecific intraventricular conduction delay.
- The finding of peri-infarction block may result in a greater propensity for ventricular arrhythmias as demonstrated in this patient.

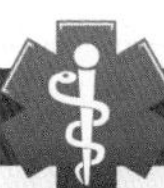

BOARD EXAMINATION ESSENTIALS

This is a board exam relevant electrocardiogram focusing on the difference between myocardial infarction–related intraventricular conduction delay and a LBBB complete. In the presence of LBBB complete, Q waves should not be identifiable in the lateral leads. For this electrocardiogram, diagnostic codes include normal sinus rhythm; left atrial abnormality/enlargement; inferior myocardial infarction, age indeterminate; lateral myocardial infarction, age indeterminate; AV block, first degree; and intraventricular conduction disturbance, nonspecific type. If no Q wave was present in leads V5 to V6, this electrocardiogram should be alternatively coded complete left bundle-branch block.

Electrocardiogram Case Study #133

CLINICAL HISTORY

A 72-year-old female with advanced atrioventricular block necessitating permanent pacemaker placement. The patient is presently taking digitalis on a daily basis.

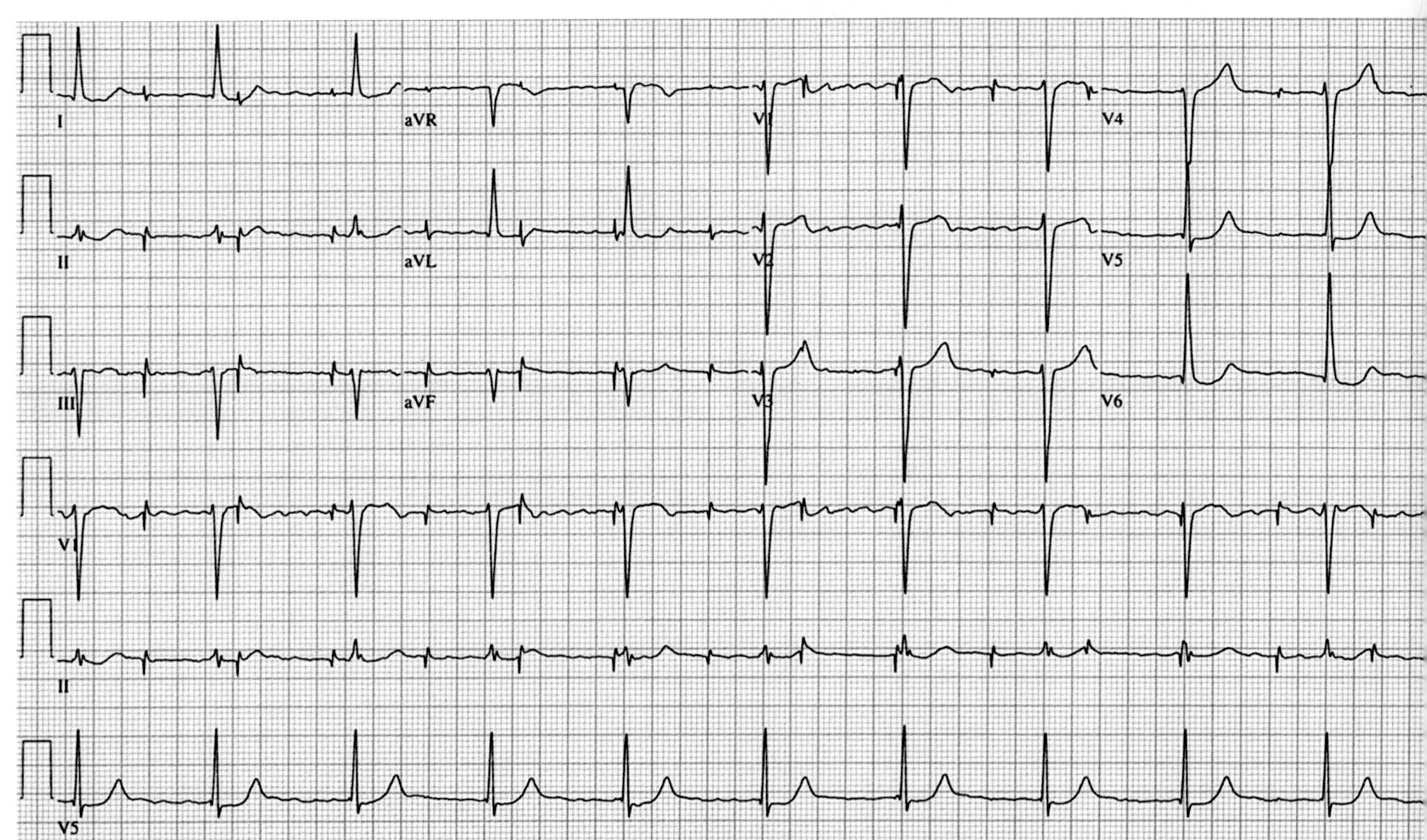

Interpretation Notes:

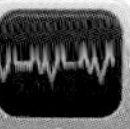

ELECTROCARDIOGRAM INTERPRETATION

The electrocardiogram baseline is devoid of discrete atrial activity. This represents atrial fibrillation. The QRS complexes occur at regular R:R intervals at a ventricular rate slightly >60 per minute. This is an unexpected finding in the presence of atrial fibrillation. This represents an accelerated junctional rhythm and atrioventricular dissociation. Ventricular pacemaker deflections occur at regular intervals throughout the electrocardiogram with no clear relationship to the QRS complexes. This represents pacemaker sensing failure. Lateral and high lateral nonspecific ST-T changes are demonstrated. The scooping of the ST segments supports the presence of digitalis effect.

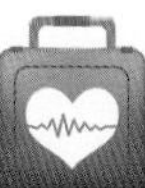

KEY DIAGNOSES

- Atrial fibrillation
- Accelerated junctional rhythm
- Atrioventricular dissociation
- Ventricular pacemaker
- Ventricular pacemaker sensing failure
- Nonspecific ST-T changes
- Digitalis effect

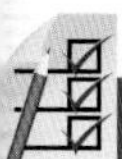

KEY TEACHING POINTS

- This electrocardiogram demonstrates abnormal pacemaker function necessitating further evaluation. This may represent pacemaker lead dislodgment.
- In the presence of atrial fibrillation, it is important to evaluate the electrocardiogram for a second independent cardiac rhythm. The important clue on this electrocardiogram is the constant R:R interval.
- Both atrioventricular dissociation and accelerated junctional rhythm support the possible presence of digitalis toxicity, requiring further clinical investigation.

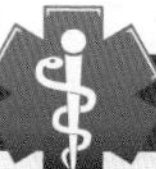

BOARD EXAMINATION ESSENTIALS

Diagnostic codes for the board exam include atrial fibrillation, AV junctional rhythm, A-V dissociation, pacemaker malfunction, not constantly sensing (atrium or ventricle), and nonspecific ST- and/or T-wave abnormalities. A code for digitalis effect is not an option and thus not coded. Complete heart block may be present but in the presence of an accelerated AV junctional rhythm, coding AV dissociation is best unless additional clinical data such as electrophysiology study results are available.

Electrocardiogram Case Study #134

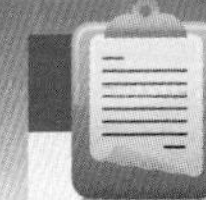

CLINICAL HISTORY

A 61-year-old male status post two prior coronary artery bypass graft operations who presents for an outpatient follow-up evaluation after a recent hospitalization for congestive heart failure.

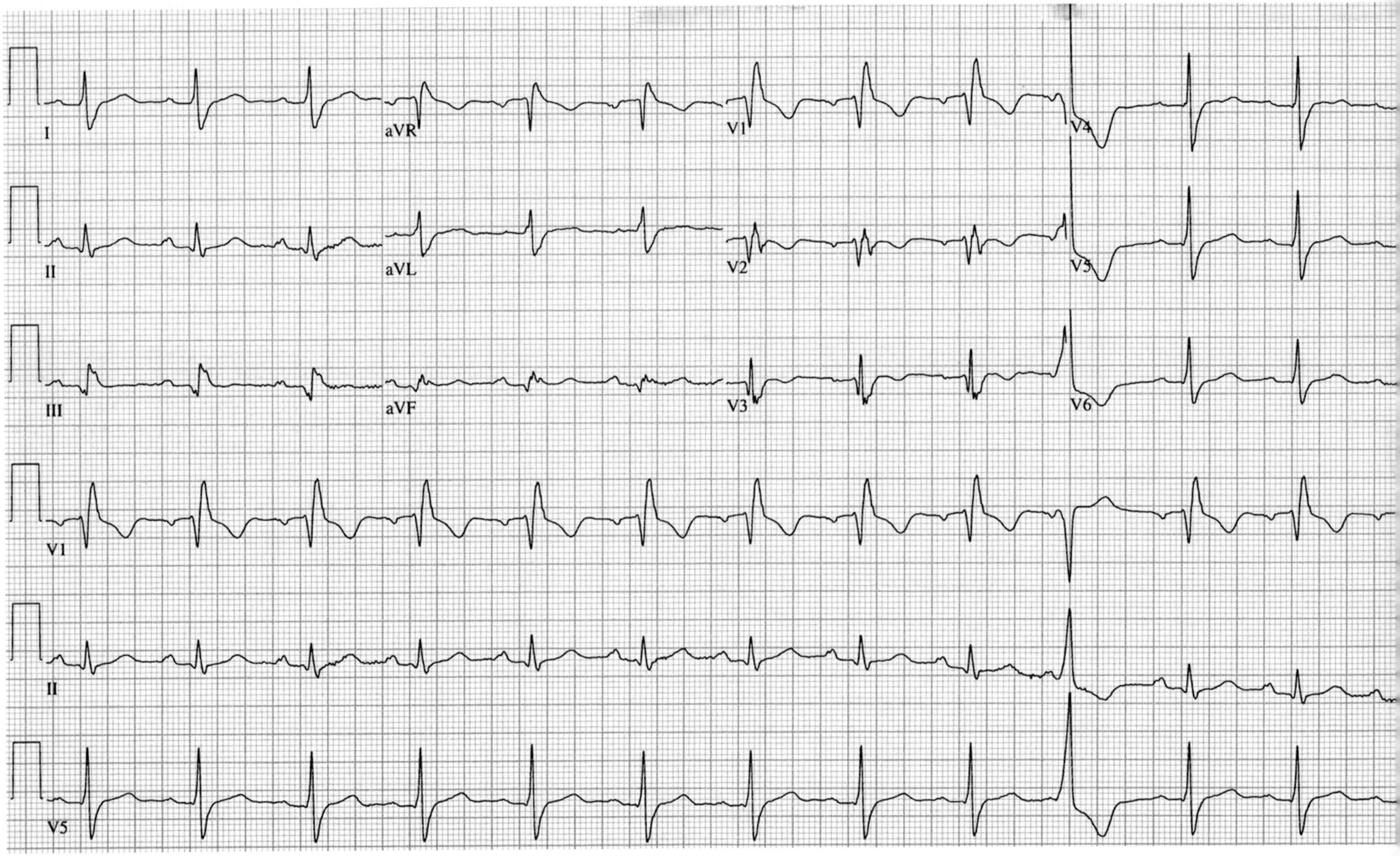

I aVR V1 V4
II aVL V2 V5
III aVF V3 V6
V1
II
V5

Interpretation Notes:

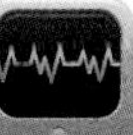

ELECTROCARDIOGRAM INTERPRETATION

This electrocardiogram demonstrates normal sinus rhythm with a prolonged PR interval slightly >200 milliseconds satisfying the criteria for first degree atrioventricular block. The QRS complex is prolonged at 120 milliseconds in the setting of terminal S-wave QRS complex slowing as seen in the high lateral and the lateral precordial leads. An rSR′ QRS complex is present in lead V1. These findings denote complete right bundle-branch block. A 40-millisecond Q wave is seen in leads II, III, and aVF without associated ST-segment elevation. This represents an inferior myocardial infarction, age indeterminate. A small R wave is present in leads V1 to V2 with R-wave regression and Q-wave formation in lead V3. This supports an anteroseptal myocardial infarction, age indeterminate. The last QRS complex is a premature ventricular complex. A terminally negative P wave is present in lead V1 and a bifid P wave is seen in lead II supporting left atrial abnormality.

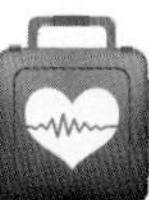

KEY DIAGNOSES

- Normal sinus rhythm
- Premature ventricular complex
- Complete right bundle-branch block
- Inferior myocardial infarction, age indeterminate
- Anteroseptal myocardial infarction, age indeterminate
- First-degree atrioventricular block
- Left atrial abnormality

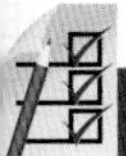

KEY TEACHING POINTS

- This electrocardiogram Q-wave pattern may represent one myocardial infarction best termed an inferoapical myocardial infarction. This is seen in patients who possess a dominant right coronary artery that also supplies the left ventricular cardiac apex.
- The left anterior descending coronary artery in this coronary artery anatomic variant generally stops before the left ventricular cardiac apex. Angiographic correlation would be necessary as this is only suggested by this electrocardiogram.

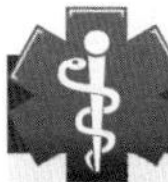

BOARD EXAMINATION ESSENTIALS

Board exam diagnostic codes include normal sinus rhythm; A-V block, first degree; left atrial abnormality/enlargement; inferior myocardial infarction, age indeterminate; anteroseptal myocardial infarction, age indeterminate; and right bundle-branch block, complete. Note the Q wave solely in lead V3. This is a contiguous lead to the inferior leads given this anatomic variant and, therefore, it is still appropriate to code for an anteroseptal myocardial infarction, age indeterminate.

Electrocardiogram Case Study #135

CLINICAL HISTORY

An 18-year-old male recently status post open heart surgery including aortic valve repair for moderately severe aortic insufficiency.

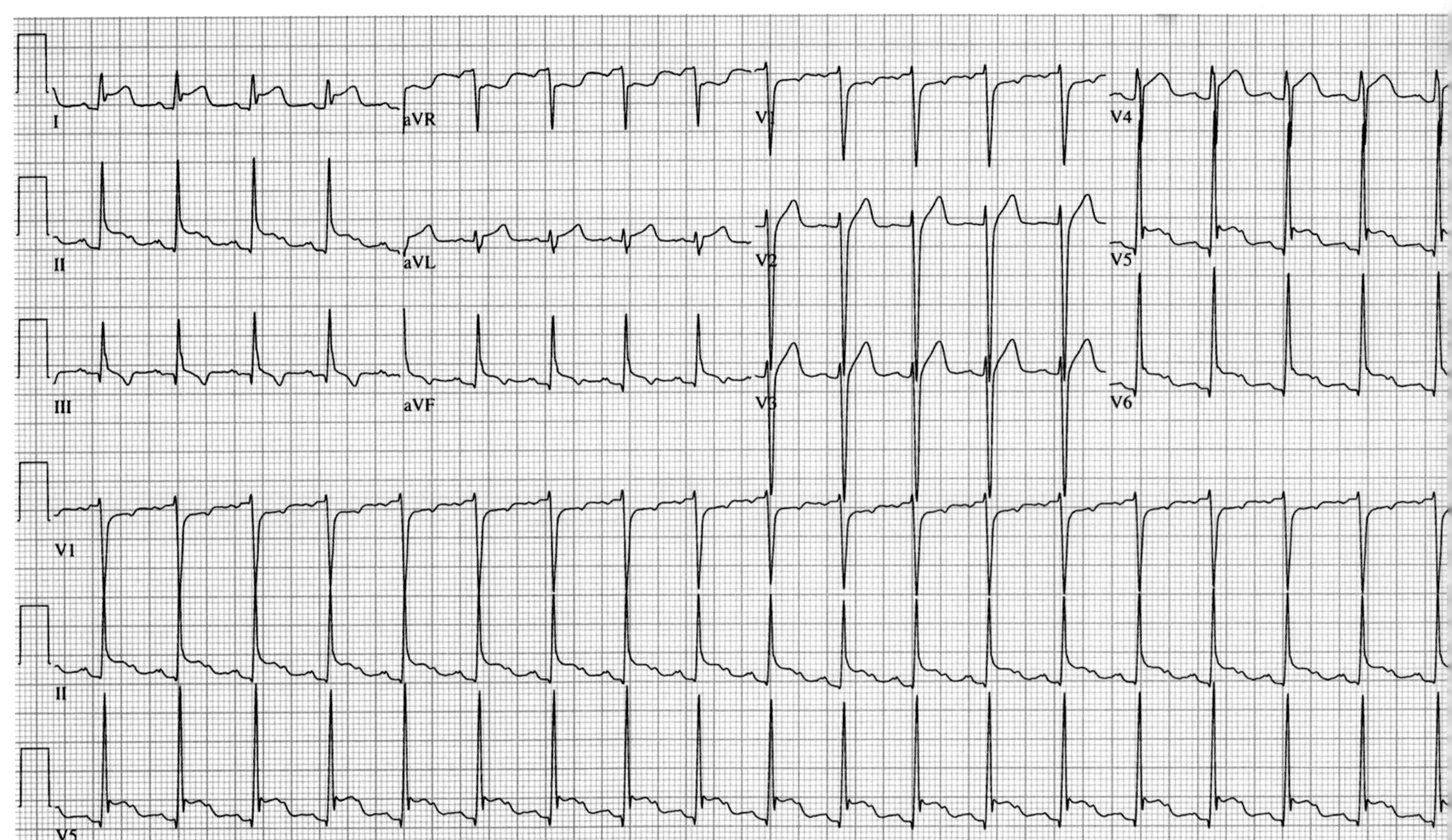

Interpretation Notes:

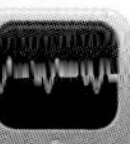

ELECTROCARDIOGRAM INTERPRETATION

This electrocardiogram demonstrates sinus tachycardia as the atrial rate is regular and >100 per minute. Diffuse ST-segment elevation is seen with marked elevation of the atrial repolarization segment in lead aVR. These findings are consistent with postoperative pericarditis. Inferior nonspecific ST-T changes are noted.

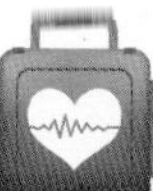

KEY DIAGNOSES

- Sinus tachycardia
- Pericarditis
- Nonspecific ST-T changes

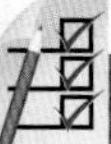

KEY TEACHING POINTS

- These findings should not be confused with acute myocardial injury as this represents a diffuse process not explainable by one coronary artery territory.
- Cardiac surgery is the most common form of pericarditis in an acute care hospital.

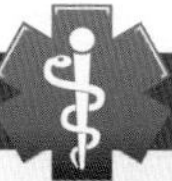

BOARD EXAMINATION ESSENTIALS

This electrocardiogram will likely appear on the board exam. Diagnostic codes include sinus tachycardia and acute pericarditis. ST-T changes are also present and they are secondary to pericarditis. One might consider coding ST- and/or T-wave abnormalities suggesting myocardial injury. Pericarditis reflects epicardial injury and thus, myocardial injury associated ST-T changes are not typically coded. There is no evidence of electrical alternans; thus, it is not coded. Pericardial effusion as a clinical diagnosis is also not coded in the absence of a supporting clinical history or electrocardiogram evidence of electrical alternans.

Electrocardiogram Case Study **#136**

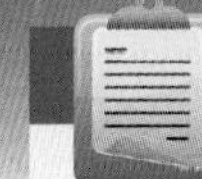

CLINICAL HISTORY

A 20-year-old male with a presumed viral cardiomyopathy and resultant severe left ventricular systolic dysfunction admitted for evaluation of recurrent palpitations and syncope.

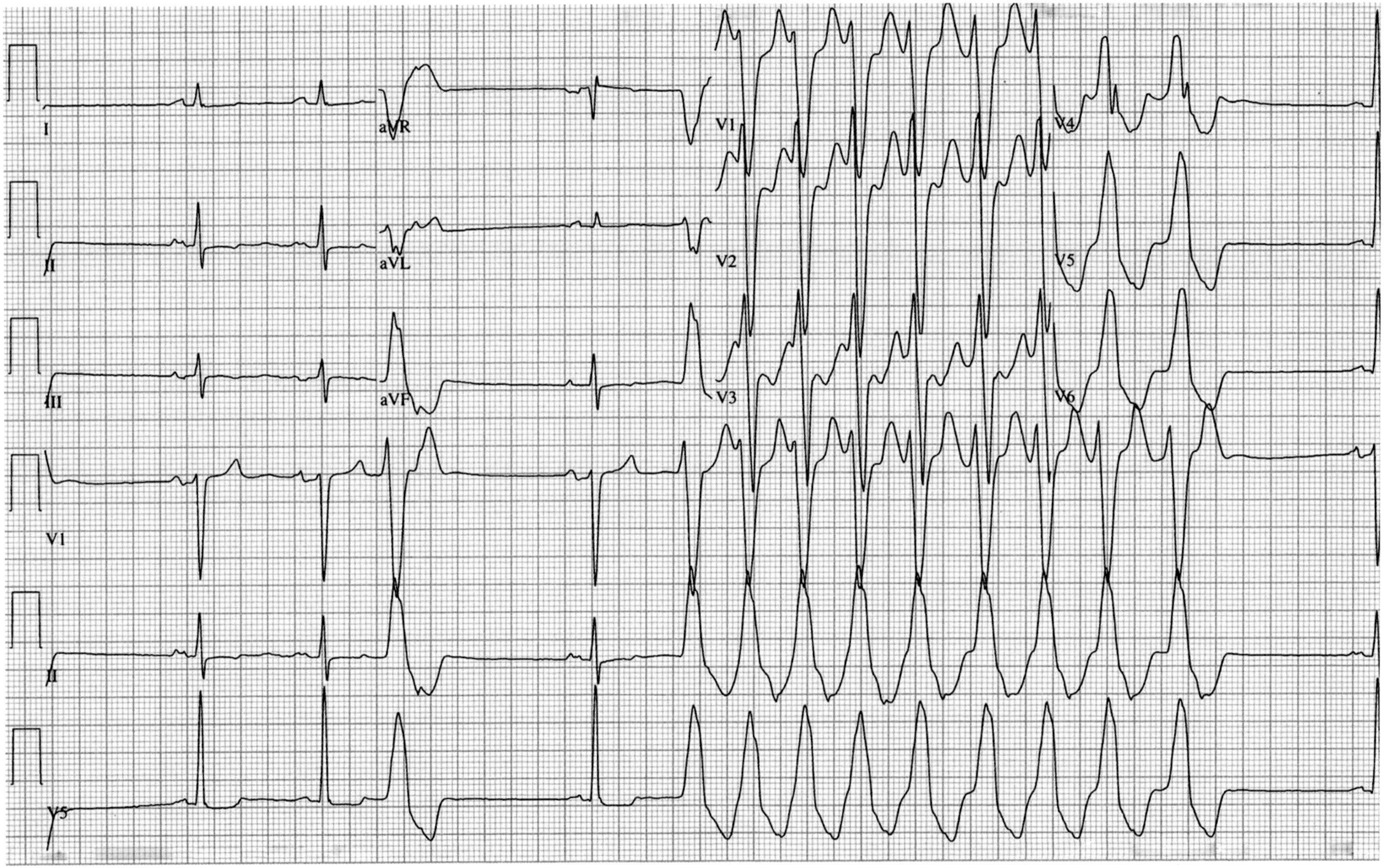

Interpretation Notes:____________________

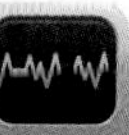

ELECTROCARDIOGRAM INTERPRETATION

The initial two QRS complexes are preceded by P waves of normal axis with a constant PR interval. The atrial rate is 65 per minute and represents normal sinus rhythm. A bifid P wave is seen in lead II suggesting left atrial abnormality. Nonspecific ST-T changes are also seen. The third QRS complex is a premature ventricular complex with a retrograde P wave seen at the nadir of the ST segment. A wide complex tachycardia is seen toward the right-hand portion of the electrocardiogram similar in morphology to the premature ventricular complex. This represents a paroxysm of ventricular tachycardia. A post-tachycardia sinus pause ensues.

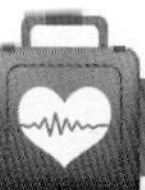

KEY DIAGNOSES

- Normal sinus rhythm
- Premature ventricular complex
- Left atrial abnormality
- Nonspecific ST-T changes
- Ventricular tachycardia
- Sinus pause

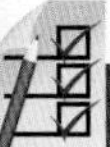

KEY TEACHING POINTS

- The differential diagnosis of a wide complex tachycardia includes supraventricular tachycardia with aberrant conduction versus ventricular tachycardia.
- When a premature ventricular complex is present on an electrocardiogram soon followed by a period of either nonsustained or sustained ventricular tachycardia of similar morphology, this provides an invaluable clue to differentiate these two diagnostic possibilities.

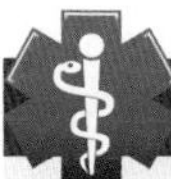

BOARD EXAMINATION ESSENTIALS

Diagnostic codes for this electrocardiogram include normal sinus rhythm, ventricular premature complex, ventricular tachycardia (three or more consecutive complexes), left atrial abnormality/enlargement, sinus pause, and nonspecific ST- and/or T-wave abnormalities. The QRS complex is slightly prolonged but remains <100 milliseconds in total duration.

Electrocardiogram Case Study #137

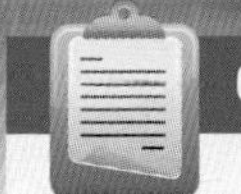

CLINICAL HISTORY

A 60-year-old male who presents acutely to the hospital with a 1-hour history of severe chest discomfort.

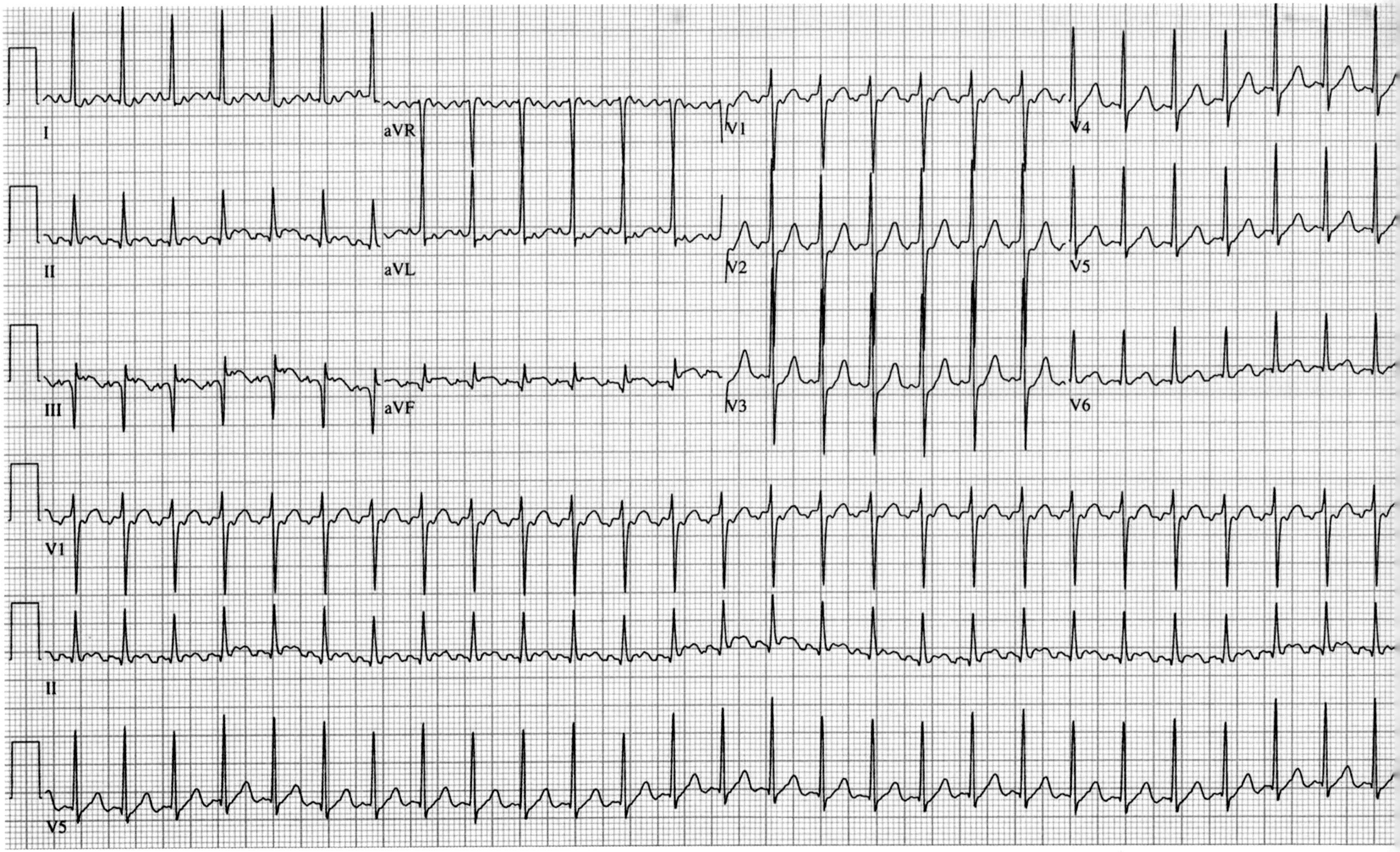

Interpretation Notes:

Electrocardiogram Case Study #137

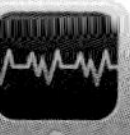

ELECTROCARDIOGRAM INTERPRETATION

Discrete P waves are not readily identified on this electrocardiogram. In rhythm strip lead V1, a negative deflection is seen preceding each QRS complex and is also present within the proximal ST segment immediately following each QRS complex. This occurs at an atrial rate slightly >300 per minute. This reflects atrial flutter. Two atrial flutter deflections are seen for each QRS complex denoting 2:1 atrioventricular conduction. 40-millisecond Q waves are present in leads III and aVF with 1.0 to 1.5 mm ST-segment elevation. This represents an inferior myocardial infarction, acute and associated acute myocardial injury.

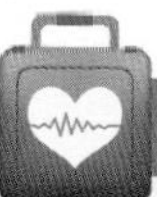

KEY DIAGNOSES

- Atrial flutter
- 2:1 atrioventricular conduction
- Inferior myocardial infarction, acute
- Acute myocardial injury

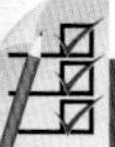

KEY TEACHING POINTS

- This atrial dysrhythmia is secondary to acute myocardial injury and requires urgent attention given the increased myocardial oxygen demand secondary to the elevated heart rate.
- This dysrhythmia may represent atrial ischemia and/or infarction that portends a worse prognosis.

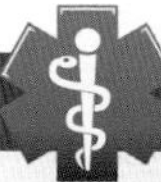

BOARD EXAMINATION ESSENTIALS

Anticipate less-than-obvious atrial arrhythmias on the board exam. Combining atrial arrhythmias with additional abnormal findings such as ischemic heart disease should be expected. This example delineates a narrow complex tachycardia of supraventricular origin. Two atrial deflections are present for each QRS complex at an atrial depolarization rate slightly >300 per minute. Diagnostic board exam codes include atrial flutter and AV block, 2:1. Additional codes include inferior myocardial infarction, acute and ST- and/or T-wave abnormalities suggesting myocardial injury.

Electrocardiogram Case Study #138

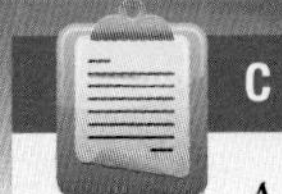

CLINICAL HISTORY

A 47-year-old male with a history of episodic atrial dysrhythmias who underwent a recent radiofrequency ablation procedure.

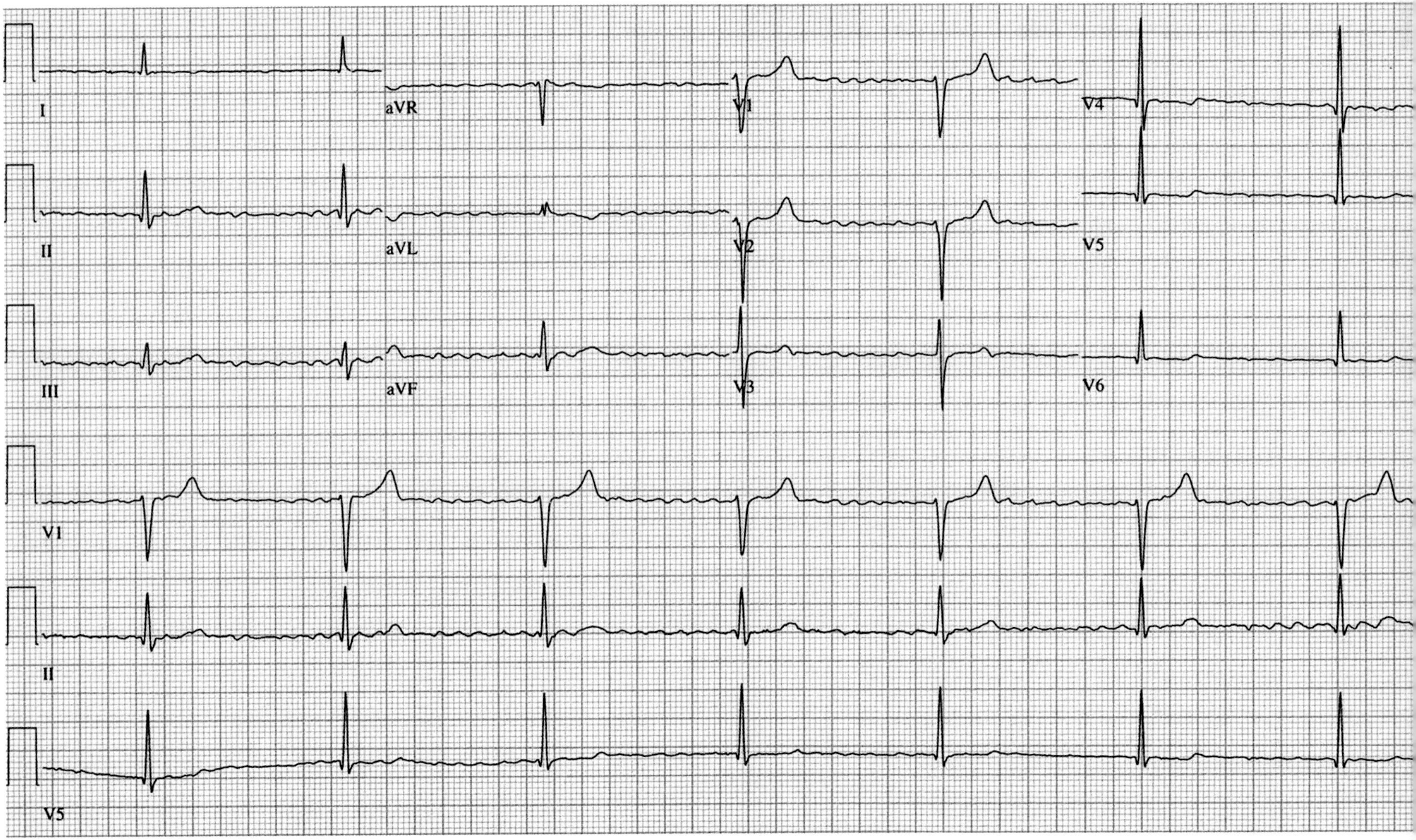

I aVR V1 V4

II aVL V2 V5

III aVF V3 V6

V1

II

V5

Interpretation Notes:

Electrocardiogram Case Study #138

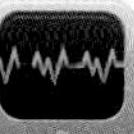

ELECTROCARDIOGRAM INTERPRETATION

This electrocardiogram demonstrates an undulating baseline without identifiable atrial activity reflecting atrial fibrillation. The ventricular response is bradycardic and regular, which is unusual in the setting of atrial fibrillation. The ventricular rate is approximately 40 per minute and the QRS complex is narrow most consistent with junctional bradycardia or more likely a junctional escape rhythm. This junctional escape rhythm is not normal in the setting of atrial fibrillation and is compatible with complete heart block. Diffuse nonspecific ST-T changes are present.

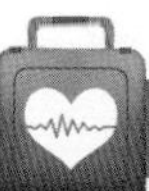

KEY DIAGNOSES

- Atrial fibrillation
- Junctional escape rhythm
- Complete heart block
- Nonspecific ST-T changes

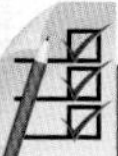

KEY TEACHING POINTS

- In the setting of atrial fibrillation, it is important to assess the R:R interval. With atrial fibrillation and intact atrioventricular conduction, the R:R intervals are irregularly irregular. When the R:R intervals are constant, this suggests a coexistent heart rhythm.
- Another possibility is a ventricular escape rhythm. Not favoring a ventricular escape rhythm are the normal duration QRS complexes.

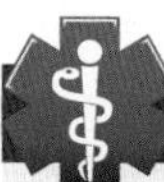

BOARD EXAMINATION ESSENTIALS

This is another example where it is important to differentiate between atrial fibrillation and atrial flutter. Given the inconsistent morphology of the atrial depolarization pattern, atrial fibrillation is favored despite a regular ventricular response. Diagnostic board exam codes include atrial fibrillation, AV junctional rhythm, complete heart block, and nonspecific ST- and/or T-wave abnormalities. This electrocardiogram favors complete heart block over AV dissociation given the bradycardic AV junctional rhythm.

Electrocardiogram Case Study #139

CLINICAL HISTORY

A 68-year-old male with severe chronic obstructive pulmonary disease, chronic renal insufficiency, and hypertension who presents with severe weakness and dyspnea upon exertion.

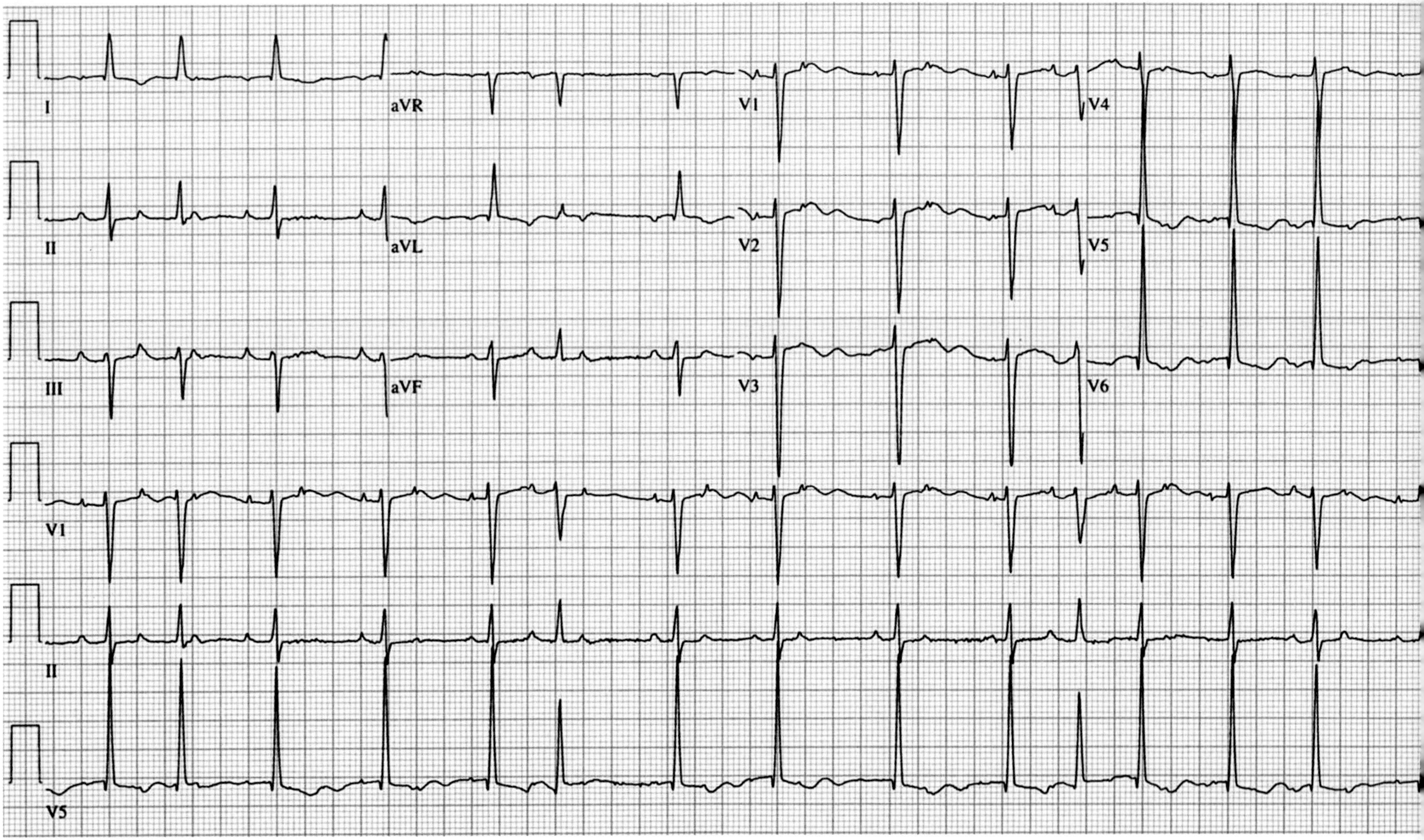

I aVR V1 V4
II aVL V2 V5
III aVF V3 V6
V1
II
V5

Interpretation Notes:

Electrocardiogram Case Study #139

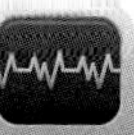

ELECTROCARDIOGRAM INTERPRETATION

The atrial rhythm is best assessed in the lead V1 rhythm strip. P waves of differing morphology occur prematurely and without predictability throughout the electrocardiogram. Some P waves conduct to the ventricle whereas others demonstrate blocked atrioventricular conduction secondary to extreme prematurity and conduction system refractoriness. This is an example of multifocal atrial tachycardia and variable atrioventricular conduction. The sixth QRS complex demonstrates aberrant conduction. Left ventricular hypertrophy with secondary ST-T changes is also seen.

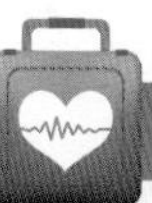

KEY DIAGNOSES

- Multifocal atrial tachycardia
- Variable atrioventricular conduction
- Aberrant conduction
- Left ventricular hypertrophy with secondary ST-T changes

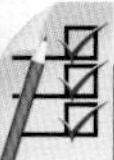

KEY TEACHING POINTS

- Unlike atrial fibrillation, with multifocal atrial tachycardia, identifiable atrial activity is seen with at least three different P-wave morphologies. This dysrhythmia is most commonly seen in patients with advanced chronic lung disease.
- The best treatment for this cardiac dysrhythmia is to aggressively treat the underlying lung disease.

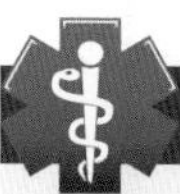

BOARD EXAMINATION ESSENTIALS

This electrocardiogram is an example of multifocal atrial tachycardia. Identifiable discrete P waves permitting differentiation from atrial fibrillation are present. Multifocal atrial tachycardia should also be differentiated from frequent conducted and nonconducted atrial premature complexes. Board exam diagnostic codes include atrial tachycardia, multifocal, aberrant conduction, left ventricular hypertrophy, ST- and/or T-wave abnormalities secondary to hypertrophy and the clinical diagnosis of chronic lung disease.

Electrocardiogram Case Study **#140**

CLINICAL HISTORY

A 20-year-old female who underwent a recent appendectomy. In the operating room, she was difficult to oxygenate and upon further clinical questioning she had been noting a blue appearance to her lips with exertion.

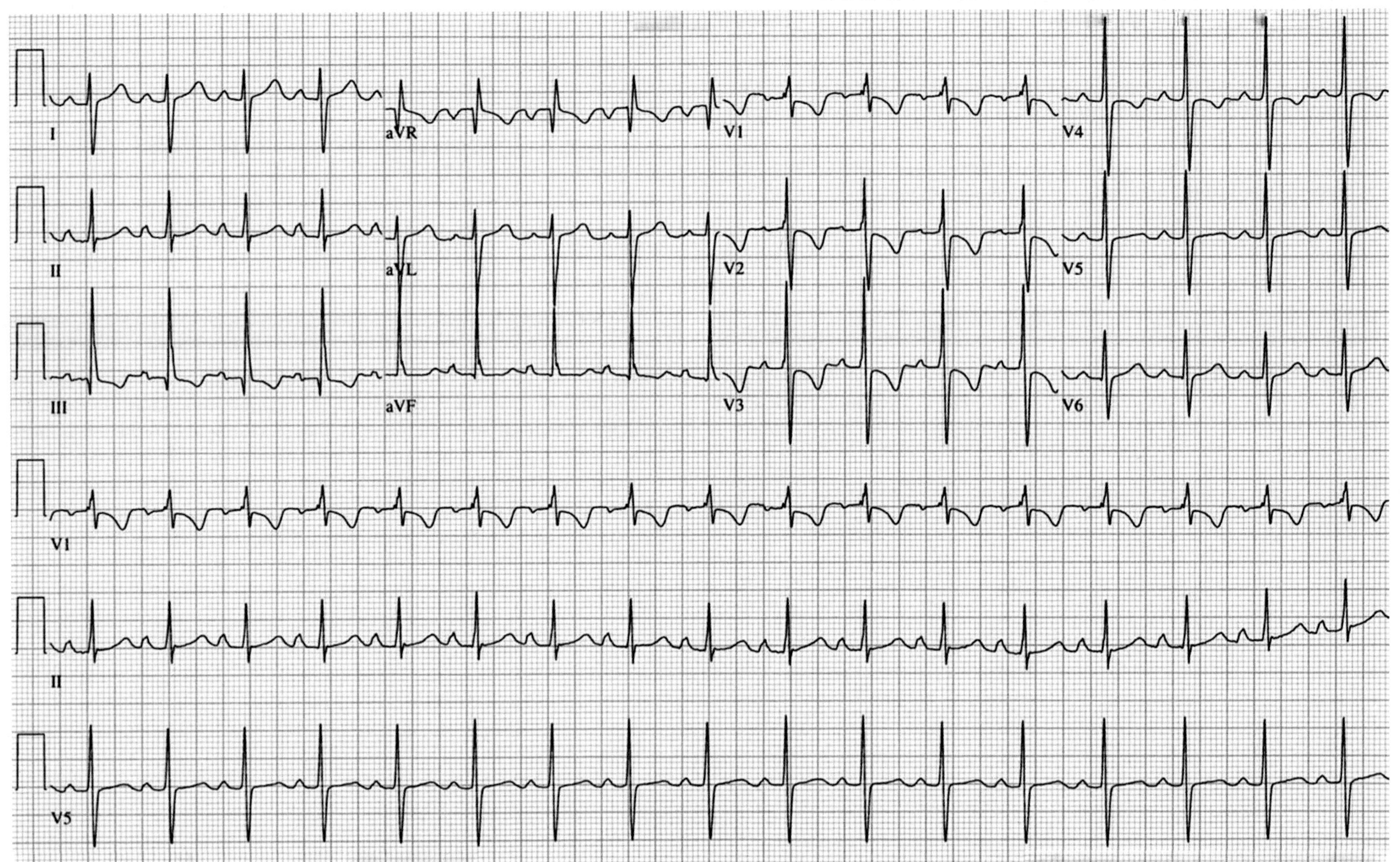

Interpretation Notes:

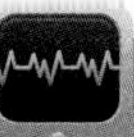

ELECTROCARDIOGRAM INTERPRETATION

Sinus tachycardia is present as a P wave of normal axis precedes each QRS complex with a normal PR interval. The atrial rate is slightly >100 per minute. The QRS complex frontal plane axis demonstrates right-axis deviation as the QRS complex vector is negative in lead I and positive in the inferior leads. A dominant R wave is seen in leads V1 to V2 with asymmetric ST-segment depression and T-wave inversion. In the setting of QRS complex frontal plane right-axis deviation, these QRS complex findings reflect right ventricular hypertrophy with secondary ST-T changes.

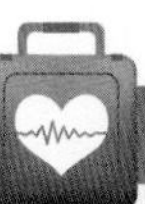

KEY DIAGNOSES

- Sinus tachycardia
- QRS complex right-axis deviation
- Right ventricular hypertrophy with secondary ST-T changes

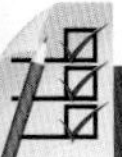

KEY TEACHING POINTS

- A dominant R wave in lead V1 in the setting of QRS complex frontal plane right-axis deviation and asymmetric T-wave inversion in leads V1 to V2 suggest right ventricular hypertrophy and a pressure overload pattern signifying pulmonary hypertension
- Further supporting this, albeit not conclusively, is the peaked P wave in lead II of approximately 0.2 mV. This suggests but does not meet the diagnostic criteria for right atrial abnormality.

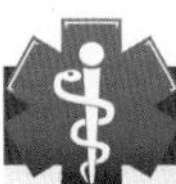

BOARD EXAMINATION ESSENTIALS

Diagnostic codes include sinus tachycardia, right-axis deviation (greater than +100 degrees), right ventricular hypertrophy, and ST- and/or T-wave abnormalities secondary to hypertrophy. There is no definitive evidence of right atrial abnormality/enlargement.

Electrocardiogram Case Study #141

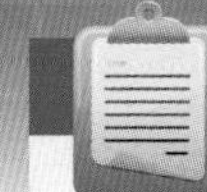

CLINICAL HISTORY

A 55-year-old male with a history of hepatic cirrhosis accepted in hospital transfer for evaluation of increasing abdominal girth and suspected ascites.

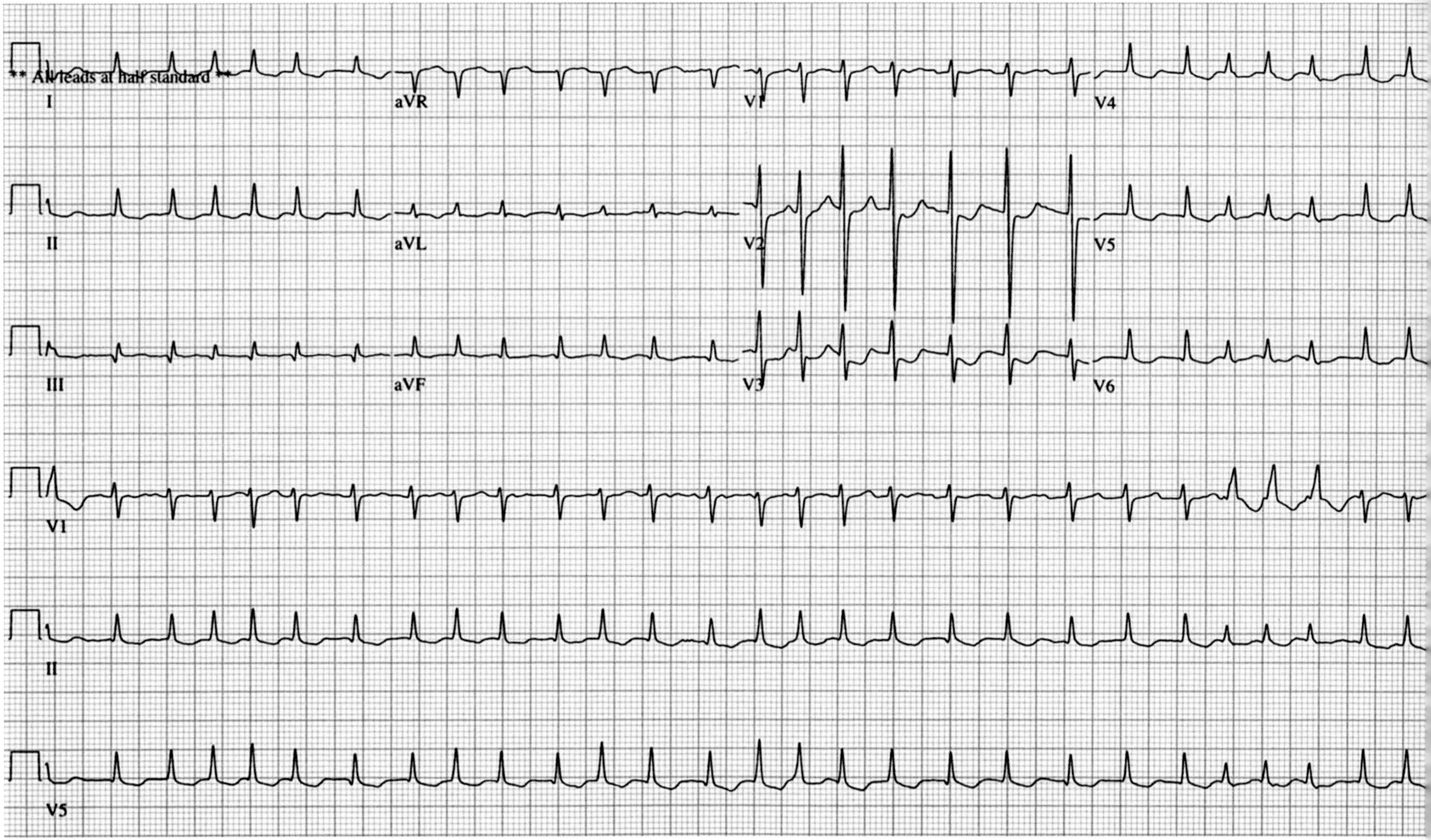

** All leads at half standard **

I aVR V1 V4

II aVL V2 V5

III aVF V3 V6

V1

II

V5

Interpretation Notes:

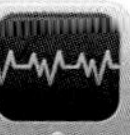

ELECTROCARDIOGRAM INTERPRETATION

This electrocardiogram is recorded at half standardization. The QRS complexes occur at a rapid rate and demonstrate irregularly irregular timing. No identifiable discrete atrial depolarizations are seen and this supports atrial fibrillation with a rapid ventricular response. Diffuse nonspecific ST-T changes are noted. On the right-hand portion of this electrocardiogram, three QRS complexes are conducted with an incomplete right bundle-branch block morphology. This represents the Ashman phenomenon and intermittent incomplete right bundle-branch block aberration. Voltage criteria for left ventricular hypertrophy are also present.

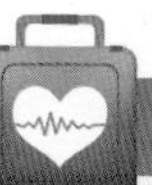

KEY DIAGNOSES

- Half standardization
- Atrial fibrillation
- Rapid ventricular response
- Ashman phenomenon
- Nonspecific ST-T changes
- Left ventricular hypertrophy

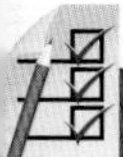

KEY TEACHING POINTS

- The Ashman phenomenon with right bundle-branch block aberration is frequently seen in the setting of atrial fibrillation with a rapid ventricular response. This is reflective of normal cardiac physiology and refractoriness of the right bundle branch at a rapid heart rate.
- It is important to distinguish the Ashman phenomenon from premature ventricular complexes. The complexes on this electrocardiogram are not premature ventricular in origin and do not represent nonsustained ventricular tachycardia.

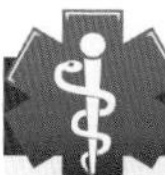

BOARD EXAMINATION ESSENTIALS

Diagnostic board exam codes include atrial fibrillation, aberrant conduction, nonspecific ST-and/or T-wave abnormalities, and left ventricular hypertrophy. Keep in mind when assessing the QRS complex voltage that the electrocardiogram was obtained at half standardization. Without taking this into account, the presence of left ventricular hypertrophy may be overlooked.

Electrocardiogram Case Study #142

CLINICAL HISTORY

A 73-year-old male with coronary artery disease who is status post four-vessel coronary artery bypass graft surgery 2 years prior to this electrocardiogram.

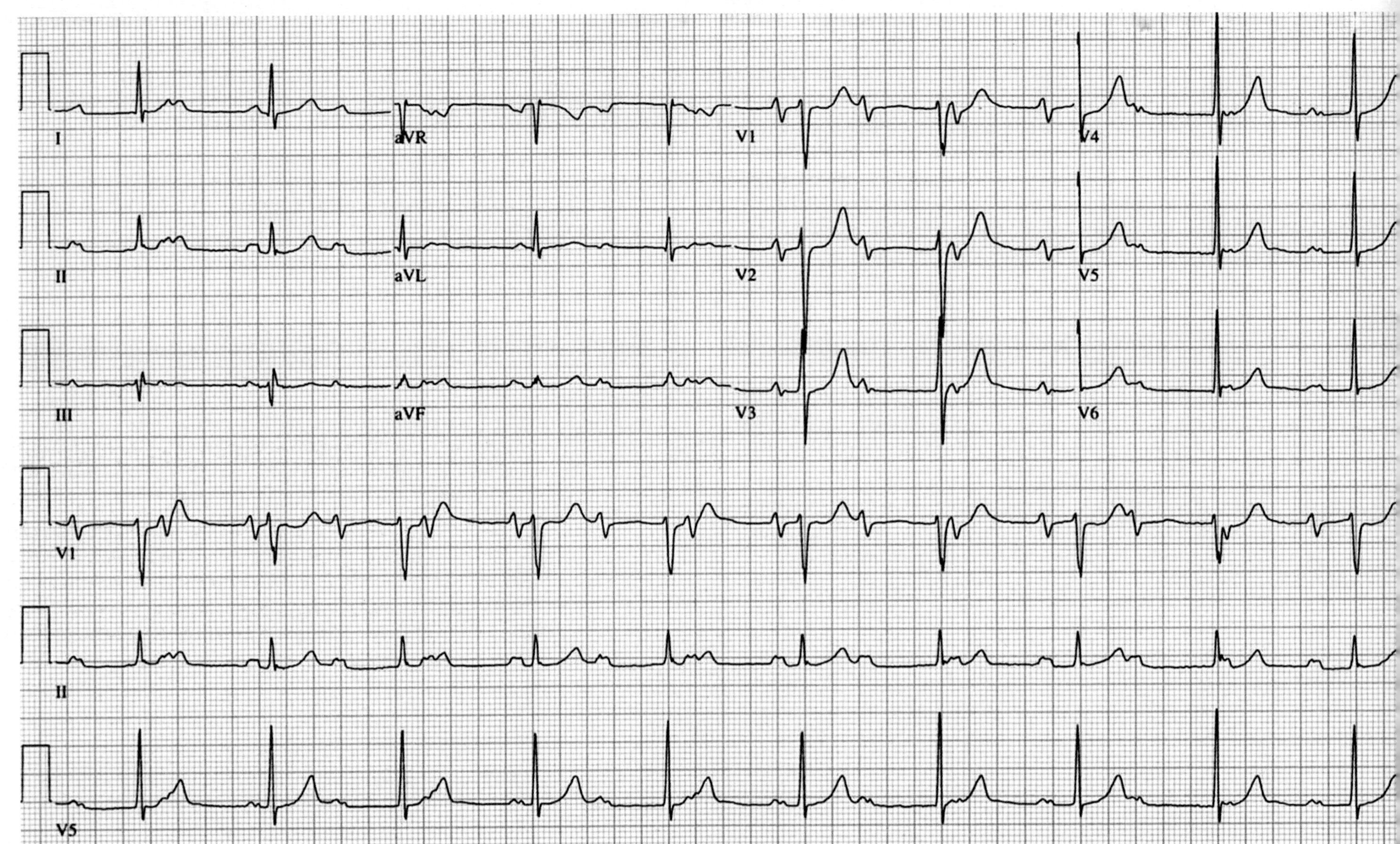

Interpretation Notes:

Electrocardiogram Case Study #142

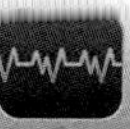

ELECTROCARDIOGRAM INTERPRETATION

P waves occur at a regular interval with a normal P-wave axis at an atrial rate of approximately 90 per minute representing normal sinus rhythm. A bifid P wave is seen in lead II with marked terminal T-wave negativity in lead V1 supporting left atrial abnormality. QRS complexes occur at regular intervals at a rate slightly >60 per minute. In lead V1, the P waves are not associated with the QRS complexes and do not demonstrate constant PR intervals. This supports the presence of complete heart block and an accelerated junctional rhythm given the normal duration QRS complex.

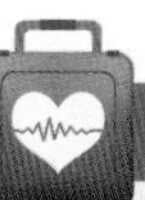

KEY DIAGNOSES

- Normal sinus rhythm
- Accelerated junctional rhythm
- Complete heart block
- Left atrial abnormality

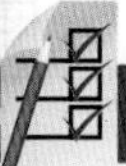

KEY TEACHING POINTS

- This patient did not have a permanent pacemaker implanted as the accelerated junctional rhythm occurred at a sufficient heart rate to maintain hemodynamic stability without symptoms of fatigue or cerebral hypoperfusion.

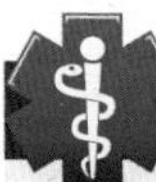

BOARD EXAMINATION ESSENTIALS

This electrocardiogram is highly likely to appear on the board exam. Board exam diagnoses include normal sinus rhythm, left atrial abnormality/enlargement, AV junctional rhythm, and complete heart block. The narrow QRS complex suggests the atrioventricular junctional origin of the QRS complex. No definitive ST-T changes or Q waves are identified.

Electrocardiogram Case Study #143

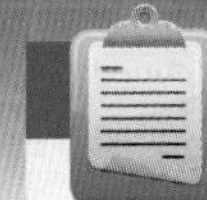

CLINICAL HISTORY

A 44-year-old male admitted to the hospital with worsening bilateral lower extremity edema. His past cardiac history includes aortic valve replacement secondary to severe aortic insufficiency and coronary artery bypass grafting surgery.

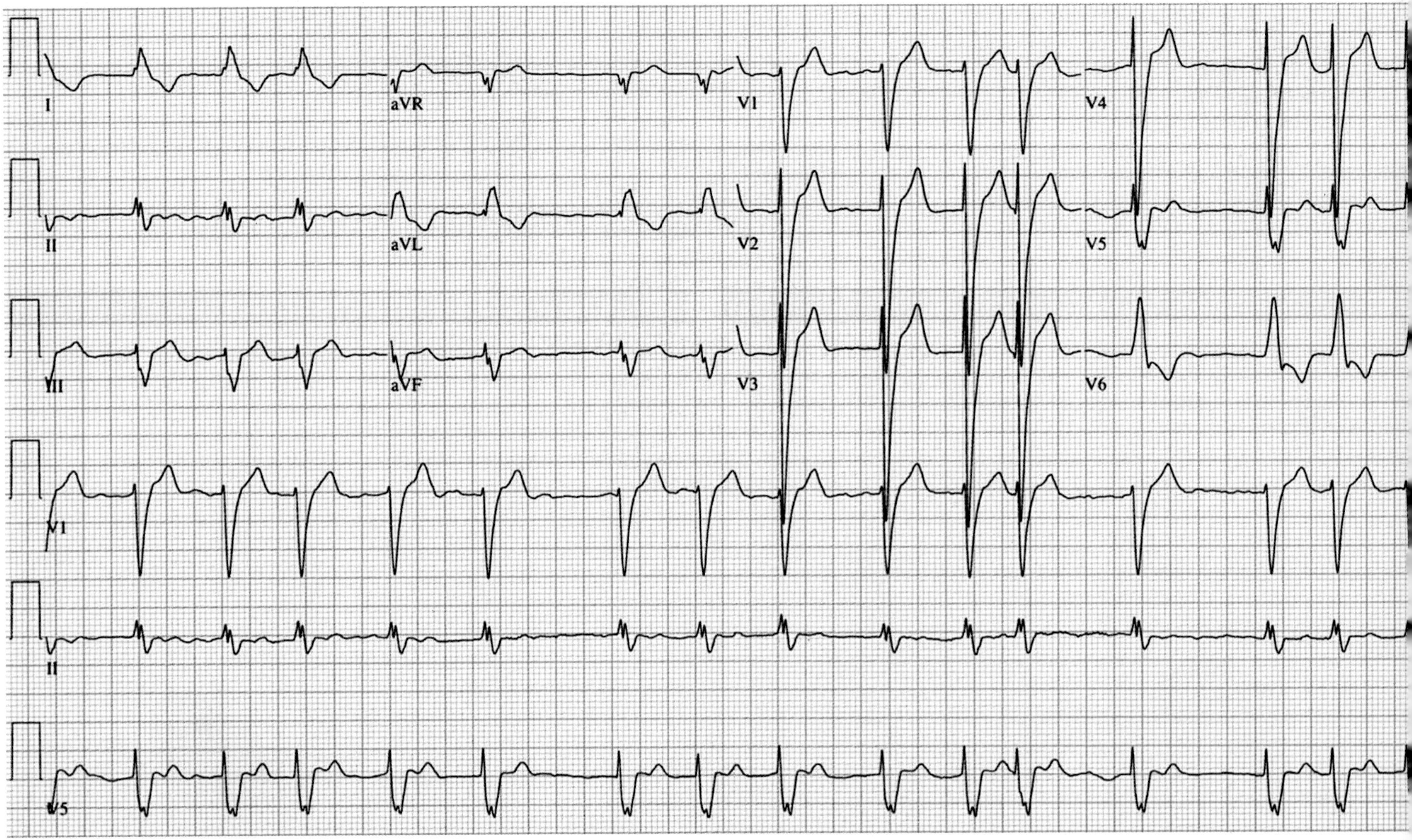

I aVR V1 V4

II aVL V2 V5

III aVF V3 V6

V1

II

V5

Interpretation Notes:

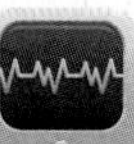

ELECTROCARDIOGRAM INTERPRETATION

Atrial fibrillation is present as no identifiable atrial activity is demonstrated. The QRS complex is widened to >120 milliseconds with complete left bundle-branch block morphology.

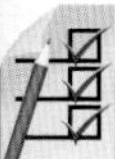

KEY TEACHING POINTS

- The finding of complete left bundle-branch block is abnormal and reflects underlying cardiac pathology. In this circumstance, it is secondary to chronic aortic insufficiency, coronary artery disease, and associated left ventricular systolic dysfunction.
- Complete left bundle-branch block may also appear in the immediate post-operative period given aortic valve replacement and close proximity of the left bundle branch to the operative field.
- Atrial fibrillation, similar to left ventricular systolic dysfunction, is most likely related to longstanding valvular heart disease.

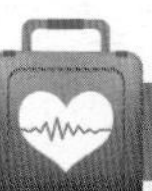

KEY DIAGNOSES

- Atrial fibrillation
- Complete left bundle-branch block

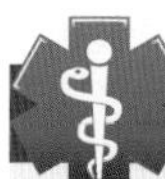

BOARD EXAMINATION ESSENTIALS

Diagnostic codes for the board exam include atrial fibrillation and left bundle-branch block complete. Another consideration would be a ventricular pacemaker. There is no evidence to support ventricular pacing. For the board exam, when a widened QRS complex is identified, carefully inspect each QRS complex for the possibility of a pacemaker deflection.

Electrocardiogram Case Study #144

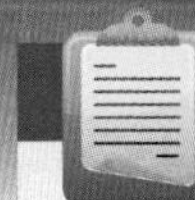

CLINICAL HISTORY

A 29-year-old female 37 weeks pregnant admitted to the hospital for close observation in the setting of pregnancy-induced hypertension.

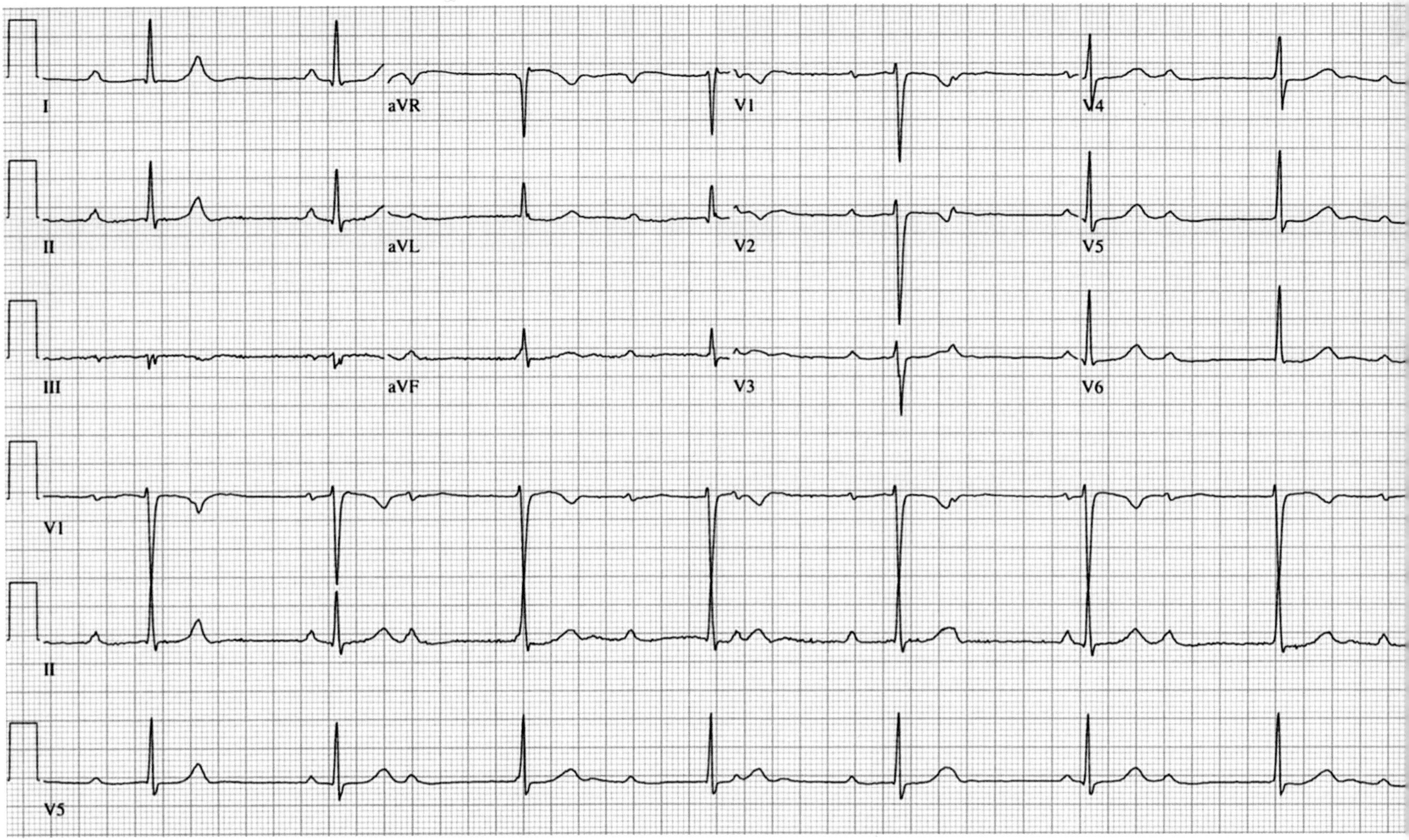

I aVR V1 V4
II aVL V2 V5
III aVF V3 V6
V1
II
V5

Interpretation Notes:

Electrocardiogram Case Study #144

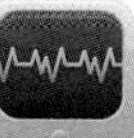

ELECTROCARDIOGRAM INTERPRETATION

For this electrocardiogram, the cardiac rhythm is best discerned in the lead V1 rhythm strip. P waves occur at regular intervals at an atrial rate of approximately 85 per minute. The P-wave axis as ascertained in leads I, II, and aVF is upright and normal. This suggests normal sinus rhythm. The PR interval varies and supports a lack of association between the P waves and the QRS complexes. The QRS complexes are normal duration and occur regularly at a rate of approximately 45 per minute. These findings collectively support normal sinus rhythm, junctional bradycardia, and complete heart block.

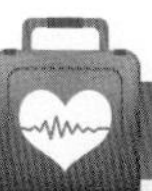

KEY DIAGNOSES

- Normal sinus rhythm
- Junctional bradycardia
- Complete heart block

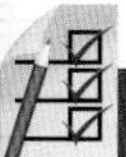

KEY TEACHING POINTS

- Electrocardiogram criteria for complete heart block include two independent cardiac rhythms, lack of atrioventricular association, and a noncompeting ventricular rhythm slower than the atrial rhythm.

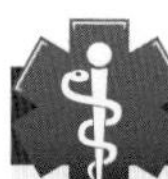

BOARD EXAMINATION ESSENTIALS

This is another electrocardiogram with profound AV conduction system disease. Board exam codes include normal sinus rhythm, AV junctional rhythm, and complete heart block. Right atrial abnormality/enlargement is suggested in lead II, but this is not definitive and therefore not coded.

Electrocardiogram Case Study #145

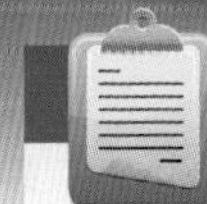

CLINICAL HISTORY

A 66-year-old female admitted to the hospital after a same-day cardiac catheterization demonstrated severe three-vessel coronary artery obstructive disease.

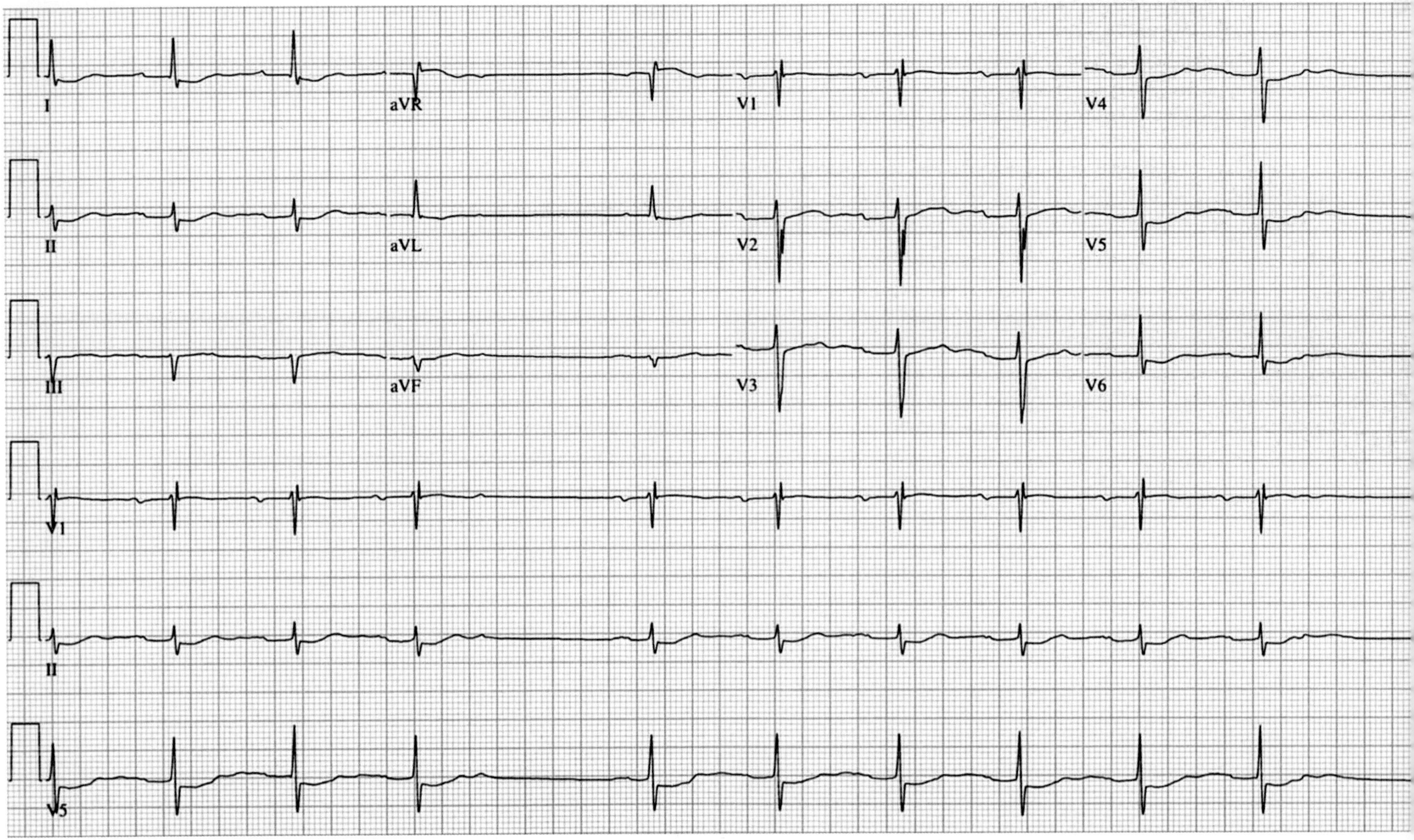

I aVR V1 V4

II aVL V2 V5

III aVF V3 V6

V1

II

V5

Interpretation Notes:

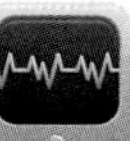

ELECTROCARDIOGRAM INTERPRETATION

This electrocardiogram demonstrates normal sinus rhythm with first-degree atrioventricular block. An apparent pause occurs on the left-hand portion of the tracing. In rhythm strip lead V1 following the fourth QRS complex, a positive deflection is seen representing a nonconducted premature atrial complex. This creates an apparent pause and is repeated toward the end of the electrocardiogram. Diffuse nonspecific ST-T changes and prominent positive U waves are seen. This suggests the possibility of hypokalemia and requires further clinical correlation. The positive U waves otherwise remain unexplained. This may be partly contributed to by a low-normal serum potassium level measured at 3.7 mEq per L.

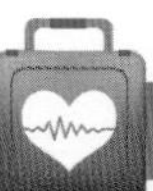

KEY DIAGNOSES

- Normal sinus rhythm
- First-degree atrioventricular block
- Nonconducted premature atrial complexes
- Nonspecific ST-T changes
- Positive U waves

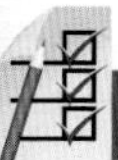

KEY TEACHING POINTS

- Nonconducted premature atrial complexes are an important source of electrocardiogram pauses. It is important to evaluate for nonconducted premature atrial complexes as these are a benign cause of electrocardiogram pauses and do not require further evaluation or treatment unless extremely frequent and symptomatic.

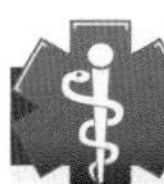

BOARD EXAMINATION ESSENTIALS

This electrocardiogram highlights an important diagnostic code distinction for the board exam. Diagnostic codes include normal sinus rhythm; AV block, first degree; atrial premature complexes; nonspecific ST- and/or T-wave abnormalities; and prominent U waves. The other important diagnostic consideration is AV block, second-degree Mobitz type I Wenckebach. After the nonconducted atrial premature complex, the PR interval is slightly shorter. This reflects the preceding longer RP interval and does not support a more advanced form of heart block such as Mobitz type 1 Wenckebach. Additionally, do not code a sinus pause or sick sinus syndrome as nonconducted atrial premature complexes do not definitively equate with sinus node disease. The QT interval is not prolonged; instead the QT-U interval is prolonged. Therefore, QT interval prolongation is not coded.

Electrocardiogram Case Study #146

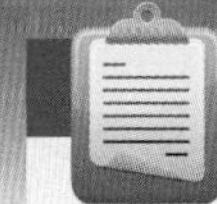

CLINICAL HISTORY

A 72-year-old female admitted acutely to the hospital in the setting of perceived rapid heart beating and profound lightheadedness.

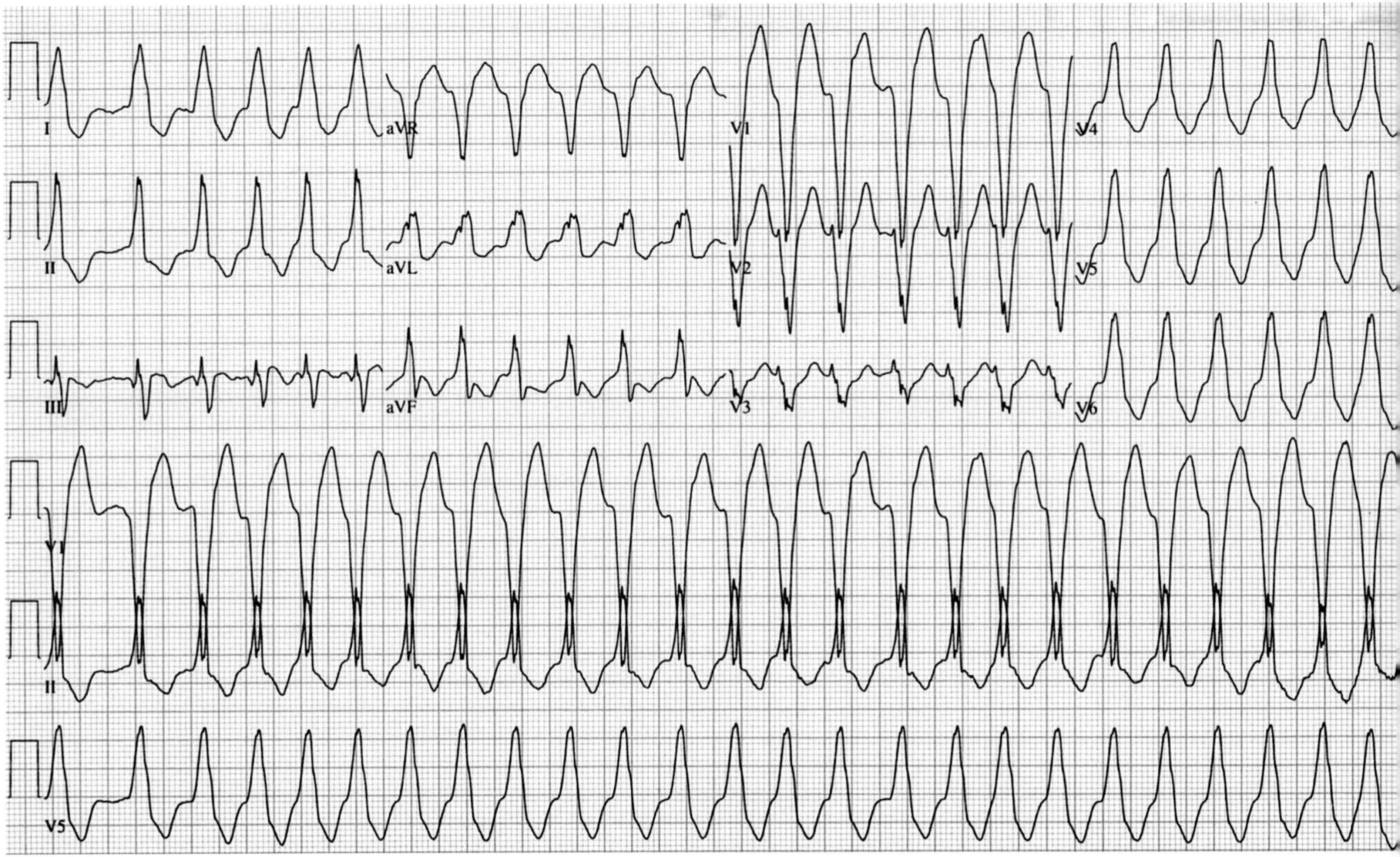

I aVR V1 V4
II aVL V2 V5
III aVF V3 V6
V1
II
V5

Interpretation Notes:

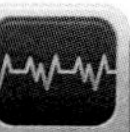

ELECTROCARDIOGRAM INTERPRETATION

The QRS complexes demonstrate a wide complex tachycardia with an irregularly irregular rhythm. Analysis of the lead V1 rhythm strip fails to demonstrate discrete atrial activity. This represents atrial fibrillation with a rapid ventricular response and complete left bundle-branch block.

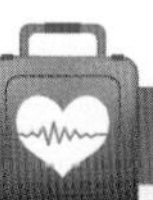

KEY DIAGNOSES

- Atrial fibrillation
- Complete left bundle-branch block
- Rapid ventricular response

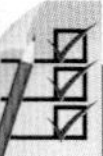

KEY TEACHING POINTS

- A diagnostic consideration for this electrocardiogram is ventricular tachycardia. What differentiates this electrocardiogram from ventricular tachycardia is the presence of an irregularly irregular ventricular response, concluded only after careful evaluation of consecutive R:R intervals.
- A prior electrocardiogram for comparison would be helpful. In this case, complete left bundle-branch block with a similar QRS complex morphology was a known finding.

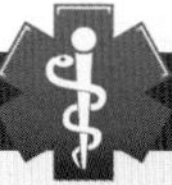

BOARD EXAMINATION ESSENTIALS

This electrocardiogram presents an important concept for the board exam. Initial assessment suggested wide complex tachycardia with complete left bundle-branch block morphology. The far left-hand portion of the electrocardiogram demonstrates an irregular baseline consistent with atrial fibrillation. Diagnostic codes for the board exam include atrial fibrillation and left bundle-branch block, complete. Do not code ventricular tachycardia in this circumstance. While coding for left bundle-branch block, complete, is appropriate for this electrocardiogram, restoration of normal sinus rhythm and slowing of the ventricular rate may unmask the QRS complex widening as functional (rate-related) aberrancy. If so, that can be beneficial as native QRS complex morphology can then be interpreted providing further insight into possible underlying cardiac pathology.

Electrocardiogram Case Study #147

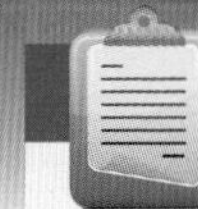

CLINICAL HISTORY

A 56-year-old male with severe ischemic left ventricular systolic dysfunction admitted to the hospital for evaluation of recent-onset shortness of breath. Serum cardiac biomarkers were negative for acute myocardial injury.

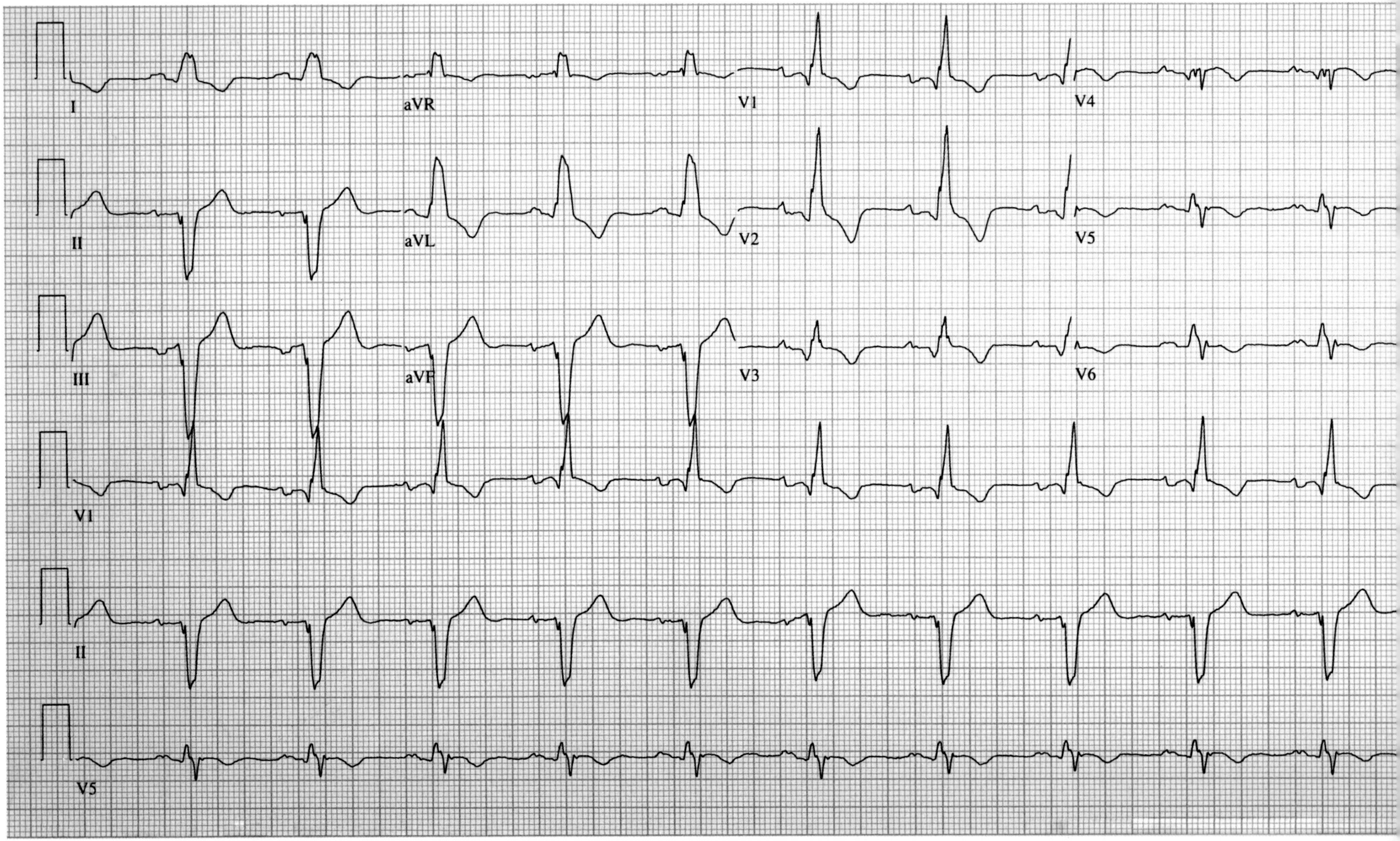

I aVR V1 V4
II aVL V2 V5
III aVF V3 V6
V1
II
V5

Interpretation Notes:

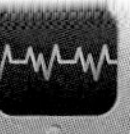

ELECTROCARDIOGRAM INTERPRETATION

The atrial rhythm is regular with an abnormal P-wave axis including a negative P-wave vector in leads III and aVF at a rate slightly >60 per minute supporting an ectopic atrial rhythm. The QRS complex duration is significantly prolonged >120 milliseconds and best characterized in the limb leads as complete left bundle-branch block. The QRS complex demonstrates left-axis deviation. In the precordial leads, the QRS complex appears to possess complete right bundle-branch block morphology. This is best termed a masquerading bundle-branch block typically identified as complete left bundle-branch block morphology in the limb leads and a complete right bundle-branch block morphology in the chest leads. Invariably, this finding is associated with significant left ventricular systolic dysfunction. Q waves are present in leads V1 to V4 and are diagnostic of an anterior myocardial infarction, age indeterminate. On the basis of this finding, the presumed advanced left ventricular systolic dysfunction is ischemic in origin.

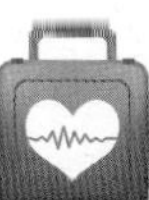

KEY DIAGNOSES

- Ectopic atrial rhythm
- Masquerading bundle-branch block
- Anterior myocardial infarction, age indeterminate
- Left ventricular aneurysm
- Left-axis QRS complex deviation

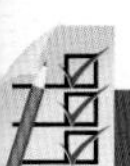

KEY TEACHING POINTS

- The finding of masquerading bundle-branch block suggests advanced left ventricular systolic dysfunction. It is not possible to differentiate a primary cardiomyopathy from ischemic left ventricular systolic dysfunction unless specific electrocardiogram findings such as diagnostic Q waves are present.
- ST-segment elevation is seen in leads V3 to V4. Without clinical correlation, this suggests an acute myocardial injury pattern. This patient was asymptomatic at the time of this electrocardiogram. The presence of persistent ST-segment elevation and Q-wave formation was consistent with the patient's known left ventricular aneurysm.

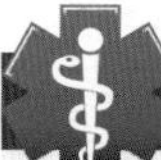

BOARD EXAMINATION ESSENTIALS

Board exam diagnostic codes for this electrocardiogram include normal sinus rhythm as a code for ectopic atrial rhythm is not available; intraventricular conduction disturbance, nonspecific type; left-axis deviation (greater than −30 degrees); and anterior myocardial infarction, age indeterminate. There is no board exam code for left ventricular aneurysm.

Electrocardiogram Case Study **#148**

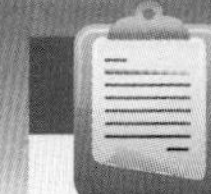

CLINICAL HISTORY

A 35-year-old male with ischemic left ventricular systolic dysfunction and a recent history of syncope scheduled for implantable cardiac defibrillator placement.

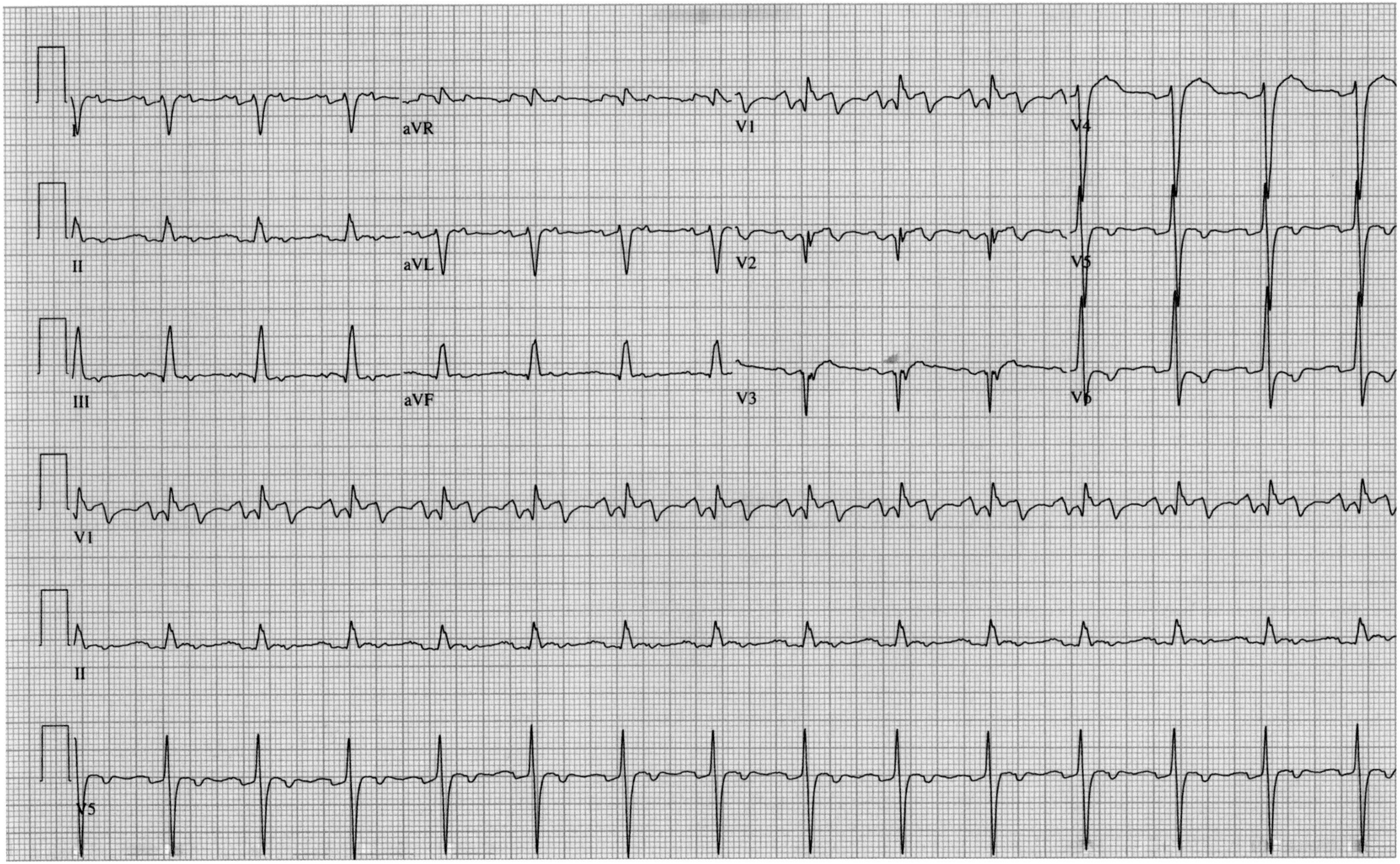

Interpretation Notes:

Electrocardiogram Case Study #148

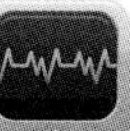

ELECTROCARDIOGRAM INTERPRETATION

Regular occurring P waves are best seen in lead I at an atrial rate of approximately 170 per minute representing an ectopic atrial tachycardia. Two P waves are present for each QRS complex reflecting 2:1 atrioventricular conduction. The QRS complex frontal plane axis demonstrates right-axis deviation as the QRS complex vector is negative in lead I and positive in leads II, III, and aVF. The QRS complex duration is prolonged at approximately 100 milliseconds with an rsR′ QRS complex pattern in lead V1 suggesting incomplete right bundle-branch block. Q waves are seen in leads V2 to V3 consistent with an anteroseptal myocardial infarction, age indeterminate.

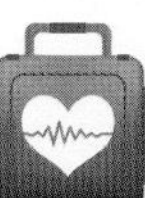

KEY DIAGNOSES

- Ectopic atrial tachycardia
- 2:1 atrioventricular conduction
- QRS complex right-axis deviation
- Anteroseptal myocardial infarction, age indeterminate
- Pseudoinfarction pattern
- Incomplete right bundle-branch block

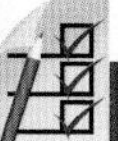

KEY TEACHING POINTS

- Atrial dysrhythmias are common in the presence of left ventricular systolic dysfunction irrespective of the cause.
- This demonstrates a pseudoinfarction pattern. By history, this patient had normal coronary arteries and there was no clinical evidence of a prior myocardial infarction.

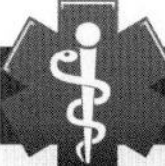

BOARD EXAMINATION ESSENTIALS

Board exam diagnostic codes include atrial tachycardia; AV block, 2:1; right-axis deviation (greater than +100 degrees); right bundle-branch block, incomplete; and anteroseptal myocardial infarction, age indeterminate. Provided the clinical history, there is no indication to code acute myocardial injury. The ST-T segments are not normal and coding for nonspecific ST- and/or T-wave abnormalities is appropriate. The apparent ST-segment elevation in leads V1 and V2 is due to superimposed ectopic atrial depolarizations.

Electrocardiogram Case Study #149

CLINICAL HISTORY

A 35-year-old female with primary pulmonary hypertension admitted to the hospital with increasing shortness of breath.

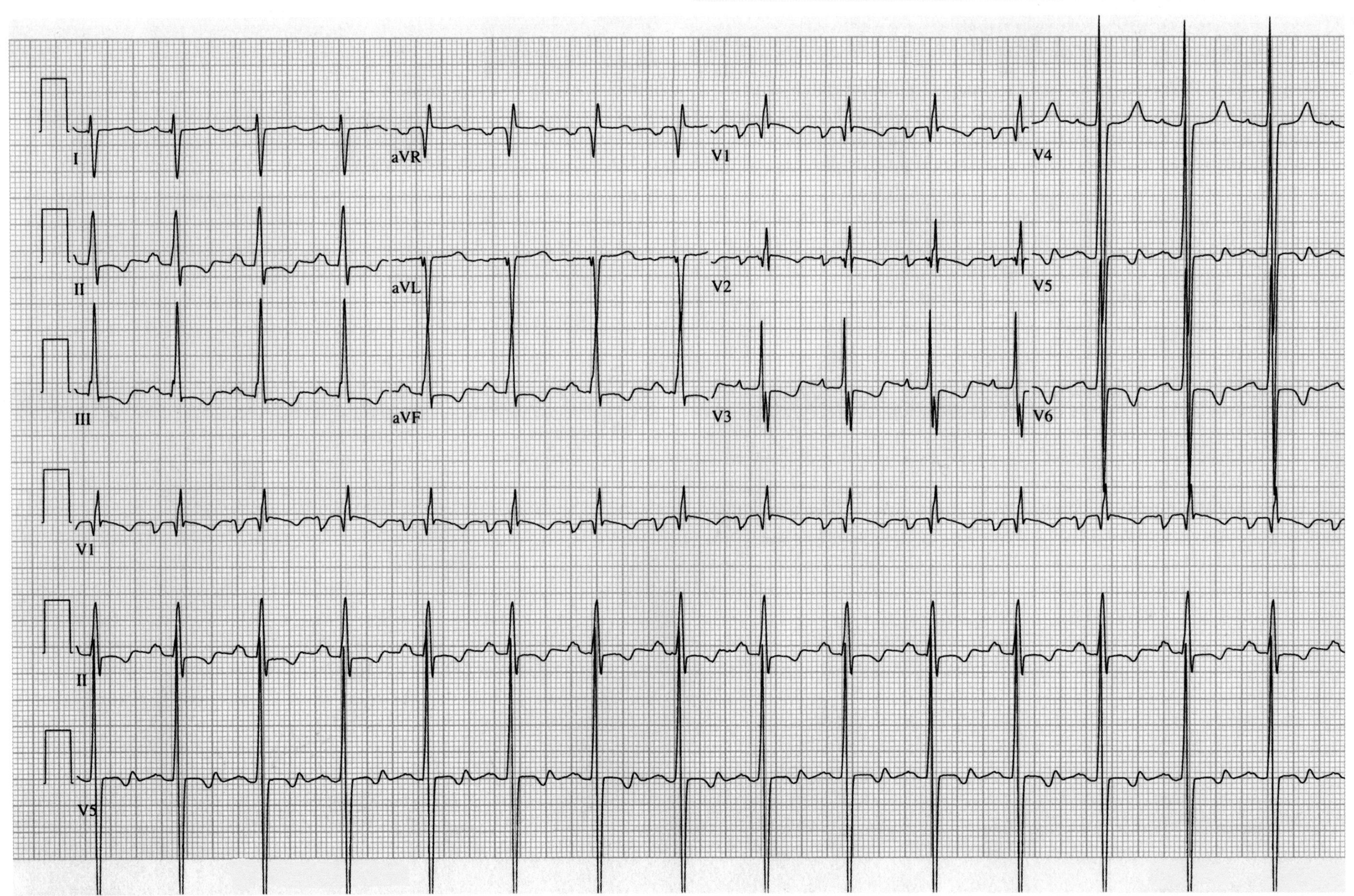

Interpretation Notes:

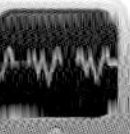

ELECTROCARDIOGRAM INTERPRETATION

This electrocardiogram demonstrates normal sinus rhythm. The QRS complex frontal plane axis demonstrates right-axis deviation as the QRS complex vector is negative in lead I and positive in leads II, III, and aVF. A qR QRS complex configuration is seen in lead V1 and in the setting of right-axis QRS complex deviation is consistent with right ventricular hypertrophy with secondary ST-T changes. The QRS complex precordial voltage is elevated with asymmetric T-wave inversion satisfying the criteria for left ventricular hypertrophy with secondary ST-T changes. This electrocardiogram satisfies the criteria for biventricular hypertrophy with secondary ST-T changes. The P wave is terminally negative in lead V1 and prolonged in lead II supporting left atrial abnormality.

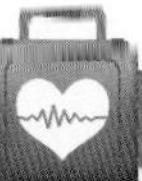

KEY DIAGNOSES

- Normal sinus rhythm
- Left atrial abnormality
- Left ventricular hypertrophy with secondary ST-T changes
- Right ventricular hypertrophy with secondary ST-T changes
- Biventricular hypertrophy with secondary ST-T changes
- QRS complex right-axis deviation
- Primary pulmonary hypertension

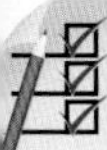

KEY TEACHING POINTS

- The right ventricular hypertrophy demonstrated on this electrocardiogram is secondary to primary pulmonary hypertension.
- The left ventricular hypertrophy is secondary to a known right to left inter-atrial shunt resulting in left atrial and left ventricular volume overload and prominent QRS complex voltage.
- The patient was cyanotic on examination given the advanced pulmonary hypertension and right to left shunt at the atrial level.

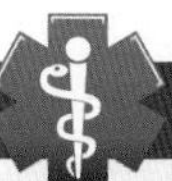

BOARD EXAMINATION ESSENTIALS

This electrocardiogram is consistent with severe pulmonary hypertension. Board exam diagnostic codes include normal sinus rhythm, left atrial abnormality/enlargement, right-axis deviation (greater than +100 degrees), right ventricular hypertrophy, ST- and/or T-wave abnormalities secondary to hypertrophy. Normally, right ventricular conduction delay patterns are not coded in this circumstance. Right atrial abnormality/enlargement is not definitively identified and therefore not coded. For the board exam, make sure to assess for this diagnosis in the presence of right ventricular hypertrophy.

Electrocardiogram Case Study #150

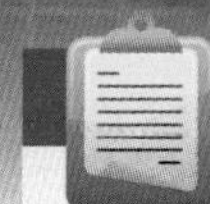

CLINICAL HISTORY

A 72-year-old male admitted urgently to the hospital with a 3-hour history of severe central chest pressure.

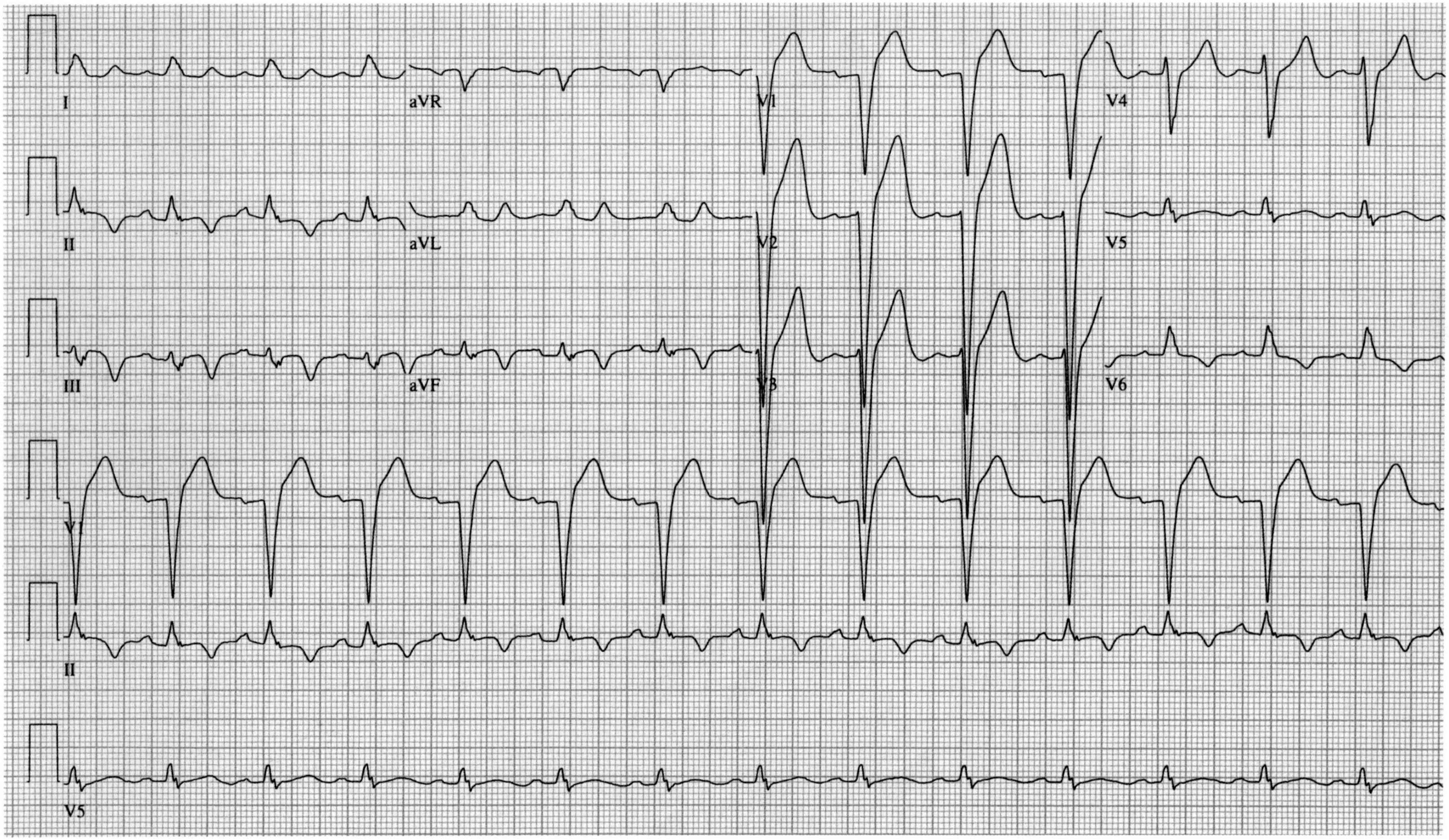

I aVR V1 V4
II aVL V2 V5
III aVF V3 V6
V1
II
V5

Interpretation Notes:

Electrocardiogram Case Study #150

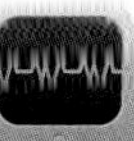

ELECTROCARDIOGRAM INTERPRETATION

The cardiac rhythm is normal sinus rhythm at a rate of approximately 85 per minute. The QRS complex is widened greater than 120 milliseconds with complete left bundle-branch block morphology. Subtle ST-segment elevation and more prominent terminal T-wave inversion are present in leads II, III, and aVF with reciprocal ST-segment depression seen in lead aVL. This is consistent with inferior acute myocardial injury in the setting of complete left bundle-branch block.

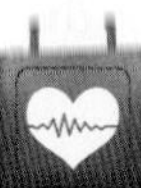

KEY DIAGNOSES

- Normal sinus rhythm
- Complete left bundle-branch block
- Acute myocardial injury

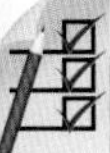

KEY TEACHING POINTS

- In the presence of complete left bundle-branch block, ST-segment deviation and T-wave inversion are readily identified and interpreted. This electrocardiogram localizes the acute myocardial injury to the inferior leads and likely, the right coronary artery distribution.

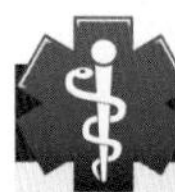

BOARD EXAMINATION ESSENTIALS

Diagnostic codes for the board exam include normal sinus rhythm; left bundle-branch block, complete; and ST- and/or T-wave abnormalities suggesting myocardial injury. Remember not to code a myocardial infarction pattern in the presence of left bundle-branch block, complete. The PR interval measures exactly 200 milliseconds and thus, AV block, first degree, is not coded.

Keys to a Passing Score

American Board of Internal Medicine (ABIM)

Cardiovascular Medicine Certifying Exam—Electrocardiogram Subsection

While electrocardiogram interpretation is an important daily component of patient care, it is also a fundamental aspect of the American Board of Internal Medicine (ABIM) Cardiovascular Medicine Certifying Exam. As presently structured, a passing score on this examination in essence requires two passing scores: one on the overall examination and the other on the electrocardiogram subsection.

To pass the electrocardiogram subsection component of the ABIM exam, a thorough understanding of electrocardiography is required. After all, achieving a passing score equates with board certification to practice cardiovascular medicine, thereby achieving requisite certification to be deemed an expert in the field. The goal of the electrocardiography subsection from the examiner's perspective is to distinguish between an expert and a nonexpert. That is why this testing component needs to be approached both seriously and systematically.

Optimal exam preparation is comprised of the following components:

1. A thorough understanding of 12-lead electrocardiography
2. A complete familiarization with the ABIM Cardiovascular Medicine Certifying Exam electrocardiogram scoring sheet content and structure
3. A comprehensive understanding of each electrocardiogram ABIM diagnostic code with the ability to recognize and diagnose each abnormality on the 12-lead electrocardiogram.

To achieve a thorough understanding of 12-lead electrocardiography requires practice and repetition. Presumably during residency and fellowship training, an electrocardiogram interpretation curriculum was an integral part of a structured didactic program. Additionally, several excellent books and interactive CD-ROM programs are available with a multitude of electrocardiogram examples, each providing necessary 12-lead electrocardiogram interpretation exposure.

Prior to sitting for the ABIM Cardiovascular Medicine Certifying Exam, an electrocardiogram scoring sheet is provided for each test taker. It is also available online on the ABIM Web site. It is absolutely essential to review the diagnoses, their location on the scoring sheet, and how they are grouped. Please remember that this examination, similar to other board examinations, is a time-limited test. As an examinee, you should aim to minimize your time locating a specific diagnosis on your scoring sheet. To maximize your performance, almost all of your time should be spent on 12-lead electrocardiogram interpretation. The bottom line is to study the diagnostic code answer sheet and make sure you are fully familiarized with how it is organized and where each specific diagnosis is located. This is an indispensable up-front investment of your time.

Now that you have an understanding of 12-lead electrocardiography and complete familiarization with the diagnostic code scoring sheet, it is next best to cross-check your 12-lead electrocardiogram knowledge with the diagnoses listed on the scoring sheet. Ensure that you are familiar with the criteria for each diagnosis and make certain that you can recognize each on the 12-lead electrocardiogram. For specific clinical diagnoses such as left ventricular hypertrophy, it is essential that you familiarize yourself with the criteria necessary to fulfill this diagnosis. Some clinical diagnoses, such as a secundum atrial septal defect or dextrocardia, require pattern recognition with the characteristic right ventricular conduction delay as seen in lead V1 and R-wave regression as the QRS complex transitions from leads V1 to V6, respectively. These are examples where reviewing numerous electrocardiograms will be of enormous assistance.

Keep in mind that the examiners will include both straightforward and complex 12-lead electrocardiograms. Each 12-lead electrocardiogram, at a minimum, will require a heart rhythm diagnosis. Many of the electrocardiograms will require three or more diagnoses to achieve full interpretation credit. Given the complexity of these 12-lead electrocardiograms, it is best to approach each 12-lead electrocardiogram similarly beginning with the heart rate, followed by the heart rhythm, a calculation of the P wave axis and QRS complex axis, and an assessment of the cardiac intervals. Next evaluate the P wave, QRS complex, ST segment and T-wave morphologies. With this structured approach, you will less likely overlook an abnormality and ensure a comprehensive interpretation of each 12-lead electrocardiogram presented.

Additionally, many of the 12-lead electrocardiograms will be accompanied by a clinical history. Carefully use the clinical history to your interpretive advantage as oftentimes, valuable diagnostic clues, especially as it pertains to potential clinical diagnoses are embedded. For example, a renal failure patient may be more apt to have left atrial abnormality/enlargement, left ventricular hypertrophy, hyperkalemia, and hypocalcemia. In other words, the clinical history should automatically place a group of potential coding diagnoses on your "interpretation radar screen" even before you begin interpreting the electrocardiogram. As part of your electrocardiogram interpretation, your task is to either confirm or refute your *a priori* diagnoses remaining flexible enough to discard those not found to be present.

For a list of the Cardiovascular Medicine Certifying Exam scoring sheet diagnostic codes, please visit the ABIM Web site. What follows is a list of the diagnoses and their group headings as found on the scoring sheet.

The ABIM Cardiovascular Medicine Certifying Exam 12-lead electrocardiography scoring sheet is divided as follows:

General Features

- Normal electrocardiogram (ECG)
- Normal variant
- Incorrect electrode placement
- Artifact

P Wave Abnormalities

- Right atrial abnormality/enlargement
- Left atrial abnormality/enlargement

Atrial Rhythms

- Sinus rhythm
- Sinus arrhythmia
- Sinus bradycardia (<60)
- Sinus tachycardia (>100)
- Sinus pause or arrest
- Sinoatrial exit block
- Atrial premature complexes
- Atrial tachycardia
- Atrial tachycardia, multifocal
- Supraventricular tachycardia
- Atrial flutter
- Atrial fibrillation

Atrioventricular (AV) Junctional Rhythms

- AV junctional premature complexes
- AV junctional escape complexes
- AV junctional rhythm/tachycardia

Ventricular Rhythms

- Ventricular premature complex(es)
- Ventricular parasystole
- Ventricular tachycardia (three or more consecutive complexes)
- Accelerated idioventricular rhythm
- Ventricular escape complexes or rhythm
- Ventricular fibrillation

AV Conduction

- AV block, first degree
- AV block, second degree—Mobitz type I (Wenckebach)
- AV block, second degree—Mobitz type II
- AV block, 2:1
- AV block, third degree
- Wolff-Parkinson-White Pattern
- AV dissociation

Abnormalities of QRS Voltage or Axis

- Low voltage, limb leads
- Low voltage, precordial leads
- Left axis deviation (greater than negative 30 degrees)
- Right axis deviation (greater than positive 100 degrees)
- Electrical alternans

Ventricular Hypertrophy

- Left ventricular hypertrophy
- Right ventricular hypertrophy
- Combined ventricular hypertrophy

Intraventricular Conduction

- Right bundle branch block (RBBB), complete
- RBBB, incomplete
- Left anterior fascicular block

- Left posterior fascicular block
- Left bundle branch block (LBBB), complete
- LBBB, incomplete
- Aberrant conduction (including rate-related)
- Intraventricular conduction disturbance, nonspecific type

Q-Wave Myocardial Infarction

- Anterolateral—Age recent, or probably acute
- Anterolateral—Age indeterminate, or probably old
- Anterior or anteroseptal—Age recent, or probably acute
- Anterior or anteroseptal—Age indeterminate, or probably old
- Lateral—Age recent, or probably acute
- Lateral—Age indeterminate, or probably old
- Inferior—Age recent, or probably acute
- Inferior—Age indeterminate, or probably old
- Posterior—Age recent, or probably acute
- Posterior—Age indeterminate, or probably old

ST-, T-, U-Wave Abnormalities

- Normal variant, early repolarization
- Normal variant, juvenile T waves
- Nonspecific ST- and/or T-wave abnormalities
- ST- and/or T-wave abnormalities suggesting myocardial ischemia
- ST- and/or T-wave abnormalities suggesting myocardial injury
- ST- and/or T-wave abnormalities suggesting electrolyte disturbances
- ST- and/or T-wave abnormalities secondary to hypertrophy
- Prolonged Q-T interval
- Prominent U waves

Clinical Disorders

- Brugada syndrome
- Digitalis toxicity
- Torsades de pointes
- Hyperkalemia
- Hypokalemia
- Hypercalcemia
- Hypocalcemia
- Dextrocardia, mirror image
- Acute cor pulmonale including pulmonary embolus
- Pericardial effusion
- Acute pericarditis
- Hypertrophic cardiomyopathy
- Central nervous system disorder
- Hypothermia

Pacemaker Function

- Atrial or coronary sinus pacing
- Ventricular demand pacemaker (VVI), normally functioning
- Dual-chamber pacemaker (DDD), normally functioning
- Pacemaker malfunction, not constantly capturing (atrium or ventricle)
- Pacemaker malfunction, not constantly sensing (atrium or ventricle)
- Paced morphology consistent with biventricular pacing or cardiac resynchronization therapy

American Board of Internal Medicine (ABIM)

Cardiovascular Medicine Certifying Exam—Electrocardiogram Subsection

What follows are interpretation tips specific to many of the scoring sheet diagnostic codes. When reviewing, picture in your mind which diagnoses are apt to be grouped together such as left atrial abnormality/enlargement and left ventricular hypertrophy. Once you solidify these likely combinations in your mind, they can be embedded in your diagnostic approach as you interpret each board exam electrocardiogram tracing.

- If you are provided a normal electrocardiogram, it is important to code the tracing as normal. This is often overlooked.
- A normal variant electrocardiogram may include diagnostic codes such as a juvenile T-wave pattern or early repolarization.
- Incorrect electrode placement can involve the limb leads, precordial leads, or both. For the limb leads, the most common error is reversed arm leads, resulting in a negative P-wave vector in leads I and aVL. When this is present, it is important to distinguish between incorrect limb lead placement and dextrocardia. In contrast to dextrocardia, incorrect limb lead placement demonstrates normal R-wave precordial progression as one transitions from lead V1 to lead V6.
- Artifact can take several forms such as an undulating irregular baseline due to patient motion or a much faster, regularized artifact, the so-called 60-Hz artifact.
- Remember, each electrocardiogram possesses a heart rhythm and, at the least, it should be coded. In patients with atrioventricular dissociation or complete heart block, typically two heart rhythms—atrial and ventricular—necessitate coding. This is also true for ventricular pacing. An atrial rhythm should be coded, if identifiable, in the presence of a ventricular pacemaker.
- Sinus pause or arrest reflects cessation of sinus activity. It is not a multiple of the intrinsic P to P interval. This is a manifestation of sick sinus syndrome and these diagnoses should be coded together. If profound, presyncope or syncope may result with a helpful clue possibly included in the clinical history.
- Sinoatrial exit block is often a manifestation of sick sinus syndrome and therefore also consider coding these diagnoses together. Sinoatrial block is divided into type I and type II. In type I, the P-P interval shortens with the sequence terminating in a dropped P wave. In type II, the P-P intervals reflect an exact multiple of the sinus cycle length with the sequence once again terminating in a dropped P wave. For the purpose of the board exam, it is less important to specify the type of sinoatrial block.
- Differentiating between atrial tachycardia with either regular or variable conduction block and slow atrial flutter can be difficult. Atrial tachycardia most often demonstrates discrete atrial depolarizations, whereas atrial flutter, in its typical form, is reflected by a saw-toothed pattern. Atrial tachycardia can also conduct with AV block, second degree—Mobitz type I (Wenckebach) and, if present, should be additionally coded. Should atrial tachycardia with regularized conduction block be present, consider digitalis toxicity in the context of a supporting clinical history.
- Multifocal atrial tachycardia and atrial fibrillation are easily confused. It is important to critically evaluate the atrial rhythm and not be influenced by an irregularly irregular ventricular response. Multifocal atrial tachycardia, unlike atrial fibrillation, possesses discrete atrial depolarizations differentiating it from atrial fibrillation. Should multifocal atrial tachycardia be confirmed, consider coding chronic lung disease as this is the most commonly associated clinical setting.
- An accelerated idioventricular rhythm will typically be depicted as a transient 12-lead electrocardiogram finding in the setting of acute myocardial injury. This helps to distinguish this rhythm from an accelerated junctional rhythm with a preexisting bundle branch block. Make certain to code the underlying atrial rhythm, if identifiable, and code a Q-wave infarction, if present, in addition to ST- and/or T-wave abnormalities suggesting acute myocardial injury.
- In the presence of more advanced forms of atrioventricular block, first-degree atrioventricular block is typically not coded. For instance, in the presence of AV block, second degree—Mobitz type I (Wenckebach), this would be coded and

first-degree atrioventricular block should a prolonged P-R interval be present would not be coded.

- A Wolff-Parkinson-White pattern can be present with a normal or prolonged P-R interval. This can be seen in patients with preexisting slowed intra-atrial conduction or, for instance, a left lateral accessory bypass tract where intra-atrial conduction times are prolonged. Make sure that you code the atrial rhythm. It is not necessary to code intraventricular conduction disturbance, nonspecific type. It is also not necessary to localize the accessory pathway with regard to anterior, posterior, septal, lateral, left, or right ventricular.
- Atrioventricular dissociation and third-degree atrioventricular block can be difficult to differentiate. When in doubt, especially when the dominant secondary heart rhythm is accelerated, favor coding atrioventricular dissociation. In either case, make sure that you code both the atrial and ventricular rhythms. If a narrow complex junctional rhythm is identified, coding with reference to QRS complex duration, QRS complex morphology such as the presence of diagnostic Q waves, and repolarization abnormalities are all valid.
- Low-voltage QRS, limb leads can be coded if the limb lead QRS complexes are ≤0.5 mV.
- Low-voltage QRS, precordial leads can be coded if the QRS complexes are ≤1.0 mV in amplitude. When coding low-voltage QRS complexes, for the purposes of the coding sheet, consider the clinical diagnosis of pericardial effusion.
- Left axis deviation and left anterior hemiblock can be difficult to distinguish. With a widened QRS complex >100 msec in duration and a QRS complex axis greater than −30 degrees, code left axis deviation. With a narrow QRS complex <100 msec in duration coupled with a QRS complex axis greater than −30 degrees and less than −45 degrees, code left axis deviation. With a narrow QRS complex <100 msec in duration coupled with a QRS complex axis greater than −45 degrees, code left anterior hemiblock.
- In left and right ventricular hypertrophy, ST- and/or T-wave abnormalities secondary to hypertrophy may or may not be present. Do not overlook coding the associated ST-T changes when identified. Additionally, left and/or right atrial abnormality/enlargement are also frequently identified as is QRS complex axis deviation. Be aware of this combination of findings.
- In combined ventricular hypertrophy, oftentimes the QRS complex frontal plane axis is normal, with right and left ventricular hypertrophy "balancing" the electrical axis to within the normal range. Similarly, left and/or right atrial abnormality/enlargement are also frequently identified as are QRS complex axis deviation and ST-T changes. Be aware of this combination of findings.
- Right bundle branch block, complete requires a RSR' pattern in lead V1 with a total QRS complex duration of 120 msec or greater. Under normal circumstances in the presence of complete right bundle branch block, the T waves are discordant (negative) in leads V1 and V2. When upright, this is considered a primary T-wave change. If present, assess for a tall R wave in leads V1 and V2 and also Q waves supporting a myocardial infarction either in the inferior or lateral myocardial distributions. The primary T-wave change may indicate a posterior myocardial infarction.
- Right bundle branch block, incomplete requires an R' (terminal positive QRS complex deflection) ≥30 msec in duration, best identified in lead V1.
- Left posterior fascicular block is a complex diagnosis to conclude with certainty as it can be mimicked by underlying structural heart disease such as pulmonary hypertension and right ventricular failure. This diagnosis is unlikely to be tested on the board exam unless two electrocardiograms are provided for the same patient within a short time sequence: one demonstrating a normal QRS complex axis and the other demonstrating a rightward QRS complex axis in the absence of a clinical explanation of concomitant acute right heart strain.
- Left bundle branch block, complete necessarily must demonstrate a QRS complex duration of >120 msec and the absence of septal q waves (indicative of the absence of intact left to right septal depolarization) in leads V5, V6, I, and aVL. Importantly, when left bundle branch block, complete is present, think about underlying structural heart disease and specifically either increased left ventricular mass such as hypertensive heart disease, valvular heart disease, or coronary artery disease with ischemic left ventricular systolic dysfunction. Carefully assess the P-wave morphology in leads V1 and II for evidence of left atrial abnormality/enlargement. Additionally, ST and/or T waves suggesting myocardial injury in the presence of left bundle branch block, complete is a possible board exam electrocardiogram question. Familiarize yourself with this electrocardiogram example.
- Left bundle branch block, incomplete versus intraventricular conduction disturbance, nonspecific type can be difficult to distinguish. Should the morphology of complete left bundle branch block be present but the QRS complex is <120 msec in total duration, code incomplete left bundle branch block. Should the QRS complex demonstrate a nonspecific morphology not characteristic of a bundle branch block pattern and be >100 msec in duration, code intraventricular conduction disturbance, nonspecific type. Prominent septal q waves in lead I, aVL, V5, or V6 favor an intraventricular conduction disturbance, nonspecific

type supporting intact left to right interventricular septal depolarization, less likely observed in a conduction abnormality confined to the left bundle branch.

- Aberrant conduction (including rate-related) can be seen in the presence of premature atrial and junctional complexes or in the absence of prematurity, instead with a slight increase (acceleration dependent) or decrease (deceleration dependent) of heart rate. Once the aberrancy abates, relevant electrocardiogram findings may be unmasked that should be coded including Q-wave myocardial infarction patterns as well as ST and T abnormalities. If truly rate related, do not code a conduction disturbance such as left or right bundle branch block, complete. Instead, stay with functional aberrancy as the incorrect diagnosis of a complete bundle branch block in this circumstance suggests permanency to the conduction abnormality.
- Intraventricular conduction disturbance, nonspecific type applies to a QRS complex >100 msec in duration without specific morphologic features supporting either left or right bundle branch block conduction delay.
- For Q-wave myocardial infarctions, it is important to distinguish a true myocardial infarction from a pseudoinfarction. Principle causes of a pseudoinfarction include Wolff-Parkinson-White pattern and hypertrophic cardiomyopathy. Additionally, the volume overload pattern of left ventricular hypertrophy such as occurs in aortic and mitral insufficiency can also demonstrate deep and typically narrow Q waves in leads V5 and V6, reflecting interventricular septal depolarization. Once a Q-wave myocardial infarction is identified with confidence, it is next important to localize the infarction to a specific myocardial territory. Always be on the look out for a myocardial infarction involving contiguous territories. For example, an inferior Q-wave myocardial infarction may also demonstrate posterior (prominent R wave > S wave in lead V1) involvement and also lateral involvement. In this instance, you would want to make certain to code all three separately. An anterior or anteroseptal Q-wave myocardial infarction involves leads V2, V3 (anteroseptal), and possibly lead V4 (anterior). Should the Q-wave myocardial infarction involve at a minimum lead V4 (anterior) and extend to lead V5 or V6 (lateral), this would qualify as anterolateral in location. A lateral Q-wave myocardial infarction can involve leads V5, V6, and/or leads I and aVL. Importantly, Q waves isolated to leads V1 and V2 should not be coded as a Q-wave myocardial infarction. Q waves are frequently present in these leads under normal circumstances.

  Next, you need to distinguish between "Age recent, or probably acute" from "Age indeterminate, or probably old." In this situation, it is important to assess the J point, ST segments, and T waves. In an "Age recent or probably acute" Q-wave myocardial infarction, the J point will likely be elevated as will the ST segments with the ST segments possessing an upwardly coved morphology. The T waves may be terminally inverted; the so-called biphasic T wave and the ST segments may already demonstrate a slight reduction from their peak elevation. In an "Age indeterminate, or probably old" Q-wave myocardial infarction, the ST segments have typically normalized, the T waves may be inverted or more likely, slightly flattened or even normalized.
- Normal variant, early repolarization is important to code for and also to distinguish from pericarditis. Unlike pericarditis, early repolarization is most prominently localized to the lateral precordial leads such as leads V4, V5, and V6. J-point elevation is seen in both situations. With early repolarization, lead aVR is normal, not demonstrating PR segment elevation as is seen in pericarditis. Also, early repolarization is most often identified in a younger age group. When attempting to differentiate between these two possible diagnoses, pay careful attention to the clinical history and regional versus diffuse J-point elevation, the latter favoring pericarditis.
- The juvenile T-wave pattern should not be confused with nonspecific ST and/or T waves or myocardial ischemia. Instead, this coding diagnosis should be guided by the clinical history, most commonly found in patients <25 years of age reflected as T-wave inversion and confined to leads V1, V2, and possibly lead V3. If the patient is asymptomatic, young, and demonstrates this electrocardiographic pattern, code the following: normal variant, juvenile T waves.
- Nonspecific ST- and/or T-wave abnormalities are an appropriately selected code when abnormal ST- and/or T-wave findings are present in the absence of another explainable cause. This is important to code after other possible explanations such as myocardial ischemia, myocardial injury, electrolyte disturbances, and hypertrophy patterns have been excluded.
- ST- and/or T-wave abnormalities suggesting myocardial ischemia are best coded in the context of a supporting clinical history. Think of a positive exercise stress test electrocardiographic pattern on a resting 12-lead electrocardiogram where flat or downsloping ST-segment depression is present in one or more coronary artery anatomic distributions. This pattern strongly supports myocardial ischemia or a non–ST-segment elevation myocardial infarction (NSTEMI). Since NSTEMI is not an available code, ST- and/or T-wave abnormalities suggesting myocardial ischemia are most appropriate.

- ST- and/or T-wave abnormalities suggesting myocardial injury are an important code to consider. In the setting of an acute Q-wave myocardial infarction, coding myocardial injury is appropriate. The opposite is not true. In the presence of acute myocardial injury devoid of identifiable Q waves, coding acute myocardial injury alone is best. Since Q waves of diagnostic duration are not identified, no Q-wave myocardial infarction should be coded. In the presence of acute pericarditis, epicardial myocardial injury is apparent. Coding for acute myocardial injury is optional. While acute myocardial injury is present, the clinical implications are negligible from a myocardial dysfunction perspective unless myocarditis is also present.
- ST- and/or T-wave abnormalities suggesting electrolyte disturbances should be coded with the specific "Clinical Disorders" diagnosis invoking either an elevated or depressed potassium or calcium level. Coding one without the other is considered an omission. Ensure that you remember to code both when taking the board exam.
- ST- and/or T-wave abnormalities secondary to hypertrophy pertain to asymmetric T-wave inversion (T-wave downslope is less steep compared to the upslope) as seen in left and right ventricular hypertrophy of the pressure overload type. When present, this is important to code along with the type of hypertrophy—left, right, or combined.
- Prolonged Q-T interval can be difficult to diagnose with certainty as it's determination is both heart rate and gender adjusted in clinical practice. For the purposes of the board examination, anticipate a significantly prolonged Q-T interval as one might see with a central nervous system event, a marked electrolyte disturbance or R on T phenomenon due to the adverse effect of an antiarrhythmic medication. Generally, leads I, II, and III are most helpful. Should the Q-T interval be >50% of the R-R interval, it is prolonged independent of gender or heart rate. Commonly but not always, a prolonged Q-T interval will be identified in the presence of bradycardic heart rhythms. Make sure that you code the appropriate clinical diagnosis if supported by both the clinical history and the electrocardiogram findings.
- Prominent U waves in the context of the board exam most commonly pertain to positive electrocardiogram deflections occurring immediately after the T wave, often best seen in the precordial leads. Lead V4 is a common location but other precordial leads can also demonstrate prominent U waves. Generally, the more bradycardic the heart rhythm, the more prominent the positive U wave. Positive U waves can also be seen in more advanced cases of hypokalemia where the height of the U and T waves demonstrates inverse proportionality as the potassium level decreases.
- Brugada syndrome is most typically identified in lead V1 where a characteristic pattern of right ventricular conduction delay is present, with terminal QRS complex slowing somewhat similar to a right bundle branch block configuration. Brugada syndrome distinguishes itself electrocardiographically from right bundle branch conduction delay as the terminal QRS component demonstrates greater delay and thus is reflected as a less discrete terminal upstroke. This is one of the few electrocardiographic circumstances where pattern recognition is important and anticipate seeing an example on the board exam.
- Digitalis toxicity is most often manifest electrocardiographically as increased automaticity and depressed intracardiac conduction. Extrasystoles, tachycardic atrial rhythms, and depressed atrial conduction including a prolonged P-R interval and atrioventricular block can be seen. In extreme digitalis toxicity, bidirectional ventricular tachycardia can occur. For the purposes of the board examination, additional heart rhythms found in the presence of digitalis toxicity include atrial tachycardia with atrioventricular block and nonparoxysmal automatic atrioventricular junctional tachycardia.
- Antiarrhythmic drug effects on the electrocardiogram are variable. Most often, a form of conduction slowing transpires and is evidenced by P-R interval prolongation, nonspecific QRS complex widening, and Q-T interval lengthening. These findings may not be perceptible and considered still within normal limits unless a baseline electrocardiogram is available for comparison and obtained prior to antiarrhythmic medication initiation. For the purposes of the board examination, anticipate a clinical clue in the patient history.
- Torsades de pointes is generally identified in a patient with a prolonged Q-T interval due to a profound electrolyte disturbance such as hypokalemia or secondary to an antiarrhythmic medication. It is typically a fast, wide complex tachycardia with a varying QRS complex of opposite polarity, the so-called twisting of the points.
- Antiarrhythmic drug toxicity carries antiarrhythmic drug effects to an extreme and potentially dangerous level. For the board examination, anticipate a proarrhythmia such as torsades de pointes in the setting of a markedly prolonged Q-T interval initiated by a premature ventricular complex demonstrating the R-on-T phenomenon. This could also transpire and be potentially confused with extreme hypokalemia. This is another example where the clinical history will greatly assist with differentiating these two scenarios. Depending on the duration of the cardiac intervals, consider coding first-degree atrioventricular block, an intraventricular conduction disturbance, nonspecific type and/or a prolonged Q-T interval.

- Understanding the electrocardiogram manifestations of potassium and calcium disorders is essential for the board examination and clinical practice.
  - Hyperkalemia—the key here is slowed intracardiac conduction including both the atria and ventricles. In this circumstance, with early elevation of serum potassium, the T waves assume a more symmetric, narrow-based, and peaked shape. This is particularly evident in the precordial leads. With a progressive increase in serum potassium, P-R interval prolongation, QRS complex widening, and Q-T interval lengthening are also seen. Premorbid hyperkalemia is reflected by extreme widening of the QRS complexes resembling a sine wave. This is commonly a bradycardic rhythm. Hyperkalemia is frequently seen in the presence of renal failure. Given abnormal calcium and phosphorous metabolism in renal failure patients, hypocalcemia is a common associated finding.
  - Hypokalemia—this electrolyte abnormality predominantly impacts the Q-T interval and specifically the T wave. The T wave broadens with no significant alteration of the ST segment. As the serum potassium level further decreases, the T wave reduces in amplitude, broadens further, and is usurped by a terminally positive U wave with greater amplitude and duration compared to the T wave. In extreme cases, the Q-T-U interval is markedly prolonged with a negligible T wave and an extremely positive U-wave vector. It is this markedly prolonged Q-T-U interval that renders the patient vulnerable for the R-on-T phenomenon and ventricular arrhythmias such as torsades de pointes.
  - Hypercalcemia—of the four electrolyte abnormalities under consideration, hypercalcemia is the most often overlooked. In this circumstance, the T wave remains unaltered. The ST segment is shortened and in extreme cases of serum calcium elevation, the ST segment "disappears" with QRS complex termination and T-wave onset occurring near simultaneously. This abnormality can be subtle unless specifically sought as the electrocardiogram is otherwise normal. This reinforces the important concept of a systematic and careful approach to electrocardiogram interpretation.
  - Hypocalcemia—similar to hypercalcemia, hypocalcemia impacts the ST segment, sparing the T wave. In a patient with a significantly depressed serum calcium level, ST-segment prolongation and straightening (loss of the slight upward orientation of the ST segment moving from left to right on the electrocardiogram) are both identifiable. Hypocalcemia is frequently seen in the presence of renal failure. Hyperkalemia is a common associated finding.
- Dextrocardia, mirror image is a likely board exam example. The key is to identify the inverted P waves in leads I and aVL. Once identified, next look for R-wave regression as the electrocardiogram proceeds from lead V1 to V6. If both are present, dextrocardia is confirmed. Be careful not to code an infarction pattern or abnormal QRS complex electrical axis. The precordial R-wave regression excludes switched limb lead electrodes as the cause of the inverted P waves in leads I and aVL.
- Acute cor pulmonale for the purpose of the board exam pertains to an acute pulmonary embolism. This should be suggested by and consistent with the accompanying clinical history. Electrocardiogram findings support the presence of but are not diagnostic of an acute pulmonary embolism. These findings may include right atrial abnormality/enlargement, QRS complex right axis deviation, right ventricular conduction delay (right bundle branch block, incomplete or complete), subtle ST-segment elevation in lead V1 indicative of acute right ventricular myocardial injury, and the so-called S_I Q_{III} T_{III} QRS complex morphologic pattern where a dominant S wave is observed in lead I, a Q wave is noted in lead III, and T-wave inversion is also noted in lead III. These findings are likely acute if not present on a recent electrocardiogram prior to the index event if available for review. In this circumstance, avoid coding left posterior fascicular block as the electrocardiogram appearance is secondary to acute cor pulmonale and not secondary to conduction block.
- Pericardial effusion like other diagnoses reflects several potential coding opportunities. When addressing the diagnosis of pericardial effusion for the board examination, consider coding for low-voltage QRS complex and electrical alternans. In the presence of low-voltage QRS, be careful not to code a Q-wave myocardial infarction unless Q waves are present and are of diagnostic duration. Pericarditis in the form of diffuse ST-segment elevation may also be present.
- Acute pericarditis is manifest as J point and ST-segment elevation present diffusely across the electrocardiogram, typically not confined to a single myocardial territory. Reciprocal ST-segment and T wave changes are typically not observed. When reciprocal ST-segment and T-wave changes are present, they favor acute myocardial injury. PR-segment elevation is frequently identified in lead aVR, helping to secure the diagnosis of pericarditis. Sinus tachycardia may also been seen. As mentioned previously, ST- and/or T-wave abnormalities suggesting myocardial injury (in this circumstance epicardial myocardial injury) remain a coding option.
- Hypertrophic cardiomyopathy will often be suggested by the clinical history as it pertains to the physical exam, paroxysms of unexplained heart palpitations, exertional symptomatology such as chest discomfort, shortness of breath, and light-headedness, or unexplained syncope. The key differentiator is to recognize

what appears to be otherwise diagnostic Q waves spanning multiple coronary artery distributions not typical of a Q-wave myocardial infarction pattern. Prominent ST- and T-wave repolarization changes may be seen. It is extremely important not to code for a Q-wave myocardial infarction as these findings instead reflect a myopathic process, not coronary in etiology. Either nonspecific ST- and/or T-wave abnormalities or ST- and/or T-wave abnormalities secondary to hypertrophy may be applicable, dependent upon if voltage criteria satisfy a ventricular hypertrophy diagnosis. In the setting of hypertrophic cardiomyopathy, criteria may exist for the diagnosis of combined ventricular hypertrophy. Also be attuned to left and right atrial abnormality/enlargement as possible accompanying diagnostic codes.

- Central nervous system disorder is most often reflected electrocardiographically as a prolonged Q-T interval and/or symmetric deep T-wave inversion, especially in leads V2 to V6. The clinical history should be of significant value. Coding a prolonged Q-T interval and central nervous system disorder along with the appropriate heart rhythm should be sufficient. The ST- and/or T-wave abnormality options are not applicable to this diagnosis. Most closely would be nonspecific ST- and/or T-wave abnormalities, but, in practicality, the findings are truly specific. Bradycardic and junctional heart rhythms may be seen. It is important to distinguish a central nervous system disorder from myocardial ischemia as both can present with deep symmetric T-wave inversion, especially if the myocardial ischemia is due to profound systemic hypotension and multivessel coronary artery disease. Once again, the clinical history should greatly assist.
- Hypothermia is an important electrocardiogram diagnosis best addressed by memory and pattern recognition. Terminal QRS complex conduction delay at the junction of the QRS complex and beginning of the ST segment is evident possessing a characteristic pattern termed an Osborne wave. It is important not to confuse this electrocardiogram pattern with acute myocardial injury. The clinical history can help discriminate between these two diagnostic possibilities. Additionally, given the presence of profound hypothermia, bradycardic heart rhythms are often identified and should be coded when present.
- Pacemaker heart rhythms on the board exam are typically straightforward. It is important to recognize which chamber (atria or ventricles) or chambers (atria and ventricles) are paced as three separate coding options exist including the following:
  - Atrial or coronary sinus pacing—depicted as a discrete electrocardiogram deflection prior to atrial depolarization followed by a P-R interval and ventricular depolarization.
  - Ventricular demand pacemaker (VVI), normally functioning—depicted as a discrete electrocardiogram deflection prior to ventricular depolarization. This may be preceded by a P wave. Make certain that the atrial rhythm is coded should it be identifiable. This could include abnormal atrial rhythms such as atrial tachycardia, atrial flutter, or atrial fibrillation. Additionally, a ventricular pacemaker may be identified in the setting of heart block, such as atrioventricular block, second degree—Mobitz type I (Wenckebach), or complete heart block. When present, the type of heart block should also be coded.
  - Dual-chamber pacemaker (DDD), normally functioning—depicted as a discrete electrocardiogram deflection prior to atrial depolarization followed by a preset P-R interval and a subsequent discrete electrocardiogram deflection prior to ventricular depolarization.
- Pacemaker malfunction is captured by two separate codes, including the following:
  - Pacemaker malfunction, not constantly capturing (atrium or ventricle)—manifests as an atrial or ventricular pacemaker spike, appropriately timed, and not followed by either an atrial or ventricular depolarization, not due to atrial or ventricular refractoriness.
  - Pacemaker malfunction, not constantly sensing (atrium or ventricle)—manifests as an inappropriately timed atrial or ventricular pacemaker discharge that may or may not depolarize the atrium or ventricle depending upon atrial and ventricular refractoriness.
  - Paced morphology consistent with biventricular pacing or cardiac resynchronization therapy demonstrates atrioventricular sequential pacing with a narrow QRS complex reflecting prompt simultaneous depolarization of the left and right ventricles.

Index

***NOTE: The entries to this index refer to the Electrocardiogram Case Study numbers, not to the page numbers.**

*NOTE: The entries to this index refer to the Electrocardiogram Case Study numbers, not to the page numbers.